BEYOND BODYBUILDING

MUSCLE AND STRENGTH
TRAINING SECRETS
FOR THE RENAISSANCE MAN

BY PAVEL

BEYOND BODYBUILDING

MUSCLE AND STRENGTH
TRAINING SECRETS
FOR THE RENAISSANCE MAN

BY PAVEL

Published in the United States by:
Dragon Door Publications, Inc
P.O. Box 4381, St. Paul, MN 55104
Tel: (651) 487-2180 • Fax: (651) 487-3954
Credit card orders: 1-800-899-5111
Email: support@dragondoor.com • Website: www.dragondoor.com

ISBN10: 0-938045-66-0   ISBN10: 978-0-938045-66-3

First edition published in January, 2005. This edition published in April, 2011

Printed in China

Book design, Illustrations and cover by Derek Brigham
Website http//www.dbrigham.com • (763)208-3069 • Email: bigd@dbrigham.com
Photographs unless otherwise credited by Ralph DeHaan
Gym, courtesy World Gym, Lake Forest, CA.

DISCLAIMER

The author and publisher of this material are not responsible in any manner whatsoever for any injury that may occur through following the instructions contained in this material. The activities, physical and otherwise, described herein for informational purposes only, may be too strenuous or dangerous for some people and the reader(s) should consult a physician before engaging in them.

TO CLARENCE BASS

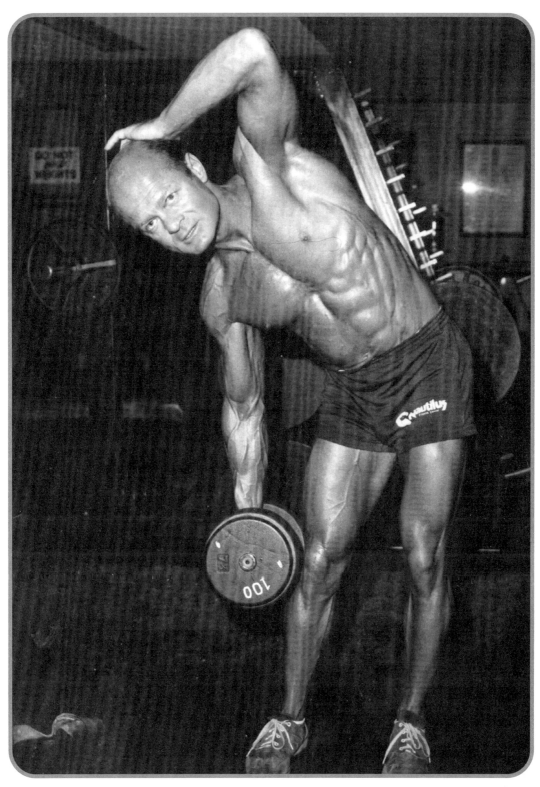

Photo courtesy CBass.com

BEYOND BODYBUILDING
TABLE OF CONTENTS

Section One: Power Training
Articles

Questions and Answers

Section Two: Training Planning
Articles

Beyond Bodybuilding
Table of Contents

BEYOND BODYBUILDING
TABLE OF CONTENTS

Section Six: Arms
Articles

Questions and Answers

Section Seven: Chest
Articles

Questions and Answers

Section Eight: Naked Warrior
Strong Anywhere, Anytime with Bodyweight Exercises
Articles

Questions and Answers

Index

INTRODUCTION

"Do we have a man here?"

I have the privilege of acquaintance with men like Clarence Bass, Dave Draper, Larry Scott, and Dennis Weis. Bodybuilders of the golden age. I have great respect for these men. Not for their physiques because, to be blunt, I have no interest in that sort of thing. I respect them for everything today's bodybuilders are not.

The old-timers are men's men. They kept their pursuit of bodybuilding in perspective, unlike the modern generation of catty beauty queens. They despised muscles that were for show only. The golden age knew true renaissance men like Tommy Kono and Bill March who went to the top in both strength and physique competition. With the exception of Ronnie Coleman and Dorian Yates, I am hard pressed to name today's bodybuilders who are as strong as they look.

We go to a bodybuilding expo every year. Last few years we ran a challenge at our booth. A one-arm military press with an eighty-eight pound kettlebell. The rules are simple: the fist must be lower then the chin at the start of the press and the knees must remain locked. You don't even have to clean the bell because I do not want any of the 'this is all technique' whining. We'll hand it to you if you insist.

Let us face it, pressing eighty-eight pounds overhead is not a feat of strength. Definitely not for a two hundred-fifty pound man. Yet the overwhelming majority of the big sissies just can't do it. And that is the ones who at least try. Most are plain scared. I call out to the passing muscleheads: "Do we have a man here?" Most flinch and keep walking. One year there was a Jazzercise booth across the isle. Whenever my challenge was ignored I would smile sweetly and say, "Sir, I understand. Not all forms of exercise are right for all people. Perhaps you would like to check out Jazzercise over there?"

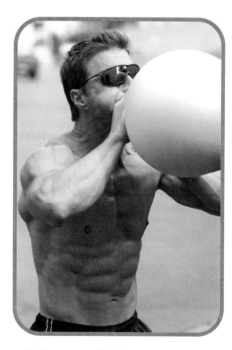

Clark Bartram of ClarkBartram.com.
As strong as he looks.

The purpose of this collection of articles is to make today's bodybuilder ashamed of his weakness and narcissism and get him as strong as he looks. Appropriately, I asked Clark Bartram to model for the photos. Not just because he is a friend but because this Marine vet is as strong as he looks. And because he used to write and model for Muscle Media, a great magazine.

Most of the articles in this anthology first appeared in MM. My friend and colleague Steve Maxwell used to cut them out and put them in a binder for his trainers at Maxercise in Philly. It was Steve who suggested that I publish them in one volume.

These articles made many bodybuilders catch the strength bug. If you are a musclehead unfamiliar with 'the Party methods' I hope this volume will do the same for you. If you are with the choir, ignore my strength preaching and pay attention to the training advice. A ton of work and research went into this volume. Think of it as a sequel to Power to the People! You will get the answers to many questions you may have had. For instance:

- What are the top Russian set and rep schemes for power?
- How to use the High-Tension Techniques outside the gym?
- What is the best way to build strength with singles?
- How to peak strength in two weeks?
- How to make the most out of the classic 'countdown to power' method?
- Powerlifters 'lift the weight'. Bodybuilders 'feel the muscle'. What is the PTP way?
- Are there other simple and effective power cycles to be used with PTP?
- Are there other simple and effective set and rep schemes to be used with PTP?
- What if I want to squat rather than deadlift?
- Under what circumstances should I explode rather than grind my deadlifts?
- Are there benefits to lowering my deadlifts slowly?
- I live in an apartment. I can't deadlift heavy and I can't drop my deadlifts. What should I do?
- Are lay-offs any good?
- Is twice-a-day training worth the trouble?
- How to convert accidental overtraining into great strength gains?
- Does being a training minimalist have exercise variety?
- What is the best neck strength routine of all time?

Plus a lot more.

Power to you!

Pavel

December 2004

**Santa Monica,
California –
where it all began**

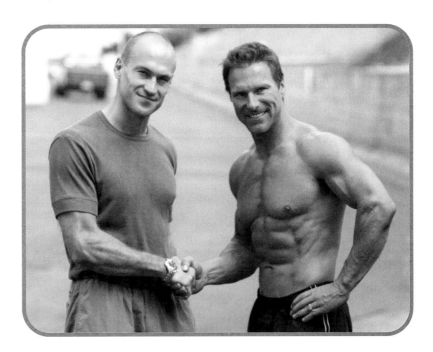

SECTION ONE

POWER TRAINING

CONTENTS

Articles

POWER TRAINING CONTENTS

Questions and Answers

POWER TRAINING CONTENTS

Questions and Answers

MIND OVER MUSCLE: THE 5X5X5 PROGRAM

Contrary to the bodybuilding mythology, true strength training is not about your muscles but about your mind.

In any endeavor mental focus delivers more than any physical transformation, a concept clearly understood by martial arts masters. "Focus is the ability to control the muscles of the body in a coordinated effort and then contract them to their maximum degree..." explains Jack Hibbard, a Green Beret vet and expert in tameshiwari, the ancient art of breaking boards and bricks bare-handed, "The deeper the concentration, the tenser the contraction of the muscle; and the tenser the contraction, the stronger the muscle grows."

Like I said before, it all boils down to tension. Effective 'mind over muscle' strength training can be summed up as **honing your skill to contract your muscles harder.** In Russian sports science there is even a term, *skill-strength*.

Some bodybuilders are quick to argue: "But it's all technique!" So what if it is? "The most important aspect one can learn to improve strength is to learn proper technique,' bench press champion George Halbert sets the record straight. "There is a mode of thinking out there that I describe as "He's not strong, he's just got good technique." This is just confused thinking... Have you ever heard anyone say, "he is not a good shooter, he just has good technique" or "he's not really fast, he just has good technique"?"

An important point to drive home: 'technique' does not refer just to the groove of a particular exercise! There are two generalized strength skills that apply to and fortify all displays of strength: **staying tight** and **power breathing.**

"Keep every body part tight during the entire movement." This is one of Ernie Frantz's famous Commandments of Powerlifting. Frantz, whose book had the rare honor of being translated into Russian, is a legend of powerlifting and a successful bodybuilder with a rugged physique along the lines of Franco Columbo's. He swears that practicing tightening up his entire body throughout the day has helped his strength. Practice. That loaded word again.

I have addressed Power Breathing in many of my writings. In a nutshell, if you compare your brain to a CD player and your muscles to its speakers, your abdominal cavity is the amplifier, the volume control. The greater the pressure inside your belly – the greater your strength in any effort. Unless you have health restrictions, practice high-pressure breathing in the context of bodybuilding exercises and by itself, and you will get stronger in every lift.

Then, of course, there is the specific practice of your pet lifts. But all strength practice follows the same laws that govern the practice of any skill. How do you improve your tennis serve? Do you hit the court once a week and keep on serving until your balls could not knock out a sick mosquito and you can barely lift your arm? No, you come to the court as often as possible, ideally more than once a day, and slam those little yellow balls until you feel that your serves are about to slow down. Why not do the same for your iron games? It worked for old-timer Arthur Saxon, who put up 400 pounds overhead with one arm.

The basic tenet of motor learning is specificity. Applied to strength, it means heavy weights. But not super heavy! As they say, practice does not make perfect; perfect practice does. An ugly, shaky, max is not perfect; a 70-80% 1RM controlled lift is. Never train to failure for the same reason, always leave a rep or two in the bank.

Heavy weights imply low reps. The perfect reps for strength are 1-6. A narrower 4-6 range is even better. Fives build muscle in addition to strength. Get plenty of rest between your sets and exercises. Long breaks will enable you to keep lifting 'perfect' heavy poundages. No pump and burn here!

Here is another axiom of motor learning: frequent brief practices are superior to infrequent long ones. Russian researchers discovered that breaking up a strength workout into smaller units is very effective. In other words, one set of five every day is better than five sets of five every five days. Very counterculture in the bodybuilding community, but I presume that you are more interested in making gains than in fitting in.

With all of the above in mind, here is the program.

THE 5X5X5 MIND OVER MUSCLE PROGRAM

1. Select five basic exercises for your whole body.
2. Perform all of them five days a week, Monday through Friday.
3. Do only one work set of five per exercise, leaving a couple of reps in the bank.
4. Focus on staying tight, power breathing, and the perfect groove.
5. Taper in week four, peak your 1RM in week five, and switch to a different type of routine.

Select five basic exercises for your whole body, for instance, the three powerlifts, pullups, and dumbbell side bends. Or clean-and-presses, deadlifts, dips, barbell curls, and Janda situps. You get the idea.

Perform all of them five days a week, Monday through Friday. Do only one work set of five per exercise. It will feel very odd to wrap up a workout when you still feel so good, but that is the way neural training is. Steve Justa, a supremely strong and muscular man, once said, "You should feel stronger at the end of every workout."

The weight is ideal if you have managed it with a couple of reps to spare. To establish that perfect poundage start every workout with a couple of lighter singles. For instance, yesterday you squatted 300x5 and felt that you could have done 300x7. Today squat 225x1, 255x1, and 275x1. The feel of 275 should tell you whether you should stay with 300, go up, or go down. And don't sweat it too hard if you do not hit it right, occasional easier and harder sets will do you good by introducing more variety. The usual 5x5x5 pattern is a very strong start on Monday, a PR on Tuesday, Wednesday could go either way. Thursday and Friday are downhill as fatigue builds up. By Monday you will be rested and ready to smash new records.

Powerlifters and weight lifters have learned the hard way that trying to continuously go up does not work. Through trial and error, they have figured out that if one takes it easy for a week, after three weeks of hard training, week five will be awesome. So unload in week four. Use this simple technique: work up in singles to establish the poundage for your usual set of five, then do only three reps with it.

In week five work up to a comfortable single on Monday. That means whatever you can put up without getting psyched up, usually in the ballpark of 90% 1RM. Russians call this poundage 'the training max' and Bulgarians lift it daily. Your Monday deadlift workout might be 315x1, 365x1, 385x1, 405x1.

Go for a max single on Tuesday. Repeat his Monday ramp-up and finish it with a new PR or PRs. The lifter in the above example would pull 425x1, possibly 435x1, and, if he feels unstoppable, 445x1.

THE MIND OVER MUSCLE TAPER AND PEAK

1. Do a triple with the weight you would have normally used for a set of five in week four.
2. In week five work up to a comfortable, around 90% 1RM, single on Monday and max on Tuesday.
3. Take the rest of the week off and switch to a different type of routine the week after.

Take the rest of the week off and switch to a different type of program the week after. You will be strong, confident, and raring to go back to volume training.

You may never admit it in public, but you know that the number one reason you are bodybuilding is to improve your self-esteem. Face the music: no amount of meat will give you true confidence. The following Internet post caught my eye: "I've found something remarkable about my [strength] training. I'm a lot more confident than I was as [just] a bodybuilder. When all I cared about was getting my muscles bigger and bigger, I still had horrible self-esteem problems. With strength training, though... I feel myself getting stronger, and it's had a profound impact on how I see myself." Strength gives confidence that does not go away when your muscles shrink after a missed meal.

THE '3 TO 5' METHOD: STRENGTH TRAINING FOR SPECIAL WEAPONS AND TACTICS TEAMS

There are many effective ways to build strength, but they all boil down to low rep non-exhaustive training. I designed the program outlined here for my S.W.A.T. clients in the Western states. "...I have tried all the conventional methods being taught for 10 years now, with little to no gain in strength. This training, in one week, has already done more for me than all the others put together..." observed a Range Master/Advanced Instructor from one of the agencies in New Mexico at the end of one of my courses.

THE '3 TO 5' METHOD:

STRENGTH TRAINING GUIDELINES FOR SPECIAL WEAPONS AND TACTICS TEAMS

3-5	Exercises (total for the whole body)
3-5	Sets
3-5	Repetitions
3-5	Minutes of rest between the sets
3-5	Days of rest for each exercise

The simplicity is obvious. If you cannot remember the program's guidelines turn in your driver's license and do not operate heavy machinery. Start out by selecting three to five exercises for the whole body. Three of these must be 'big' lifts such as deadlifts or squats. Variations are many; you have twelve to choose from in the table below.

TWELVE POWER DRILL COMBINATIONS RECOMMENDED WITH THE '3 TO 5' METHOD

- Squat
- Bench press
- Deadlift

- Pullup
- 'Pistol' or one-legged squat
- Double kettlebell snatch

- Clean-&-press (reclean the bell before each press)
- Extended deadlift (use small plates or stand on a box and squat low)
- Hanging leg raise

- One arm dumbbell clean and push press (reclean the bell before each press)
- Towel pullup
- Split squat

TWELVE POWER DRILL COMBINATIONS RECOMMENDED WITH THE '3 TO 5' METHOD

- Pullup
- Dip
- Dumbbell snatch

- Power clean
- Incline bench press
- Front squat

- Squat
- Barbell shrug
- Dips

- One arm pushup
- Good morning
- One arm lat row

- Double kettlebell or dumbbell C&P (reclean the bells before each press)
- Sumo deadlift
- Janda situp

- Close grip bench press
- One arm deadlift
- Jump shrug with two kettlebells or dumbbells

- Power snatch
- Squat
- Handstand pushup

- High pull
- Side press
- Box squat

Bodybuilders may add two exercises of their choice. You can pick isolation exercises if you wish but you must stick to the low rep power format specified for the whole program.

TWELVE SECONDARY BODYBUILDING EXERCISE COMBINATIONS RECOMMENDED WITH THE '3 TO 5' METHOD

- Barbell curl
- Incline close grip bench press

- Floor fly
- Preacher curl

- Lateral raise
- Bent over lateral raise

- Alternate dumbbell bench press
- Alternate dumbbell curl

- Incline fly
- Hammer curl

- Concentration curl
- French press

- Janda situp
- Incline bench alternate dumbbell curl

- Alternate dumbbell military press
- Reverse curl

- EZ bar curl
- EZ bar skull crusher

- Arnold press
- Cable crunch

- Rope curl
- Triceps pushdown

- Thick bar curl
- Thick bar close grip bench press from power rack pins

Military, law enforcement, and other hard living types should pick two secondary drills for the forearms, neck, or midsection instead of the above bodybuilding exercises. For instance, heavy gripper work plus neck harness exercises. Or thick bar reverse curls plus Janda situps.

TWELVE TACTICAL STRENGTH SECONDARY DRILL COMBINATIONS RECOMMENDED WITH THE '3 TO 5' METHOD

- Sledgehammer leverage drill
- Hanging leg raise

- Front half bridge
- Barbell finger rolls

- Janda situp
- Reverse curl with a thick bar

- Rolling bridge
- Heavy-duty gripper work

- Straddle style one arm deadlift
- Finger extensions against a rubber band or in a bucket of sand

- Wrist roller
- Headstand leg raise

- Neck harness work
- Full contact twist

- One finger partial deadlifts (all finger pairs)
- Suitcase style one arm deadlift

- One-legged deadlift
- Fingertip pullups

- Wrist extension with an EZ curl bar
- Wrist flexion with an EZ curl bar

- Thick bar deadlift
- Neck harness work

- Bent press
- Pinch gripping two barbell plates

Do 3-5 sets of 3-5 reps with 3-5 minutes of rest in between. These powerlifting rest periods will seem like eternity to a busy bodybuilder. Deal with it. You may alternate – not superset! – sets of two or more exercises. For instance, C&P – 2min – DL – 2min – C&P, etc.

The high-tension techniques I have written about in my books *Power to the People!* and *The Naked Warrior* are essential. Train tight and heavy but pull the plugs on your sets when you still have one or two reps in the bank. Ignore the bodybuilding intensity folklore about 'doing as many reps as you can and then two more' and gain!

"I used to be enthralled at 'the Barbarians' and Dorian Yates and their balls to the wall training style," writes US Military Powerlifting National Champion Jack Reape in his article on dragon-door.com. "Getting those hard fought last couple reps were the key to getting bigger and stronger I believed. WRONG! Intensity is not a grimace and a backwards baseball cap, it is a mathematical formula! That Mathematical formula is based on all the reps you do above about 40-50% of 1RM…"

All you need is to train heavy and stay tight; failure is unnecessary and counterproductive. And if you disdainfully blow this bit of advice off as 'sissy', do it in 500-pound bencher Jack Reape's face. It will be amusing to watch you fly.

Add weight when you can, without training on the nerve. Practice each exercise every three to five days. How you split them up is up to you. If you are short on time follow the split by Igor Sukhotsky, M.S. Comrade Sukhotsky, a Russian nationally ranked weightlifter turned full contact karate fighter, squats, bench presses, deadlifts, and practices good mornings and full contact twists three times in two weeks. Monday-Friday-next week's Wednesday.

Or you could train three times a week and alternate two workouts. To use Sukhotsky's workout as an example, do squats, good mornings, and full contact twists on Monday. Bench and pull on Wednesday. On Friday do your SQ & Co. again.

Experienced lifters can practice more sophisticated splits within the same three to five days of rest formula. For instance, you could train three times a week, squat and pull three times in two weeks and bench twice a week:

Monday	Squat, bench press
Wednesday	Deadlift
Friday	Squat, bench press
Monday	Bench press, deadlift
Wednesday	Squat
Friday	Bench press, deadlift

It is also fine, if you want to split the workout further to train almost every day. The '3 to 5' setup offers enough choices to suit anyone.

Waving the training load up and down is essential for progress. There are many complex periodization systems out there that would put a Ph. D. to sleep. Just say no and keep it simple. After three weeks of hard training just reduce your volume or the total reps by 40-50%. In the traditional Ostapenko model practiced by many Russian powerlifters, the sets get reduced. 4x4 becomes 2 sets of 4 reps. 5 sets of 5 reps taper to 3 sets of 5 reps.

I prefer cutting the reps instead of the sets: 4 sets of 2, 5 sets of 3. With the weight you used on your last heavy week; you are tapering and this is supposed to be easy! "I pushed myself hard for three weeks, to the point where I was really getting fatigued," reports David Valentiner, RKC. "Then… I really reduced my volume…during the 4th week… and I felt better than ever." In the first week of the next month you are guaranteed to see great gains in strength.

Power to you!

MAKE A QUANTUM STRENGTH LEAP WITH 'PROGRESSIVE MOVEMENT TRAINING'

There are two kinds of vodka: good and very good. A simple Russian lad named Misha was too preoccupied with his thoughts to notice which kind he had been consuming. He scratched his head: why do automatic weapons have to be so complex and unreliable? Unburdened by formal education and too stupid to know that a more straightforward design was impossible, Mikhail Kalashnikov put together a weapon that would become the choice of many armies and most terrorists for years to come: the AK-47.

About the same time a poor boy, Paul from Georgia, came up with the Kalashnikov assault rifle equivalent in the iron game: Progressive Movement Training. Paul Anderson would do partial repetitions in the squat, with a weight he could not full squat. Over a period of time he gradually lengthened the movement until he worked his way down to parallel with a new record.

The science behind Progressive Movement Training and the results this method delivered were decades ahead of their time. It took generations of Ph.D. bearing geeks to clue in how PMT produced Paul Anderson's 1,200-pound squat sans powerlifting gear, a mark that will remain untouched way into this millennium. That might give you a hint why the hard to impress Russians called Paul 'the Wonder of Nature'.

Paul Anderson recommended to start squatting from a pin about four inches below the lockout, with a weight about one hundred pounds over your one rep max full squat. "I realize that this is a very light weight in comparison to what you can quarter squat with," admits Big Paul, "but this is part of the plan." Burning out on max singles is not.

Two sets of twenty to twenty five reps are performed. "I would say the secret lies in taking a lighter weight that you can do many repetitions with and just working it down that way." It is amusing that in his recommendation to do high reps in the Progressive Movement Training routine Paul again beat the science geeks to the punch. Much later Meyers (1967) discovered that the greater is the number of contractions, the higher is the transfer of strength to the untrained part of the exercise ROM.

Ironically, in Paul's day scientists did not believe that such carryover was possible at all. Strength gains were thought to be highly joint angle specific, that is limited to the exercise range at which you train (Williams & Stutzman, 1959; Gardner, 1963, etc.). Only a few years before Paul's death the lab rats caught up with his instinctive knowledge. The new generation of scientists realized that while most gains indeed occur at the specific training angles, there is a transfer to the untrained angles as well. In fact, most carryover of strength takes place in the range of plus-minus twenty degrees from the exercised angle (Knapik, Mawdsley & Ramos, 1983). By the way, the scientific term for Paul Anderson's method is *neurological carryover training*. It was coined by 900-pound squatter and Powerlifting World Record Holder Dr. Fred Clary.

Every three workouts – once in three days for Paul, and once in three weeks for mere mortals – lower the power rack pins three inches and knock off three reps. You may want to experiment with smaller drops, one or two inches. Anderson recommended one-inch sheets of plywood for precise movement graduation. It is not the only way. Paul's mentor and 'world's best deadlifter' Bob Peoples would pull his deads standing in a hole he had dug in the ground and fill it up with dirt as his strength grew! Peoples' deadlift was another remarkable success of neurological carry-over training: 725 at 178 pounds of bodyweight in the days before steroids, speed, industrial strength powerlifting belts, and canvas underwear!

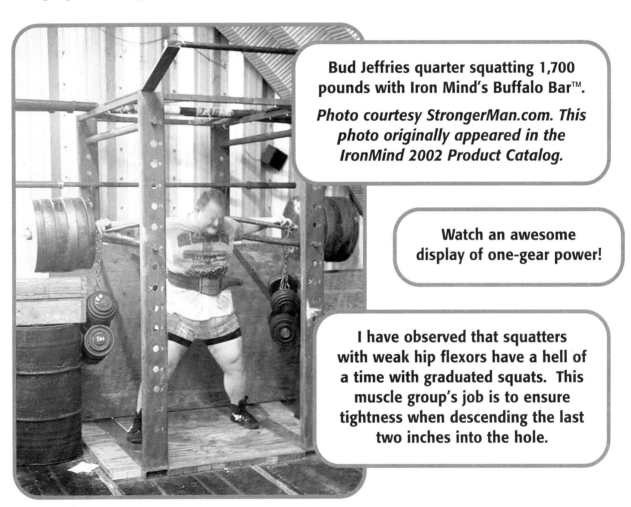

Bud Jeffries quarter squatting 1,700 pounds with Iron Mind's Buffalo Bar™.

Photo courtesy StrongerMan.com. This photo originally appeared in the IronMind 2002 Product Catalog.

Watch an awesome display of one-gear power!

I have observed that squatters with weak hip flexors have a hell of a time with graduated squats. This muscle group's job is to ensure tightness when descending the last two inches into the hole.

Keep lengthening the movement and knocking off reps until you are down to two repetitions. Then take a few days off – Paul himself rested for two or three days – and try for a new personal best in the full squat. "I believe that you will find that you have gained quite a bit of strength during this drawn out Progressive Movement routine," promised the 'Wonder of Nature'.

When you are down to two reps, most likely you are not going to be all the way in the hole. Don't fret. Neither was Paul. Your max will still go up because you will have worked down to your sticking point.

According to Dr. Fred Clary, the reason you are not likely to get all the way down, is a sharp transition from one muscle group to another, at some point of the lift. "I have found that whether I be pressing, bench pressing, squatting, etc., I seem to have to change gear as the bar travels," admits Big Paul himself. "On the other hand, I have seen fellows who rammed a press to arms length or stood straight up with a dead lift in an almost sudden gesture, without any evidence of this "changing gears".

From my coaching experience I can tell you that the latter lifters are more likely to work a heavy partial into a full movement. Generally they squat with a wide stance. You will do yourself a favor if you get Bud Jeffries' *How I Squatted 900 Pounds* video from Strongerman.com. Watch Bud squat and deadlift: a smooth display of one-gear power.

I have observed that squatters with weak hip flexors have a hell of a time with graduated squats. This muscle group's job is to ensure tightness when descending the last two inches into the hole. When a bodybuilder with weak hip flexors reaches this depth with a bar bending weight, he just collapses. If that is you, learn to 'pull' yourself down into the hole with your 'situp muscles', before embarking on the Paul Anderson program. Rock bottom front squats would also come in handy.

Anderson and Peoples' unique program will work even better on the deadlift. It is easier to perform a shorter movement without 'changing gears'. To make neurological carryover training work on the bench, you must change your groove – so the bar travels in a straight line from your sternum slightly towards your feet, rather than arcs toward your face. That will ensure that the pecs do not suddenly surrender the weight to the shoulders and triceps, but dominate the whole movement with constant assistance from the latter. You should also sort of push the bar from your elbows rather than your hands. It is a subtle point, but it will make a huge difference in the quality of your pec workout and the amount of weight you are going to put up.

These days there is an exercise far superior to the power rack bench press – the board press. Lifters used to press from the pins set in a cage at the sticking point level. The problem was, unlike the deadlift, the BP does not start from a dead spot. So, even if one got stronger in the power rack, he did not always get a carryover to his regular bench groove.

A few years ago a so-called 'board press' has emerged from the powerlifting Westside Barbell Club in Columbus. Set a couple of boards, two, four, or six inches thick depending on your sticking point, on your chest. Lower the bar to the boards, pause while staying tight, and press back. The exercise has a feel very similar to the regular bench and thus has a great transfer of strength.

Champion bencher J.M. Blakley warns not to bounce the bar off the boards. He mentions another innovative cheating technique to avoid: letting the bar and the boards sink into the chest, then heaving the works up with a chest push. Treat the board press they way you should the conventional BP – and you will do fine.

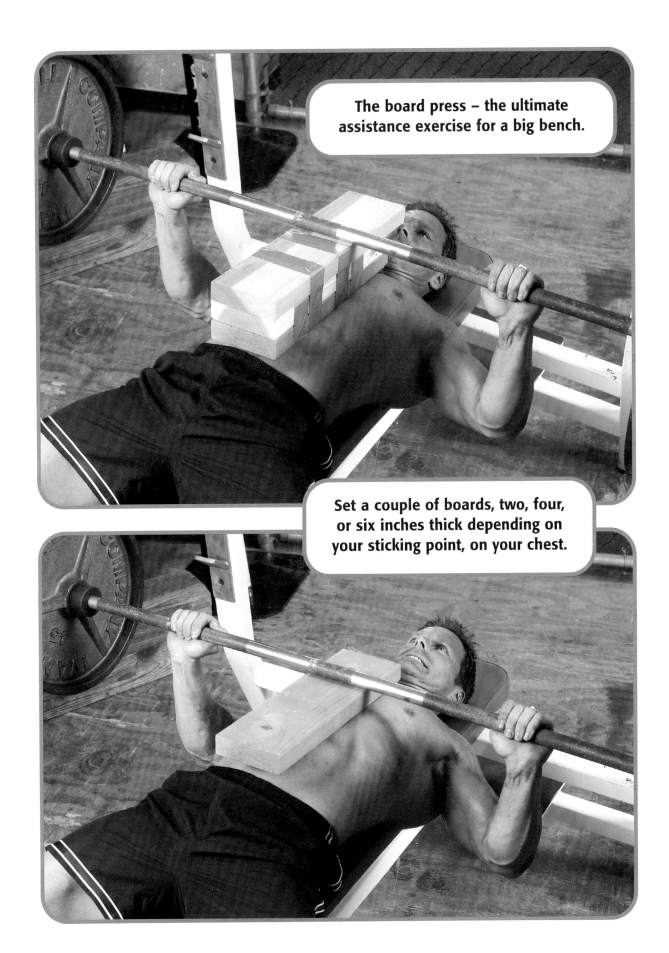

The board press – the ultimate assistance exercise for a big bench.

Set a couple of boards, two, four, or six inches thick depending on your sticking point, on your chest.

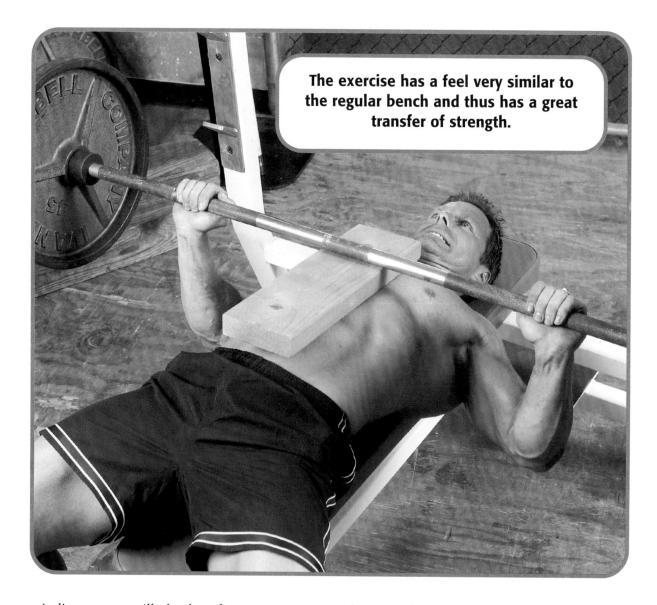

The exercise has a feel very similar to the regular bench and thus has a great transfer of strength.

A direct grove will also benefit your one rep max because changing the direction of the movement with a maximal weight tends to stall it and lead to a failed attempt (Rodionov, 1967). As Nietsche put it a century earlier, "formula for success, a straight line."

By no means should you limit the application of neurological carryover training to 'big' compound exercises like the powerlifts. Because the same muscles start and finish the movement, in isolation drills like the barbell curl, you would do yourself a favor by applying the Progressive Movement principles to one joint moves as well. Start the graduated standing barbell curl in a power rack with a one-inch movement and work your way down. Make a point of keeping your abs tight and don't lean back. It helps to think of pulling yourself towards the barbell rather than the other way around.

Just like I said before, don't accept 'the full range of motion' as dogma. Try Paul Anderson's quantum alternative and you might leapfrog from a 500 squat to 550 without even bothering with anything in between!

HARDGAINER? — I'LL FIX IT.
A DELORME METHOD INSPIRED SIX WEEK HYPERTROPHY CYCLE

Russian sports science is crystal clear on the roles of volume and intensity in training. Intensity delivers short-term strength gains for peaking, largely due to neural adaptations. Volume makes lasting changes in the muscles and other tissues. With that in mind, here is a high tonnage program that will easily pack ten to fifteen pounds of beef on your frame in two months, provided that other gaining variables such as nutrition and rest are taken care of.

Surprisingly, the routine will not take much of your time. On a couple of Mondays you will suffer for over 90 min, but on the rest of the training days you will be in and out in no time flat, sometimes in as little as twenty minutes and fresh as a daisy. This is purposeful; workouts greatly varying in length and difficulty are a lot more effective than conventional flatliners.

One of the most efficient ways to crank up the volume, while simultaneously refining your lifting technique and sparing your nervous system, is a modified DeLorme Method.

Right after World War II Dr. Thomas DeLorme of the Harvard Medical School devised an effective set-rep scheme for building muscle and might. Deceptively simple, the DeLorme Method called for a set of ten reps with half your ten rep max, then, after a brief rest, another tenner with three quarters of your top ten, and finally an all out set of whatever you can get with the ten rep maximum (DeLorme, 1945, 1946).

The DeLorme Method causes significant strength increases when employed for a short term (DeLorme & Watkins, 1948; Leighton et al., 1967). Although more effective strength training protocols do exist, DeLorme's ascending sets build an excellent foundation for heavy power training. A friend of mine, Mike, progressed from hardly being able to pick up his toddler without back pain to pulling 475 after I put him on a routine that rotated the original DeLorme with working up to a heavy single every other workout. What might interest you more than Mike's powerlifting exploits is the fact that ladies refer to him as 'a hunk of a man'. The 50-75-100 approach builds slabs of beef quicker than you can say 'moo'!

In the Soviet military, a few of my brothers-in-arms dug a bigger than regulation size physique and made spectacular gains, with a modified DeLorme workout – despite excessive exercise, sleep deprivation, stress, and a limited protein intake.. Ironically, even though you can find references to DeLorme's work in most Russian university weightlifting textbooks, these bodybuilders in uniform had never heard of the American scientist and the 50-75-100 percentages were a pure coincidence. The Red Army trained with 'kettlebells', cast iron balls with handles that came in fractions of a pood or 16kg. Standard K-bells came in three sizes, one, one and a half, and two poods; 16, 24, and 32kg respectively.

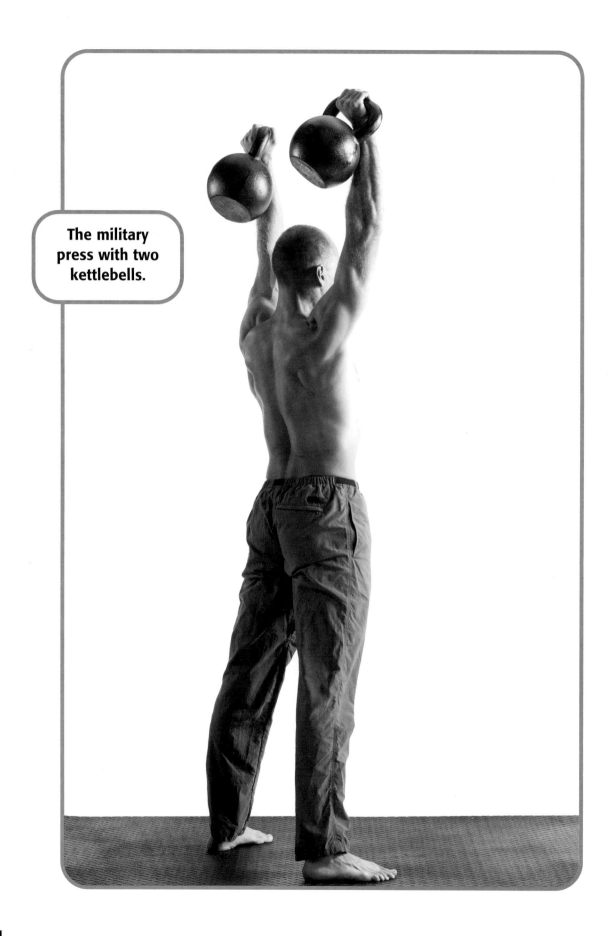

The military press with two kettlebells.

A Russian soldier would strip down to 'uniform two', BDU pants and boots, and start with a few repetitions with the lightest, 16kg, kettlebell or bells. After a brief rest, anywhere from a few seconds to a minute, he would repeat the drill for the same number of reps with the next kettlebell up, or 24kg. Then 32kg, and after a brief rest start all over with 16kg.

The technique was called 'a weight ladder'. *Salagi*, or greenhorns, were specifically instructed not to pyramid like this: 16, 24, 32, 32, 24, 16. A pyramid quickly burned out the muscles whereas a ladder pushed and backed off, thus maximizing anabolic workload: 16, 24, 32; 16, 24, 32; 16, 24, 32; 16, 24, 32; 16, 24, 32... Longer rest periods were usually recommended between each series. Sometimes another exercise was inserted between series or a number of series. For the record, a *series* is defined in Russian textbooks and gyms as a specified sequence of sets that would be performed more than once, e.g. (16kg x 5, 24kg x 5, 32kg x 5).

You were supposed to try to stick to the same rep count – whatever you could hack on your top sets without going into the do or die mode – for the light, medium, and heavy sets. You were not supposed to rep out with the lighter bells. It goes without saying, five repetitions with 32kg are twice as hard as the same with 16kg, but that was intentional. Constant loading and unloading is easier on your head and spurs greater gains. You can think of the DeLorme method as a miniature powerlifting cycle compressed from weeks into minutes.

Naturally, with fixed weights, rigidly sticking to the classic ten-rep protocol was not an option. You were stronger on one legged front squats than military presses and your buddy was in a league of his own. Troopers improvised. Sets of five happened to be in big favor – and indeed they had been tested successfully in a clinical setting by E. Krusen (1949), in a protocol similar to DeLorme's.

Fives is exactly what you are going to do on the following DeLorme inspired program. They are safer and more effective than higher reps. The numbers will still be based on your 10RM to give you a running start.

Another modification of the original protocol is the introduction of the time tested heavy-light-medium approach as an alternative to busting your chops every workout. Read Bill Starr's classic *Strongest Shall Survive* to learn the logic behind the H-L-M setup.

You will be doing only two basic drills, the bench press and the powerlifting style deadlift. Tight and bounce free. A one second pause on the chest for the press (do not relax); a one second pause on the floor for the pull. No arms, no calves, nothing else. The only acceptable addition is a couple of heavy sets of abdominal work.

Bench before deadlifting. The dead is not affected by the bench as much as the other way around. The 'rule' that states that 'bigger' exercises should always be done first does not apply when you are stressing different muscle groups.

DELORME METHOD INSPIRED SIX WEEK HYPERTROPHY CYCLE

Monday   (50% 10RM x 5, 75% 10RM x 5, 100% 10RM x 5) x max

Wednesday   (50% 10RM x 5) x the number of series performed on Monday

Friday   (50% 10RM x 5, 75% 10RM x 5) x the number of series performed on Monday

- Do two exercises, bench presses and deadlifts, in that order.

- Perform all your sets at a medium to slow tempo with a one second pause on the bottom.

- Rest for approximately 1 min or as long as it takes to adjust the poundage between sets. Rest for three minutes between series.

- On Monday perform as many series as possible in good form. When you have successfully completed five series, add five pounds to the bench press and ten pounds to the deadlift 10RM and recalculate the 50% and 75%.

You will start with a conservative ten-rep max instead of an aggressive five-rep max to meet the requirements of 'cycling'. This fundamental principle of training states that your progress will cease if you are always training at your limit. For best gains you must start easy, build up to a PR, and back off to easier training again before climbing the next peak. I know that starting out light and training not to failure will mess with your HIT brainwashed head, but that is between you and your therapist.

Assuming that your 10RM in the deadlift is 200 pounds – a rough estimate will suffice – on Monday you will perform the (100x5, 150x5, 200x5) series as many times as you can. Stop when you can barely make 200x5. The only rest you get between sets is whatever takes you to add plates. Rest for three minutes between series. Walk around and loosen up your limbs as if you are shaking water off.

Assuming you have completed four series on Monday, on Wednesday you will do only (100x5) x 4. This light session will aid recovery and painlessly increase your weekly tonnage.

Friday will see you doing another four series, this time with (100x5, 150x5). This medium day is building back up to a tough Monday workout.

On Monday you shall hopefully make five or six full size series of (100x5, 150x5, 200x5). When you have made a fiver, it is time to add weight to the 10RM you have used in planning your workouts. The deadlift calls for a ten-pound jump, unless your 10RM is higher than 400 pounds or lower than 100 pounds. 200 + 10 = 210. Recalculate your 50% and 75% sets based on 210, 105 and 160, and keep on plugging away. Add only five pounds to your bench press.

Since the souped up DeLorme workout calls for up to seventy five reps per exercise, most bodybuilders, spoiled by trendy infrequent low set training, will be totally unprepared for such a manly workload. That is why before tackling the real thing you should do a two-week long introductory cycle that gently builds up the tonnage.

INTRODUCTORY CYCLE

WEEK 1

Monday	(50% 10RM x 5, 75% 10RM x 5) x 3
Wednesday	(50% 10RM x 5, 75% 10RM x 5) x 4
Friday	(50% 10RM x 5, 75% 10RM x 5) x 5

WEEK 2

Monday	(50% 10RM x 5, 75% 10RM x 5, 100% 10RM x 5) x 2
Wednesday	(50% 10RM x 5, 75% 10RM x 5) x 7
Friday	(50% 10RM x 5, 75% 10RM x 5) x 5

You will also get a chance to get into the deadlift groove; I can bet dollars against roubles that you have not been doing those lately. By the way, Comrade, none of those 'fitness model' straight legged deads with your neck crooked to the side to watch your butt in the mirror! The good ole' powerlifting style deadlift. Conventional or sumo, your choice. Ask a PLer to show you how. And no, you are not supposed to wear a belt, so make sure to base your percentages on a beltless ten-rep max. No straps either. Chalk up and use the staggered powerlifting grip: one hand facing forward and the other back. Don't forget to switch hands to even out the load on your back. Make sure to keep your triceps flexed to avoid pulling with your arms and hurting your elbows.

The bench press, even though you think that you have it down pat, also requires a precise technique, especially when you are handling such an Olympian workload. If you do not want your shoulders to flare up, you will make a point of keeping them pressed into the bench, your shoulder blades pinched together, and your chest as high as possible. If you do not long for aching elbows, you will not snap them out at the lockout.

Off to the gym you go!

Behold the anabolic power of a cyclical high tonnage regimen! When a long lost friend bumps into you two months from now, checks out your newly bulging physique, and exclaims, "Weren't you a hardgainer?!", give him Inspector Clouseau's uppity look: "Not any more!"

'FATIGUE CYCLING': ANOTHER SECRET OF THE RUSSIAN BODYBUILDING UNDERGROUND

It was the mid-1980s, the euphoric years of Gorbachev's perestroyka and glastnost, when bodybuilding exploded in the Soviet Union. And exploded it did. Under the direction of retired weightlifters, scrawny kids from the rough part of town filled out into he-men worthy of a Charles Atlas ad. All that on a porridge and potato based diet often supplemented with soy animal feed for extra protein. Where there is a will, there is a way. Hard and ingenious training overcame cards clearly not dealt in their favor.

The following routine born in the basements of tough town Lyubertsi is unique, yet very simple, as all things that impress.* It got a two thumbs up from Sergey Zaytsev, the USSR champion in BOTH bodybuilding and powerlifting. Two workouts were alternated, usually three times a week:

RUSSIAN BODYBUILDING UNDERGROUND 'FATIGUE CYCLING' PROGRAM

WORKOUT A

1. Wide grip pullup – 4xRM
2. Bent over row – 1x12 (easy), 4x8
3. Overhead press – 1x12, 4x8
4. Squat – 1x15, 3x12
5. Bench press – 1x12, 4x8
6. Lateral raise – 4x10
7. Seated dumbbell curl –1x12, 4x8
8. Hanging leg raise – 4x12-15

WORKOUT B

1. Bench press – 1x12, 4x8
2. Lateral raise – 4x10
3. Seated dumbbell curl – 1x12, 4x8
4. Squat –1x15, 3x12
5. Wide grip pullup – 4xRM
6. Bent over row –1x12 (easy), 4x8
7. Overhead press – 1x12, 4x8
8. Hanging leg raise – 4x12-15

The exercises listed are nothing special and neither are the loading parameters. If you look at the routine carefully, you will notice that both workouts are made up of identical exercises, sets, and reps. The only difference is the order of the drills. Explains a veteran Soviet bodybuilder who gained big on this program, "As a rule, you can lift more weight in a given exercise in the beginning, rather than the middle or the end of your workout. However, if you have already conquered that weight fresh in the past and have no psychological barriers about it, you should be able to work yourself up and make the numbers late in the workout. The next workout, when you are scheduled to do the same exercise fresh, the old weight will be too light and you will definitely add more."

What is the point? – In a perfect world, you could add five pounds to all your lifts every workout and grow stronger ever after. Before you know it, you would be benching a grand. Nice try. It is too bad, but in this galaxy the physiological law of accommodation spoils all the fun in just a few short weeks. The law states that an organism gets desensitized and stops adapting to a training stimulus after a period of time. Your body figures, "Hey, it hasn't killed me, why bother to adapt?" At this point a change in the program is called for.

This is where most bodybuilders screw up. The easiest thing to do is to simply overhaul your workout completely: new exercises, sets, reps, new everything. The day after you are sore to the bone and happy as a clam. But are you making gains or just fooling yourself?

Scientists who study complex systems – the human body is one of them – know that in order to thrive, these systems must teeter 'on the edge of chaos'. To use a political analogy, a country with no structure, anarchy, is doomed. And a totalitarian state with too much structure such as the Soviet Union is bound to stagnate eventually.

If the training schedule is totally erratic, there is no structure or direction. You get very sore but you are not building much muscle and even less strength. If, on the other hand, your training hardly changes at all, you will hit the wall and stay there for years. What is required is enough change to stimulate gains but not too much, so your training does not lose its focus.

Until now the only surefire way of doing this was powerlifting style cycling. You stick pretty much to the same exercises but after reaching a PR you back off to very light weights to make your muscles get somewhat out of shape and become responsive to training again. The author of *Brawn* Stuart McRobert aptly named this process 'softening up'. Although hard to handle psychologically, cycling is the only training structure that is reliable over a long haul.

Not any more. The Russian 'fatigue cycling' technique is another dependable plateau buster in your strength and muscle building toolbox. The routine maintains the structure (the same exercises, sets, and reps) but jolts the system with the fresh stimulus of a new exercise order.

Here is a powerlift-based routine structured according to the fatigue cycling principle. Train twice a week, for instance Mondays and Thursdays, rotating the three listed workouts. Wrap up each workout with some ab work, low reps also. If you wish, you can do some light beach work such as curls on Saturdays.

FATIGUE CYCLING
POWERLIFT BASED PROGRAM

WORKOUT A	WORKOUT B	WORKOUT C
1. Bench press – 6x4	1. Squat – 3x4	1. Deadlift – 3x4
2. Squat – 3x4	2. Bench press – 6x4	2. Squat – 3x4
3. Deadlift – 3x4	3. Deadlift – 3x4	3. Bench press – 6x4

And one more routine for you to choose from. Rotate the two workouts and train three times a week.

FATIGUE CYCLING
'NEVER LIE DOWN TO TRAIN' PROGRAM

WORKOUT A	WORKOUT B
1. Deadlift – 3x3	1. Clean-and-press – 5x5
2. Weighted dips – 5x5	2. Weighted pullups – 5x5
3. Clean and press – 5x5	3. Deadlift – 3x3
4. Weighted pullups – 5x5	4. Weighted dips – 5x5

Follow any of the above routines for as long as you make gains, then switch to a basic power-lifting cycle without changing the exercise. If you have a couple of years of training under your belt do not feel the pressure to up the poundage for each 'fresh' lift in every workout. Staying with the same numbers for two or three sessions is legit for an experienced muscle head.

Here is an arm specialization routine that is built around the fatigue cycling principle. Do the workout A on Mondays and B on Thursdays. On Tuesdays and Fridays perform the infamous twenty-rep squat routine plus 5x5 of your favorite ab exercise.

FATIGUE CYCLING ARM SPECIALIZATION PROGRAM

WORKOUT A

1. EZ bar French press – 3x6
2. Incline dumbbell curl – 3x6
3. Close grip bench press – 3x6
4. Barbell curl – 3x6

WORKOUT B

1. Barbell curl – 3x6
2. Close grip bench press – 3x6
3. Incline dumbbell curl – 3x6
4. EZ bar French press – 3x6

In the Soviet Special Forces we successfully applied the fatigue cycling principle to a number of exercises we were tested on, especially pullups and snatches with a 53-pound kettlebell. In fact, we did a lot of strength training once fatigued from a ruck march, a run, or an obstacle course. You can apply this setup to your sport conditioning as well. For instance, a fighter could alternate strength training before and after his martial art practice. In addition to cutting back on plateaus, such training builds guts.

In order to get good at something you must practice it specifically. On the other hand, if you keep doing the same thing you will eventually plateau. This is the conflict between the laws of specificity and accommodation. So effective training must be 'same but different'! A puzzle for a Zen master. Solved.

* When referring to training in Lyubertsi in this and other pieces, I have used material from the book *Bodybuilding Our Way* by 'Dr. Lyuber'.

THE RUSSIAN SQUAT ASSAULT

There are many effective routines but few are powerful enough to acquire cult status. The Five-Sets-of-Five... The Twenty-Rep-Super-Squats... The Smolov...

Shortly before the fall of the Soviet Union, powerlifting coach S. Y. Smolov, Master of Sports designed what is undeniably the hardest and the most effective squat program ever. This strong statement is backed up with extraordinary gains from lifters on both sides of the pond. After I wrote up the Smolov in *Powerlifting USA* magazine a few years ago I was swamped with incredible success stories. Here is one. A drug free master lifter took his squat from 560 pounds to 665 in thirteen weeks! Then he went on to win the world lifetime drug free master title and to set a world squat record in his class! Usually, a report like this is followed by 'individual results may vary' in small print. Not in the Smolov's case! Such gains are typical. I repeat: many advanced strength athletes have added 100 pounds to their squats in just over four months!

Now for the bad news. Quoting the above powerlifter, "I have never worked harder in 25+ years of exercise." Coming from a world champion, these words carry weight. The original Smolov routine calls for four heavy squat days a week totaling 136 reps with very heavy weights!

I am a realist; most iron athletes just do not have the conditioning to survive the full Smolov. Following is a kinder, gentler version of the program adapted to two days a week.

THE RUSSIAN SQUAT ASSAULT

Week#	Monday	Thursday
1	70%x9x4*	75%x7x5
2	80%x5x7	85%x3x10
3	(70%+10lbs.)x9x4	(75%+10lbs.)x7x5
4	(80%+10lbs.)x5x7	(85%+10lbs.)x3x10
5	(70%+15lbs.)x9x4	(75%+15lbs.)x7x5
6	(80%+15lbs.)x5x7	(85%+15lbs.)x3x10

* %1RM x repetitions x sets
Double the poundage increases if you squat 1RM is greater than 300 pounds.

The percentages are based on your current, not projected, max. Review the matrix to get a feel for the routine. You will be squatting with 70, 75, 80, and finally 85% of your max on four consecutive workouts for the specified sets and reps. Make sure not to confuse the reps and the sets; it is ten sets of three and not vice versa! Put up your weights at a slow to moderate tempo; dynamic efforts do not belong here.

The fifth workout will drop back to 70%, except this time you will need to add ten pounds. If your squat max is 200 and 70% is 140, the workout number five will have you squat 150. Keep following the sequence and add ten pounds to your higher percentages as well. E.g., 75%1RM = 150. 150+10=160. 80%1RM = 160. 160+10=170. 85% 1RM =170. 170+10=180.

The routine repeats the same four-workout cycle one more time for a total of three. The third wave calls for a fifteen-pound increase in all the percentages. Pay attention that you will be adding fifteen pounds to the original 80%, 160+15=175. Do not make the painful mistake of stacking an additional fifteen pounds to the 80%+10 lbs. of the last wave. Review the following sample cycle to make sure we are on the same wavelength.

SAMPLE RUSSIAN SQUAT ASSAULT CYCLE BASED ON A 200-POUND 1RM

Week#	Monday	Thursday
1	140lbs. x 9 reps x 4 sets	150x7x5
2	160x5x7	170x3x10
3	150x9x4	160x7x5
4	170x5x7	180x3x10
5	155x9x4	165x7x5
6	175x5x7	185x3x10

If you squat three wheels or more, double the poundage jumps: twenty and thirty rather than ten and fifteen. This is how the routine would look for a bigger squatter.

SAMPLE RUSSIAN SQUAT ASSAULT CYCLE BASED ON A 400-POUND 1RM

Week#	Monday	Thursday
1	280 lbs. x 9 reps x 4 sets	300x7x5
2	320x5x7	340x3x10
3	300x9x4	320x7x5
4	340x5x7	360x3x10
5	310x9x4	330x7x5
6	350x5x7	370x3x10

If you are having a tough time making the numbers, cut the reps and up the sets to keep the weight and the total repetitions constant. For instance, if 280x9x4 is killing you do 280x4x9 instead.

The mad Commie who dreamed up this evil cycle promises that once you have survived these weeks your legs will turn into car jacks.

Rest for a week after completing the above cycle, then test your max. This stretch is usually good for fifty pounds on your squat and inches on your thighs.

Then you have some choices to make. After the above loading cycle, powerlifters usually spend two weeks recouping with light and explosive lifts – and then head into the peaking cycle to get ready for a meet. If you choose to do that, you will add another pair of big wheels to your squat but do not expect to gain a lot more muscle. This not the place to go into the intricacies of peaking, using support gear, and other purely powerlifting concerns. If inquiring minds really need to know, they can find a free reprint of my old *Powerlifting USA* article on PowerbyPavel.com.

A much more fitting choice for a power bodybuilder is to follow the Smolov application of powerlifting champion Marty Gallagher. He chose to bench as well as squat following the same Smolov format and added some arm work to top it all off. (There have been reports of impressive bench gains on this routine as well.) Here is Gallagher's weekly split:

Monday – squat   **Friday** – bench, arms

Tuesday – bench, arms   **Saturday** – off

Wednesday – off   **Sunday** – off

Thursday – squat

"This… squat/bench specialization program… lasts for 4-8 weeks. After this specialization program is over I will then hit a back specialization program for 4-8 weeks. Afterward this is all over I will roll into a standard powerlifting program. In addition, I hit the steep mountain trails 5-6 days a week for 40-60 minutes."

Please note that after the Smolov, America's top powerlifting coach goes back to conventional training. The Russian Squat Assault was designed as a shock treatment to deliver unprecedented gains when everything else fails; it was not meant to be followed on an ongoing basis!

Russian expatriate powerlifting authority Andrey Butenko spoke up about the Smolov regimen, "I've used this squat program many times and I was drug free. It gave me huge gains and that's the only program I would recommend for fast and guaranteed improvement… my weight has gone up with huge increases in the legs and the back… it is very, very, very intense… or insane, but it does work… I've done it a hundred times and it always worked… It kills but it works!"

Accept the Russian Squat Assault challenge! This brutal routine will flush every cowardly myth about 'overtraining' down the toilet and make your legs swell with muscle and power! Comrade Smolov promised that your gains will surprise you and he has not let anyone down yet. Squat till, as Soviet weightlifting great Yuri Vlasov put it, there is 'dark red twilight in your head' and 'the roaring of blood in your ears' and you will earn it. The power.

THE PRESENCE OF POWER AND THREE SUPER SQUAT TECHNIQUES TO DEVELOP IT

Bound for Columbus, where I was to speak at the Arnold Classic martial arts seminar, I changed planes in Chicago. Suddenly the usual preflight hustle of military pressing non-regulation size bags into the overhead compartments stopped and somebody whispered, "Dorian Yates!"

'Shadow' was working his way to his seat avoiding eye contact with other passengers and hopelessly trying to remain inconspicuous. Medium height, in a baggy leather jacket, and far from his peak condition, he should not have made a larger than life impression, yet he rendered everyone speechless.

Dorian exuded the quiet strength of a man with whom, as the Russians say, 'you would go on a recon mission'. That look of an old war horse who does not need his campaign ribbons to show that he has been around. That look of a hand-to-hand combat expert whose efficiency in violence is advertised, rather than hidden, by his serene composure.

You cannot fake that look. It must be earned by facing a great challenge and living up to it. A challenge like Mr. Olympia's 700-pound squats. They made him sweat blood and made him a better man for it. Heavy squats forged Dorian's physique to the point where he looked more like a rock on the Moon than a carbon based life form. More importantly, heavy squatting built the champion's inner strength. Subtle, yet irresistible like gravity, Dorian's force field made the passengers on the Columbus flight turn his way even though his Olympian guns were far from his prime. The presence of strength...

Take a hint: squat! Forget your hamstring striations and quad separations, and add a hundred pounds to your squat, even if it kills you! Forget the pump and train like a weightlifting champion. Three powerful techniques you are about to learn, two of them from my native Russia, will help you to achieve squatting greatness in the shortest time possible by conditioning your nervous system to the peak of performance. Get the power and you will have the look. Guaranteed.

PROPRIOCEPTIVE SENSITIVITY TRAINING

Robert Roman used to conquer gold for the Soviet Empire on the weightlifting platform. Today he is a top coach who has trained many young lifters to greatness using his revolutionary methods. Roman is convinced that developing superior sport specific body awareness will make a difference between being good and great!

It is not enough to have muscle, you have got to know how to use it. Soviet experiments revealed that even elite lifters made huge errors in estimating the height of the lift, the magnitude of the force, etc.[1] When special techniques for maximizing what Roman calls the 'muscle-joint sense'[2] were developed, the top guys outdid themselves and some unpromising also-rans became world class!

Robert Roman's sportsmen develop their muscle-joint sense by lifting ...blindfolded! Their coach explains that because we so heavily rely on our eyesight, we do not pay enough attention to the various sensations in our muscles, tendons, ligaments, and joints. When blindfolded, the lifter is forced to listen to his body. Contrary to what a mirror gazing bodybuilder wants to believe, this tremendously improves the technique and its stability![2]

Kick off your muscle-joint sense training by getting a pair of blindfolds. Roman does not recommend lifting with your eyes closed because it distracts you from what you are supposed to be doing. Training with the lights turned off may be an effective alternative, but the gym owner might object, at least if he finds you before he stumbles on a dumbbell and cracks his head against the Smith machine. So blindfolds it is.

Start squatting light with your eyes open, then cover your eyes. Keep alternating open and shut eye sets or reps, but do not add wheels until you own a given weight, blind. Do not just go through the motions but concentrate on the feedback your body has to offer: muscular tension, joint angles, etc. When something feels wrong, correct it and remember what you have corrected. Make a point of sinking every squat to parallel, that is the top of the knee higher than the crease on top of your thigh. Have your training partner watch your depth but ask him not to give you any feedback until you are done squatting. You must rely on your senses.

The purpose of this drill is not to make your squats pretty, but to make them heavy. The squat is a very complex lift and by finessing your skill, you are guaranteed to lift a lot more iron. Just ask four times Powerlifting World Record Holder Dr. Judd Biasiotto, who spent a lot of time developing his squatting body awareness with special techniques of his own. "...I was able to become aware of the muscles I was using during each segment of my lifts. When I got stuck at a certain part of the lift, I knew exactly which muscles to recruit and/or concentrate on to make the lift. " And stood up with 605 pounds at 130 pounds of bodyweight! Today Judd Biasiotto is a successful bodybuilder who routinely squats 330 pounds for 30 reps. Have no doubt that his proprioceptive sensitivity training paid off!

EXTENSOR REFLEX TRAINING

There is a Russian joke about a guy who wore shoes two sizes too small for him. When asked about his bizarre behavior, he complained about his miserable life and concluded that his only happiness in life was to come home and take off his shoes! You will be even happier than this dude if you lose yours – at least for a part of your squat workout.

The forcefulness of a muscular contraction is determined by the sum of the mental effort and various reflexes. When Dr. Fred Hatfield bounced out of the bottom of his 1,000-pound squat, he took advantage of the stretch reflex. Another power boosting reflex is called the *extensor reflex*. This reflex causes the leg musculature to contract in response to the pressure on the sole of your foot. It is a protective measure against loading.

Research suggests that always wearing shoes diminishes the sensitivity of the foot 3, which may turn off the squat friendly reflex. Too bad, because when the barbell is intent on squashing you like a bug on the windshield, you could use any help you can get! The rare squatter who has recognized this problem is Dr. Fred Clary, a human crane who has elevated 900 pounds! Fred regularly performs heavy, 1,000 pounds plus, walkouts barefoot 'just to fire off those receptors'.

Clary believes that such training sensitizes the extensor reflex receptors and enables him to squat heavier. And not him alone. Long before he became a Senior RKC instructor, Brazilian Jiu Jitsu Senior World Champion Steve Maxwell, M.S., read about barefoot lifting in my book *Power to the People!* He ordered all the people he coached to lose their shoes – and every one of them succeeded in knocking off a couple of extra reps on their leg exercises!

The proof is in the pudding, it pays to add barefoot walkouts or squats to your routine. But since the gym owner might object if you go native with your dirty toe nails scraping his floor, get yourself a pair of deadlift slippers. They look almost like ballet slippers and are probably available in pink. Have fun.

It is ironic that the barefoot populations of countries with nice climates and no extradition, suffer fewer running injuries than Americans and others who look up to Imelda Marcos 3. Scientists believe that running, aerobic, and other fancy shoes cause injuries that would not have happened without them [4].

The extensor reflex recruits the leg muscles in a precise pattern according to the direction of pressure from the ground [5]. Poorly designed shoes may redirect the pressure where it does not belong – and alter the proper recruitment pattern [6]. Besides, shoes with high shock absorption delay the transmission of pressure to the sole of your foot [6]. That has the effect of a devious KGB trick devised to find out if a person who pretends to be deaf really is. The men in black have the American spy suspect read a script into a microphone and feed it back to his headphones with a slight delay. This will not phase a deaf guy but will totally confuse the enemy of the state who is faking it. He will stumble and be unable to continue. The cushy soles of your workout shoes, thick as the platforms hippy girls wore at Woodstock, will play the same joke on your extensor reflex. Although the consequences, a reduced squat poundage and increased odds of injury, are less drastic than the firing squat in the Lubyanka courtyard, this is considered a problem in this land of minor inconveniences.

So lose your sneakers on steroids, once and for all! When you are not lifting barefoot, wear shoes with non-giving soles like all top powerlifters do. Quad squatters go for specialized shoes made by SAFE USA (you may have seen a picture of Tom Platz wearing them) or weightlifting shoes from Adidas. You can track both down through the *Powerlifting USA* magazine. Ditto for the deadlift slippers from Crain's Muscle World.

Supersquatters who rely on their hamstrings and glutes more than their quads prefer Chuck Taylor's Converse old-fashioned basketball shoes. Your Gramps must have worn a pair of these canvas-topped classics with a flat solid sole. You can get a pair for around thirty bucks in any athletic shoe store. The Chucks are probably the best all around shoes for strength training. An understated hard core design.

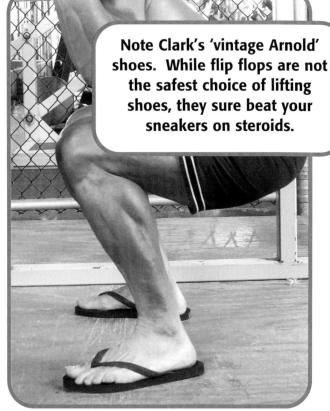

Note Clark's 'vintage Arnold' shoes. While flip flops are not the safest choice of lifting shoes, they sure beat your sneakers on steroids.

It is not unusual for modern power programs to include supramaximal walkouts, lockouts, or supports after regular lifts. They condition the body and mind for heavier weights. It works, but what if instead of walking out 600 pounds after your maximum 500 pound squat, you do the overload a couple of minutes BEFORE the heavy full squat? – 500 pounds will feel like 400 and an all time high 515 will go up like 490!

Every gym rat knows that the heavier the weight, the more muscle is recruited. Manhandling 600 pounds fires off more motor units than 500 pounds, even if you only hold the bar. This is called the Henneman's size principle [8], probably because it builds some serious size! Especially if combined with the after-effect phenomenon [9], or the fact that your nervous system is a bit slow on the uptake. Remember pushing your arms against the doorway at the summer camp and then watching them float up involuntarily? It happened because your brain had not caught on quick enough to the fact that the resistance had been removed. Good! After you have supported 600 pounds on your back, five wheels will explode to lockout!

After-effect overloads make you stronger in more than one way. In addition to boosting muscle recruitment, they lower the sensitivity of the Golgi tendon organs, spinal mechanoreceptors, and other governors of strength. After dealing with 600 pounds, these subversive sensors think, "Hey!

515 is not too bad!" and pull the brick from under your gas pedal! This type of disinhibition training has an awesome potential for reaching the final frontier in strength development.

Start your after-effect overload power squat program by deciding what personal best you would like to shoot for today. How about ten more pounds on your max single, or four reps with your all time heaviest triple? It is your call, as long as you keep your reps to five and under. After-effect overloads are strictly for power squatting!

After your last warm-up set load up the bar with 110-130% 1RM. Do not go heavier than that. This will not make the technique work any better but will certainly tire you out prematurely. Besides, an excessively heavy overload might make your regular weight feel so light that your muscles will not contract hard enough to lift it! An optimal, rather than maximal, load delivers the most powerful after-effect [7].

Safety must be considered as well. If you have not done any type of lockouts, walkouts, or supports in the past, take as many workouts as necessary to build up the poundage. When you overload, you should feel super tight and powerful, and not shaky!

Unrack the barbell, walk it out, and set up using the same stance you are about to full squat with. Hold your burden for five to ten seconds, and park. Stay tight and breathe shallow. In two to five minutes– the optimal rest time to take advantage of the aftereffect phenomenon [7]– or whenever you feel ready, go for the record!

Why, you might ask, should you bother with these powerlifting techniques? After all, you get a lot better pump doing high reps on the Smith machine! – Because no amount of pumped tissue can make you look powerful. The look comes with the power. Martial artists know the ancient Chinese wisdom: a real master does not fight. He does not have to; his humble appearance cannot hide his lethal skills from anyone. In my favorite western *The Magnificent Seven*, Yul Brynner sat at the bar stone faced while a young punk was waving his loaded Colt in a hormone fit. The deadly calm of the veteran gunfighter won the shootout before it even started. It is the presence of power. You can't fake it with a tough grimace from a cheesy action flick or vain flexing of virtual muscles pumped up with Barbie weights. It must be earned on the battlefield, be it the OK Corral, the kickboxing ring, or the squat rack.

References

1. Sokolov L. (1982). Nekotoriye voprosi sovershenstvovaniya v sportivnoy tekhnike tyazeloatletov. (Some issues in improvement of weightlifters' technique.) In: Sandalov, Y., ed. *Tyazhelay Atletika Yezhegodnik (Weightlifting Yearbook)*. Moscow: Fizkultura i Sport, 1982: 24-26.

2. Roman R. (1986). *Trenirovka Tyazheloatleta (A Weightlifter's Training)*, Moscow: Fizkultura i Sport.

3. Robbins S., Hanna A. & Gouw G. (1988). Overload protection: avoidance response to heavy plantar surface loading. *Med. & Sci. Sports Exerc.* 6: 253-259.

4. Robbins S. & Hanna A. (1987). Running related injury prevention through barefoot adaptations. *Med. & Sci. Sports Exerc.* 19: 148-156.

5. Guyton A. (1984). *Textbook of Medical Physiology*, 6th ed. Philadelphia: WB Saunders Co.

6. Verkhoshansky Y. & Siff M. (1996). *Supertraining: Special Strength Training for Sports Excellence,* 2nd ed. Witwatersrand, South Africa: M. C. Siff & Y. V. Verkhoshansky.

7. Verkhoshansky Y. (1977). *Osnovi Spetsialnoy Silovoy Podgotovki v Sporte (The Fundamentals of Sport Specific Strength Training),* 2nd ed. Moscow: Fizkultura i Sport.

8. Henneman, E., Somjen, G. & Carpenter, D. O. (1965). Functional significance of cell size in spinal motoneurons. *J. Neurophysiol.* 28: 560-580.

9. Pavlov, I. (1927). *Conditioned Reflexes.* London: Oxford Univ. Press.

BENCH PRESS TRAINING, THE RUSSIAN NATIONAL POWERLIFTING TEAM STYLE

This article was originally published in *Powerlifting USA* and later translated by its Russian equivalent, the leading powerlifting magazine in the countries of the former USSR *Mir Sili*. If you have no powerlifting background, it is likely to give you a splitting headache rather than a big bench press. If you do, it will give you a deep insight into the Russian system of training.

Eight out of the eleven gold medals at the IPF Men's Worlds went home beyond what used to be the Iron Curtain. Wouldn't you like to know how guys like Alexey Sivokon train?

Following is a bench press program designed by the Russian powerlifting mastermind Boris Sheyko. The man used to train the Kazakhstan team and today is the Chief Coach, Men's Powerlifting Team Russia. Comrade Sheyko's credentials include Sivokon, Mor, and Podtinniy. 'Nuff said.

Heavily influenced by R. Plukfelder and I. Abajiev, Sheyko believes in some serious volume. While Western PLers have gradually cut back to one weekly BP workout the Russian team coach insists on four to eight bench press sessions a week! The arms and shoulder girdle can recover a lot quicker than the legs and back, he says, so why not?! Sheyko likes to quote the expression popular among Russian weightlifters in the fifties and sixties: "To press a lot one must press a lot".

No, it is not a program just for bench specialists like Irina Lugovaya who owes it her European championship title. The following super system is every bit as effective for full meet lifters. So enjoy the pain, Comrade!

The matrix is designed for five BP workouts a week and is aimed at an advanced powerlifter, a KMS or an MS in Russian classification. The cycle is divided into preparatory and competition periods. Here is how the prep period gets kicked off:

PREPARATORY WEEK 1

Monday	1. BP – 50%x5, 60%x4, 70%x3x2, 80%x3x5 (30)
	3. BP – 44%x5, 65%x5, 75%x4x4 (26)
Tuesday	1. Incline BP – x4x6 (24)
	2. Parallel bar dips (with weight) – x6x5
Wednesday	1. BP – 50%x6, 60%x5, 70%x4x2, 75%x3x2, 80%x2x2, 85%x1x2, 80% x2x2, 75%x3x2, 70%x4, 65%x5, 60%x6, 55%x7, 50%x8 (71)
Friday	2. BP – 50%x5, 60%x4, 70%x3, 80%x2x5 (25)
Saturday	2. PBN – 5x5 (25)
	3. Parallel bar dips – x4x6

Total lifts per week: 201
Average intensity: 67.1%

Note the number in brackets following a series; it is the total number of lifts in the series. The number before an exercise denotes its position in a training session. For example, on Monday you bench first, then do some SQ or DL drill and bench again. On Friday you bench second after another lift.

More often than not, Sheyko's charges – including IPF bench press world champions Alexey Sivokon and Fanil Mukhamatyanov – press twice in one training session. There is a curious wrinkle: the two pressing series are always separated by squat or deadlift work.

Boris Sheyko points out how the Monday load is intense and the Wednesday load beats you up with high volume. Note, says the Team Russia coach, even though the athlete has worked up to 80-85% 1RM, he has done many lighter lifts and therefore the average intensity is low.

If you have a general idea of the Russian approach to strength program design, you should appreciate how this elegant and precise method relies heavily on the calculations of the volume expressed in a number of barbell lifts (NBL) in a given intensity zone, or percentage of one rep max. According to Boris Sheyko, tracking these numbers, as well as the average training weight and total tonnage – or, if you are not up on the metric system, poundage – is mandatory. The Russian coach points out how helpful the numbers are for serving the critical component of any strength training plan: variability, or rotation of heavy, medium, and light training sessions, both in a weekly and in a monthly cycle. Indeed, these calculations have been an integral part of Soviet weightlifting since 1958, when scientist Leonid Matveyev worked with coach Suren Bogdasarov on future world champion Yuri Vlasov's training plans.

PREPARATORY WEEK 2

Monday	1. BP. – 50%x5, 60%x4, 70%x3x2, 80%x2x2, 90%x1x3 (22) 3. BP. – 50%x3, 60%x3, 70%x3, 80%x2x5 (19)
Tuesday	2. Parallel bar dips. – x5x5
Wednesday	2. BP. – 55%x5, 65%x4, 75%x3x2, 85%x2x4 (23)
Friday	2. 50%x5, 60%x4, 70%x3x2, 80%x3x7 (36)
Saturday	2. BP. – 55%x5, 65%x5, 75%x4x5 (30) 4. Triceps work. – x10x5

Total lifts per week: 130
Average intensity: 71.5%

Note how the NBL has been cut back from 201 in the first week to 130 in the second. When the volume goes down, the intensity goes up; in week two Sheyko added more 85-90% 1RM lifts and thus upped the average intensity from 67.1% to 71.5%

PREPARATORY WEEK 3

Monday	1. BP. – 50%x5, 60%x4, 70%x3x2, 80%x3x5 (30) 3. BP. – 50%x5, 60%x5, 70%x5x5 (35)
Tuesday	2. BP. – 55%x4, 65%x4, 75%x3x4 (20)
Wednesday	1. BP. – 50%x8, 55%x7, 60%x6, 65%x5, 70%x4, 75%x3x2, 80%x2x2, 75%x3x2, 70%x4, 65%x6, 60%x8, 55%x10, 50%x12 (86)
Friday	2. 50%x5, 60%x4, 70%x3x2, 75%x3x6 (33)
Saturday	2. BP. – 50%x6, 60%x6, 65%x6x4 (36)

Total lifts per week: 240
Average intensity: 64.7%

In week three Sheyko gives his lifters 240 barbell lifts at a 64.7% average intensity. The increased volume in the 65-75% intensity zone has necessitated a drop in intensity. But because there is no one right way to wave the load up and down, the coach muses that he might as well have written up something like NBL 170/69.1%.

Note the brutal eighty-six rep Wednesday marathon. Sheyko warns that you will be a hurting unit and will have to have the grit to make it through. By the way, the above numbers are not the limit; Alexey Sivokon has done one hundred and twenty rep marathons while working up to 90% intensity! Naturally, he cut back on intensity the week after.

PREPARATORY WEEK 4

Monday	2. BP. – 50%x4, 60%x4, 70%x3x2, 80%x2x5 (24)
Tuesday	2. Incline BP. –x3x5 (15) 3. Parallel bar dips. – x6x5
Wednesday	2. BP. –50%x5, 60%x4, 70%x3x2, 75%x2x2, 80%x1x3, 75%x2x2, 70%x4, 60%x6, 50%x8 (44)
Friday	2. BP. – 55%x4, 65%x4, 75%x3x2, 85%x2x4 (22)
Saturday	2. PBN. – x4x5 (20) 3. Triceps work. – x10x5

Total lifts per week: 125
Average intensity: 67.2%

The following table, which should find its way into your training log, illustrates the variability in the Russian bench press program:

PREPARATORY PERIOD LOAD DISTRIBUTION

Intensity Zones	Week 1	Week 2	Week 3	Week 4	Per Month
50%	24	13	41	17	95
51-60%	31	21	54	20	126
61-70%	34	24	84	20	162
71-80%	61	61	61	27	210
81-90%	2	11	----------	8	21
91-100%	----------	----------	----------	----------	----------
NBL	152	130	240	92	614
Intensity	67.1%	71.5%	64.7%	67.2%	67.1%

In the four to six week long competition period the Russian National Team says good-bye to marathons and reduces the reps to the maximum of three per set. NBL with warm-up weights of 50-70% goes down and the number of 75-95% lifts goes up.

COMPETITION WEEK 1

Monday	2. BP. -50%x3, 60%x3, 70%x3x2, 80%x3x6 (30)
Tuesday	1. Incline BP. – x3x5 (15)
Wednesday	1. BP. – 50%x3, 60%x3, 70%x3x2, 80%x2x3, 85%x1x3 (21)
Friday	1. BP. – 50%x3, 60%x3, 70%x3x2, 80%x3x5 (27) 3. BP. – 55%x4, 65%x4, 75%x4x4 (24)
Saturday	Rest

Total lifts per week: 117
Average intensity: 71.6%

COMPETITION WEEK 2

Monday	1. BP. – 55%x3, 65%x3, 75%x3x2, 85%x2x4 (20) 3. BP. – 50%x3, 60%x3, 70%x3, 80%x3x6 (27)
Tuesday	1. PBN. – x4x5 (20)
Wednesday	1. BP. – 50%x3, 60%x3, 70%x3x2, 80%x2x8 (28)
Friday	1. BP. – 50%x3, 60%x3, 70%x3x2, 80%x2x2, 85%x2x3, 80%x2x2 (26)
Saturday	1. BP. – 55%x3, 65%x3x2, 75%x2x4 (14)

Total lifts per week: 135
Average intensity: 72.7%

COMPETITION WEEK 3

Monday	2. BP. – 50%x3, 60%x3, 70%x3x2, 75%x2x4 (20)
Tuesday	Rest
Wednesday	1. BP. – 50%x3, 60%x3, 70%x2x2, 80%x1x2, 90%x1, 95-100%x1x2-3 (16)
Friday	1. BP. – 50%x3, 60%x3, 70%x3x2, 80%x2x5 (22)
Saturday	1. BP. – 55%x3, 65%x3x2, 75%x3x4 (21)

Total lifts per week: 79
Average intensity: 70.0%

Approximately twenty days before a meet, Sheyko plans a prikidka, or a trial run. Experienced Russian National Team members just work up to 90-95% of their max to get a feel for their opener.

During the third week, a Russian lifter also cuts back to four bench days a week.
Observe how he performs a medium volume/low intensity workout on Monday and rests on Tuesday to taper before the Wednesday trial run.

COMPETITION WEEK 4

Monday	2. BP. – 50%x3, 60%x3, 70%x3x2, 80%x2x3, 90%x1x2, 80%x2x2 (24)
Tuesday	Rest
Wednesday	1. BP. – 55%x3, 65%x3, 75%x3x2, 85%x2x3, 80%x3x2 (24)
Friday	2. BP. – 50%x3, 60%x3, 70%x3x2, 80%x3x5 (27)
Saturday	1. BP. – 55%x3, 65%x3, 75%x2x5 (16)

Total lifts per week: 81
Average intensity: 71.8%

The fourth week is the last week with substantial NBL and heavy, 80-90% 1RM, poundages. It is time to taper before the competition. Next, or fifth, week the athlete will cut back to three training days a week and throttle down on volume and intensity.

COMPETITION WEEK 5

Monday	2. BP. – 50%x3, 60%x3, 70%x3x2, 80%x2x4 (20)
Tuesday	Rest
Wednesday	1. BP. – 50%x3, 60%x3, 70%x2x2, 80%x1x3 (13)
Friday	1. BP – 50%x3, 60%x3, 70%x3x2, 75%x2x4(20)
Saturday	Rest

Total lifts per week: 53
Average intensity: 67.7%

In week five the lifting frequency drops to three times a week and both the intensity and the tonnage are tapered.

COMPETITION WEEK 6

Monday	1. BP. – 50%x3, 60%x3, 70%x2x2, 75%x1x2 (12)
Tuesday	Rest
Wednesday	1. BP. – 50%x3, 60%x3x2, 70%x1x3 (12)
Thursday	Rest
Friday	Rest
Saturday	Competition

Total lifts per week: 24
Average intensity: 61.7%

Sheyko points out how the last session before the meet is similar to a pre-competition warm-up.

COMPETITION PERIOD LOAD DISTRIBUTION

Intensity Zones	Wk 1	Wk 2	Wk 3	Wk 4	Wk 5	Wk 6	Per Mo.
50%	9	9	9	6	9	6	48
51-60%	13	15	12	12	9	9	70
61-70%	22	21	22	18	16	7	106
71-80%	55	56	32	47	19	2	211
81-90%	3	14	1	8	-------	-------	26
91-100%	--------	-------	3	--------	-------	-------	3
NBL	102	115	79	91	53	24	464
Intensity	71.6%	72.7%	68.8%	72.4%	67.7%	61.7%	70.8%

If you compare the two tables you shall notice that in the competitive period the Russian coach cut back on the volume while increasing the intensity compared to the preparatory period. In the last two weeks of the competition cycle, both the intensity and the tonnage take a dive to enable the athlete to recover well before the meet.

Nothing fancy-trendy about Sheyko's cycle; just the classic Matveyev formula of progression from volume to intensity and finally the taper. You will not find any exotic assistance exercises in the Team Russia regimen either. "A golden rule is never to use more complex movements than necessary to achieve the desired result," as Bruce Lee once put it. "…To hit a worthy opponent with a complex movement is satisfying and shows one's mastery of technique; to hit the same opponent with a simple movement is a sign of greatness."

QUESTIONS & ANSWERS:

HOLISTIC BODYBUILDING? — NO, POWER BODYBUILDING!

Question: Your mass building routines are very one-dimensional. High set/low rep training does not stimulate many muscle tissues that could grow from other regimens. What do you have to say about that?

A functional and realistic physique for a drug free bodybuilder, say a hard 210 pounds at 5'10", can be easily and naturally achieved with powerlifting style training without the headaches of complicated routines. 'PL style training' does not mean an exclusive diet of squats, benches, and deadlifts but the high set/low rep loading you refer to in your question.

So your slow twitch fibers do not grow to their potential. So your mitochondria do not get enough stimulation. So your sarcoplasm, the filler goo in the muscle, does not get bloated. Who cares? Powerlifters do not – and sport more meat than you will ever have.

Power bodybuilding will reward you in three ways. First, you will start filling out your shirts very fast, often within days, provided you eat as heavy as you lift.

Second, you will get as strong as you look. Respect yourself; just say no to purely cosmetic training! The greatest karate master of all time, Mas Oyama, jibed at overgrown dysfunctional meat that "it didn't do the cow any more good than it will you."

Third, you will greatly simplify your life by reducing the number of variables you are juggling. Powerlifters successfully build great mass and strength while hardly ever changing their exercises. They just manipulate the poundages, the sets, and the reps. And the fewer moving parts a machine has, the more likely it is to reach its destination without breaking down.

'WORKOUT' OR 'PRACTICE'?

Question: I came across a book on physical culture published in the early XX century. It referred to a workout with weights as 'a practice' and so do you. Are you just being cute?

As my leatherneck father-in-law – who can take on any punk a third his age – likes to tell his son when the junior is heading to the health club, "Tell them sissies hello."

Mental toughness aside, one of the reasons Liederman, Nordquest, and their contemporaries succeeded in the game of strength is the simple fact that they treated their iron time as a *practice* rather than a *workout*. Understanding this subtle semantic difference made the physical culturists of the golden era supermen.

Recall the importance of neural adaptations in strength development. You can sum up these adaptations as honing your skill in contracting your muscles harder. Quoting Prof. Thomas Fahey, "Skill is perhaps the most important element in strength." In Russian sports science there is even a term *skill-strength* and your date with iron is referred to as 'a lesson' or 'a practice'.

Once you appreciate that strength training – as opposed to bodybuilding – is a form of skill practice, designing an effective customized strength program becomes just a matter of following the fundamental principles of motor learning. There are three.

First, practice must be specific. Do not rep out with a light weight when you are training for a heavy single.

The second rule is an extension of the first one. Practice fresh and stop before your skill starts deteriorating. That means ending your practice before you start dragging your tail – and saying no to training to failure.

Third, practice as frequently as possible while observing the first two rules.

Radical as it sounds, it is plain common sense. How do you go about improving your tennis serve? Do you go out on the court once a week and keep on serving until your balls could not knock out a geriatric mosquito and you could barely lift your arm? "Literally he has *worked himself out*," writes Earle Liederman in his classic 1925 *Secrets of Strength*, describing a man of iron who 'was ahead of his time' and trained like today's gym rats, obsessed with pump and afraid of frequent training, "and this is exactly the thing the strength-seeker cannot afford to do."

Everyone knows that you will improve your tennis game the most by coming to the court as often as possible, ideally more than once a day, and slamming those little yellow balls until you feel that your serves are about to go south.

Why not do the same for your iron games? Arthur Saxon who instinctively understood the motor learning principles did. He lifted close to his max but 'not on the nerve', he got good rest between his sets, and called it a day while he was still 'full of pep' – he did not *work himself out*. Saxon did only low rep work, and he *practiced* daily. Who was Saxon? – Oh, just some German who put up 370 pounds overhead with one arm almost a century ago.

Although the above guidelines evolved in the quest for wiry strength rather than massive muscles, a bodybuilder will do himself a favor by following them for three to four weeks every six months or so. Being as strong as you look should be worth something, even in this age of soft hands.

Be strong, stay fresh

Question: Lifting weights makes me sore and tired and my demanding sport practices are suffering. I am committed to excelling at my sport and I am contemplating quitting bodybuilding. Give me a reason not to.

Quit bodybuilding; start strength training. Traditional blitzing and blasting does not meet your needs. As I have explained in *Power to the People!*, a comrade who has to balance the iron with a sport should drastically cut back on his or her sets, reps, and exercises, increase the weight, and never train 'on the nerve' or close to failure. This type of training will make you very strong. And you will not be exhausted; just the other way around, it has been documented to have a tonic effect on your nervous system.

This is not a new idea. Charles MacMahon wrote in his 1925 *The Royal Road to Health and Strength,* "Instead of spending more time as I went along I spent less, because the more concentrated the exercise, the fewer times you have to repeat it.

"Once I was in the performer's tent of a big circus, chatting with a very famous trapeze performer. Just before it was time for him to do his act, he walked over to a nearby ring, hooked his first and second fingers to his right hand around it, and chinned himself twice with his right arm. Then he did the same with his left arm. He did this to "warm up" for his performance, and he told me that it was all the exercise he took outside his performance; except when he had to practice for a new stunt. Everybody knows that it takes more strength to chin once with one arm that it does to chin twenty-five times with two arms. The funny thing is that it causes far less fatigue. The performer knew that, and that is why he was so economical of his time and energy."

What does it mean, 'training the nervous system'?

Question: I keep hearing about 'training the nervous system'. What does the nervous system have to do with strength?

A legend of the iron game, weightlifting champion Yuri Vlasov, quipped that judging a man's strength by his size was akin to judging a book by its thickness. It is not the beef but a superior 'mind-muscle link' that enables one hundred and sixty-five pounders to squat six or seven big ones. The following crash course in neuroscience of strength shall clarify that point.

A skeletal muscle consists of thousands of muscle *fibers* that generate force when they contract.

A group of fibers is hooked up to the brain through a nerve cell called a *motor neuron*. This group is referred to as a *motor unit*, or an *MU*.

A muscle fiber either contracts, or it does not; there is no intermediate 'half contracted' state. This is the *all-or-none law*. The nervous system varies the force output of an individual motor unit by its *firing frequency*. Like the cylinders of an internal combustion engine, muscle MUs do not fire constantly, but at intervals. Firing the fibers with a greater frequency increases the muscle's force and power output, just like increasing a car engine's number of revolutions per minute.

Firing synchronization with other motor units is another way your nervous system can vary the muscle's force output. Normally motor units take turns firing to produce a smooth, controlled movement. A good analogy is running. You push off with one leg at a time. The force production is half of what you are capable of, the movement is smooth, and while one leg is working, the other one gets a chance to rest.

Long-term heavy training synchronizes the MU activation. As a result, you become what Russians call 'an elephant in a glassware store' (forget them bulls and china, Comrade). Your movement becomes more forceful, jerky, and cannot be sustained for a long period of time, like broad jumping. Fine motor control goes south. Your wife does not let you close to the dishes, which is just as well.

Only a small percentage of available MUs is used at one time. The number of active MUs, or *recruitment*, is crucial to your max force production. According to *Henneman's size principle*, the smaller and weaker the motor unit, the weaker the command required from the motor cortex to fire it. Feeble motor units, built for extended use at a relatively low intensity, are called *slow* and are said to have a low *firing threshold*.

Fast motor units are composed of fast twitch fibers. They are large, they generate high force, high velocity, and have very little endurance. Fast MUs are reserved for an occasional burst of effort. Your brain needs to send a forceful command, or *neural drive*, to recruit them. In other words, they have a high *firing threshold*.

In every day activities you mostly use your slow MUs. Faster motor units are engaged when the load increases. The biggest, baddest, and strongest MUs are reserved for *Reader's Digest* stories, mothers lifting cars off their children, that sort of thing.

MU recruitment, firing frequency, and firing synchronization are collectively referred to as *intra-muscular coordination*. As a side note, one of the reasons testosterone – and the steroids which mimic it – make you stronger is the fact that the motoneurons have receptor sites for the macho hormone. When testosterone plugs itself in, it 'closes' the muscle activating 'circuit' and increases your powah.

Another neural factor contributing to your strength is *inter-muscular coordination*. It is a skillfully orchestrated activation of all of the muscle groups within a specific movement, say the deadlift.

All of the above neural factors and a few I have not listed are critical to superstrength and can be improved through patient practice with heavy metal.

IS TRADITIONAL POWER CYCLING OBSOLETE?

Question: I was about to start a squat cycle from 'Brawn' that uses low reps and simply adds a little weight to the bar each week for three months. Then I heard that this type of cycling is obsolete. Is it true?

No. Progressive overload cycling is the most reliable muscle and strength building method, period. It has produced great champions like Marty Gallagher's star pupil Kirk Karwoski. 'Captain Kirk' squatted a grand and his legs have been compared to a T-rex's for their Jurassic muscularity. Take on the following squat cycle and see for yourself how 'obsolete' it is.

The cycle lasts sixteen weeks, one squat workout a week. For the first eight weeks you will be doing two sets of five with the same weight. Then take fifty pounds off the bar and perform two more sets. This time pause in the 'hole' where your thighs are parallel to the floor for three painful seconds. Add ten pounds per week. For the second eight cut your reps to triples.

Make a realistic estimate of how much you can improve in sixteen workouts and work back to establish the starting poundage. If you are new to power cycling, just take your current 1RM, tested or estimated, as the goal for two sets of three in the end of four months. If your max is 355, subtract 160 pounds – ten pounds multiplied by sixteen workouts – and you will get 195. This is your starting poundage. Your first workout will be 195x5x2 and 145x5x2 pause squats. It may not sound like much but this easy start is one of the secrets to the success of powerlifting cycles.

In workout number eight you should confidently put up 275x5x2 and 225x5x2 paused. Your ninth workout will be 285x3x2, 235x3x2 paused. In workout number sixteen you will squat your old max for two triples, 355x3x2 and 305x3x2 paused. You are closing in on four wheels!

You owe one to record holder Rickey Dale Crain who designed the above cycle. Get his straight shooting book *To Squat or Not to Squat* from crainsmuscleworld.com.

A STRAIGHTFORWARD POWER CYCLE

Question: I have a hit a plateau in my training. I've been benching my max for weeks and I am going backward instead of forward. Help!

It has been said that only mediocrities are always at their best. Top powerlifters display their max strength not more than a couple of times a year. The rest of the time they 'cycle', or back off into easier training and then build up to a new PR. Apply this form of periodization to your workouts and you are guaranteed to break your personal records! At least if you have the will power to say good-bye to pump and burn and reduce your reps to the one to five range.

Let us use your bench press as an example. Say, your one rep max is 225 pounds and your best set of ten reps is 185. On Monday perform 185x5, 190x4, 195x3, 200x2, 205x1. Rest for 3-5 minutes between the sets, power needs rest. Note that none of the sets come close to failure. It is intentional, a part of the periodization strategy. It may be hard psychologically to stop until you reach 'complete muscle failure' but that is between you and your therapist.

On Wednesday add five pounds to all your sets: 190x5, 195x4, 200x3, 205x2, 215x1. You will notice that not all the sets are equally hard. That is intentional, scaled down cycling within a workout.

On Friday add another fiver: 195x5, 200x4, 205x3, 210x2, 215x1. On this and any other of your bench days you may do a couple of your favorite muscle building exercises or, better yet, powerlifting assistance drills like the board presses, after your power sets.

Next Monday, back up to your last Wednesday numbers and work back up. Every week you will add fifteen pounds to your sets and then take ten pounds off and build up again. This is called 'wave cycling'. If you look at just your singles, your weeks will stack up like this: 205, 210, 215; 210, 215, 220; 215, 220, 225, etc.

You will have worked up to your previous best by the end of the third week and you will top off the month with a PR 230. If it goes up easy – and it should – you may want to try for 235 or wait for Monday and test yourself without the tiring preliminary sets. Try this: 135x5, 185x2, 205x1, 225x1, 235x1, and, if the going is good, 240x1 and even 245x1!

Spend the fifth week repping out with your pet bodybuilding moves and on Monday start another power cycle with slightly heavier weights, say 195x5, etc. A cycle does not have to last four weeks. If your gains keep on coming there is no reason why you should not take advantage of it for another week or two. Three wheels, here you come!

A LAST MINUTE PEAKING CYCLE

Question: I have spent a couple of months bringing up my weak muscle groups. I thought I was doing alright, both strength and muscle wise, until I benched for the first time since my weakness specialization program. My strength has gone well down! What happened and what did I do wrong?

You did nothing wrong. You just got out of your bench press groove. In other words, your muscles have a great potential, you just need to realize it through specific practice of your target lift. Follow this twelve-day peaking cycle:

43

Monday	– work up to a comfortably heavy triple
Wednesday	– work up to a comfortably heavy double
Friday	– work up to a comfortably heavy single
Monday	– work up to a comfortably heavy double
Wednesday	– work up to an easy single with the weight you used for your top triple nine days ago
Saturday	– work up to your new max

'Working up' refers to doing ascending sets of the same rep count. For instance, if your old max BP was 405 your first workout might look like this: 225x3, 275x3, 315x3. You probably could have put up 350 or more for three reps but don't. You are just practicing your bench technique; do not burn out by pushing the envelope too soon! Do not do any other chest, shoulder, or triceps exercises. It will be hard on your head because you will not be getting any pump. Deal with it.

Make sure to practice all of the high-tension techniques: irradiation, power breathing, etc. Note that on Wednesday of the second week your top single will equal the top triple of your first bench press session: 315 in the above example. Very easy but that is intentional and a vital part of the tapering process.

On Saturday get psyched up and hold nothing back! You are likely to be pleased with the gains. You have taken advantage of the phenomenon of 'delayed transmutation', or creating great performance potential with assistance exercises for the relevant muscle groups – and then peaking with specialized training.

POWER UP WITH SINGLES

Question: I have gotten the singles bug on my bench press but burnt out very quickly. Do you have a good singles routine?

Kurinov, a Russian world weightlifting champ of Paul Anderson's era, used to lift very heavy in training and always got emotionally worked up. After a serious of 'flat' performances in competition he learned his lesson and from then on he hit maxes only occasionally and only when he was 100% sure of making them without undue excitement.

Although lifting maximal weights brings about the quickest strength development, the great emotional stress which accompanies such training rapidly burns out the nervous system and eventually leads to a decrease in that lift (Rodionov, 1967). According to Vasiliev (1954), training with 1x1RM once a week increases strength significantly for up to six weeks. After that it is downhill, at least for mere mortals.

But training with singles does not have to mean training with max singles. Try the following program from Steve Justa's great *Rock, Iron, Steel: The Book of Strength* (available from IronMind.com). This colorful strongman from America's heartland has forgotten more about effective training than most degreed authorities will ever know.

Pick one lift and train it daily. Do no other work for the involved muscles, although you may carry on with your regular lifting for the rest of your body. On Monday do three singles with 70% 1RM and one to two minutes of rest in between. Add two sets of one daily. Five singles with the same poundage on Tuesday. Seven on Wednesday. Nine on Thursday. Eleven on Friday. Thirteen on Saturday and fifteen on Sunday. 3-5-7-9-11-13-15.

On Monday add five or ten pounds and repeat the cycle. Once a month test your max and recalculate your 70%. Everything about Steve Justa's program flies in the face of conventional wisdom but trust me, it works. A fellow I know, went from four to five wheels in the deadlift in one year without breaking a sweat. His gains are typical.

BUILD MIGHT AND MUSCLE WITH THE CLASSIC 'COUNTDOWN TO POWER'

Question: I hear a lot about the '54321 system'? How does it work?

John McKean sent me an article he wrote about the 54321 routine back in the sixties. It details how to make great gains by doing consecutive sets of 5, 4, 3, 2, and 1 repetitions.

"The countdown provides the lifter with several advantages," writes McKean who has won many titles in powerlifting and all-around lifting and started his writing career in Strength & Health under legendary John Grimek. "First of all, he is relieved of the boredom of doing set after set with the same weight or for the same number of counts. Secondly, he looks forward to each coming set because, in his mind, the decreased repetitions make it easier to perform. Of course there is more weight to contend with but those detestable reps are diminished! It can also be seen that the body acquires a gradual adjustment to an ever-increasing weight. When one can force his mind and body to accept heavier workloads, he begins to improve."

McKean gives you the freedom to decide what poundage jumps you are going to make between sets. Most experienced lifters jump ten to twenty pounds, John McKean added thirty five pounds per set to his squats, and some big dudes add as much as a hundred pounds between sets! Simple math tells that you should be putting up at least five wheels to make such jumps. Ten pound increases should be about right for the average bodybuilder, e.g. 200x5, 210x4, 220x3, 230x2, 240x1. Note that not all sets will be equally difficult; that is fine and even purposeful, 'cycling' within a workout.

John advises that your first workout should start out with the top single twenty pounds below your best. Practice the 54321 system three times a week and add five pounds to each set every workout. In two weeks you will overshoot your old max. If you keep working hard, you may end up with a forty-pound gain on your lift in one month, a typical experience for the 1960s powerlifters and bodybuilders who took on this program.

Presuming that you want to look as strong as you get, finish your 54321 routine with three to five sets of three to five reps, the standard solution by McKean's contemporaries who felt that the pure 54321 workout did not give their muscles enough stimulation to build them. You may want to do these back-off sets only on Fridays.

If you are a beginner, or the exercise you have chosen for the power countdown does not lend itself to big weights, e.g. the barbell curl, you may make only one or two jumps, e.g. 65x5, 65x4, 70x3, 70x2, 70x1. Or you could even stay with the same weight: 45x5, 45x4, 45x3, 45x2, 45x1. Naturally, take shorter rest periods between your sets if you stick with a flat poundage.

"Like a knockout punch," concludes hard man McKean, the 54321 workout "is quick and hard but extremely effective."

RUSSIAN SETS AND REPS FOR POWER

Question: I like being as strong as I look and having a dense lifter's physique. What sets and reps should I do?

In a nutshell, multiple sets of low reps. A classic Soviet weightlifting textbook by V. I. Rodionov lists seven set and rep schemes that you can choose from:

> 1. 60x2-3, 70x2-3, 80x2-3, 87.5-90x1-2x5-6, 80x2-3, 70x2-3 (percentage of the one rep max x repetitions x sets)

This format is recommended for experienced strength athletes. The first light sets get the trainee into the groove, the last light sets are meant to provide active rest before tackling the next exercise.

> 2a. 70x2-3, 80x2-3, 90x1, 100-102.5x1, (85-90x2-3x3-4), 70x2-3
> 2b. 75x2-3, 85x2-3, 95x1, 100-105x1, (85-90x2-3x3-4), 70x2-3

This scheme is recommended for a rare session when you want to go for a personal best. Rodionov warns not to perform many sets and reps before you go for a max to avoid wearing yourself out. The choice of the 90 or 95% weight preceding the max set is up to the athlete. If this weight feels light, up the projected PR by 5-10 pounds or whatever seems right.

If after the max you do not feel up for the heavy back off sets in brackets, drop them and wrap up just with a couple of light 70% sets.

> 3. 65x2-3, 75x2-3, 85x2-3, 90x1, 75x2-3x2, 65x2-3x2

This sequence is great for finessing your lifting technique. You get to critically compare your technique in both sets with each weight. This approach was a favorite of B. Farkhutdinov, weightlifting world champion from the USSR.

> 4. 65x2-3, 70x2-3, 80x2-3, 87.5-92.5x1-2x3-4, 85x2-3x3-4

This arrangement allows the power monger to perform a high volume of work with sufficiently heavy weights. Very effective for building strength and mass while honing the technique.

> 5. 60x2-3, 70x2-3, 80x1-2, 90x1, 95x1x3-4, 85x2-3, 75x2-3

This design is for an athlete whose technique tends to deteriorate when the poundage approaches maximal. Keep lifting a near maximal weight, that would be your opener if you were to compete in a strength sport such as weightlifting, powerlifting, or the bench press.

> 6. 60x2-3, 70x2-3, 80x1-2, 90x1, 95x1, 85x2-3x3-5

A great method for developing strength, technique, and hypertrophy.

> 7. 65x2-3, 75x2-3, 85x2-3x4-6, 95x1

The 95% set will feel like a true max after the 85% sets. Skip it if you are not up for it or lift 90%x1 instead.

One way to put the above schedules to work, is to pick three to four 'big', basic exercises, for instance the powerlifts plus cleans-and-presses or pullups, and train each lift two to four times a week. Vary the set and rep scheme every workout making sure not to practice the #2 that requires lifting a 1RM more than once a week. Follow the above program for three weeks, blow your old PRs out of the water, and return to your usual training.

WHAT DO THE RUSSIANS THINK OF PYRAMIDS?

Question: I read in Prof. Vladimir Zatsiorsky's book that Russian weightlifters stopped using pyramids in their training in 1964. Does it apply to bodybuilders and powerlifters?

Pyramids fatigue the muscles and the nervous system before you get to your money set or sets. That is why they are not optimal when strength is your primary objective. Things are different when you are after more mass.

Although Russian Olympic lifters said good-bye to the pyramid even before the clean-and-press bit the dust in 1972, it lives on in the regimen of the Russian National Powerlifting Team, albeit on a limited basis. In the preparatory period, when the lifters are concentrating on building up the volume, they hit it once a week, usually on Wednesday. Their typical bench press pyramid workout, referred to by the team's senior coach Boris Sheyko as 'the marathon' looks like this: 50%x8, 55%x7, 60%x6, 65%x5, 70%x4, 75%x3x2, 80%x2x2, 75%x3x2, 70%x4, 65%x6, 60%x8, 55%x10, 50%x12 (percentage of the one rep max x reps x sets). Compare it to a more typical workout for the same phase of the cycle: 50%x5, 60%x4, 70%x3x2, 80%x3x5. Note that the latter session, even though it starts light and builds up to heavier weights like a pyramid, uses lower reps – e.g. fives versus eights, with a fifty percent weight – to arrive fresh to the top sets. And it does not employ back-off sets because you are too tired to do more quality work. Besides, as the Russians put it, these descending sets 'congest the muscles', and compromise your recovery for the next bench press session.

The bottom line. Although there are much more effective set and rep schemes than pyramids for strength training, pyramids still can be recruited by a powerlifter or a bodybuilder on a part time basis for variety's sake. Just do not pyramid when you are about to peak your strength – and make sure to make the same muscle group workout following the pyramid less demanding.

A PTP/LADDER HYBRID TO JUMPSTART YOUR BENCH

Question: My bench press has stalled. Do you have any cool routines to get it going?

Try the following program by Jason Brice of Johnson City, Tennessee. Jason combined one of the power cycles from my book *Power to the People!* with 'ladders', a technique popular in the Russian military for improving pull-ups.

On June 30th, 2001 Brice started out with one set of five reps with 225 pounds, or 67% of his 335-pound max bench (naturally, you will need to plug in your own numbers). Jason did only one set of five reps per workout, adding five pounds each time. What will surprise you is that he benched five days a week, Monday through Friday. The reasoning behind such an unorthodox schedule is outside the scope of this piece; it is explained in *Power to the People!*

Since you cannot keep on adding five pounds a workout forever, even if you started the cycle with a light weight, eventually you will reach your five-rep max. When Jason reached his he switched from powerlifting style cycling to ladders. 'A ladder' means doing one rep, resting briefly, doing two reps, etc., then starting all over when you cannot top the reps of the last set. Brice did sets of 1-2-3-1-2... with his 5RM until his form started to get sloppy. He did this every other day for two weeks.

Then Jason backed off ten pounds from his 5RM established two weeks earlier and resumed a linear cycle: one set of five Monday through Friday adding five pounds a day. When he had a tough time completing his fiver Jason took two days off and tested his one-rep max, something he did every two months. Here is what he accomplished:

	June 30th	August 30th	October 31st
Bench press 1 RM	335	385	420
Bench press 5 RM	285	325	360

"After benching I did one-arm snatch pulls with dumbbells and heavy ab work, wraps up Jason Brice. "...My lifts were witnessed by my co-workers as well as a few powerlifters who compete with me. If I lied about my results they would call my bluff."

MOSCOW BENCH PRESS CHAMPION'S PROGRAM

Question: My bench press has stalled. I could use a new routine!

The following program by Moscow bench press champion Alexey Moiseev pushed his bench up by 20kg or about 45 pounds in just three months! More good news: it has enough beach work to keep the bodybuilder in you happy.

Train twice a week, for instance Mondays and Thursdays, heavy and light.

Heavy Day   1. Bench press – 3x3, 2, 1
                2. Board press – 3x3, 2, 1

Set a four to five inch thick board, for instance a sawed off 2x4, on your chest. Lower the bar down to the board and press it back up. You cannot help noticing Louie Simmons' influence in Moiseev's program.

3. Incline bench press – 3x3, 2, 1
4. Scott or preacher bench curls – 4-6x8-10
5. Triceps exercise of choice – 4x8

Light Day
1. Speed bench press – 7x3 @ 50% 1RM
Lower the barbell slow, explode up.
2. Narrow grip bench press – 4x8-10
3. Bent over lateral raises – 3x8-10
4. Lateral raises – 3x8-10
5. Scott or preacher bench curls – 4-6x8-10
6. Triceps exercise of choice – 4x8

Moiseev adds 5kg, which is in the ballpark of 10 pounds, every set of the heavy 3, 2, 1 workout. If you are not in the major league, there is no dishonor in adding only five pounds.

The powerlifting champion adds another 5kg to all three money sets every workout. Unless you can give the big guy a run for his money, a 5-lbs. increase every workout or even every other workout is just right.

When the gains stalled, Alexey temporarily switched to 3x3 but periodically attempted to put up heavier weights. I believe you will be better off back cycling your poundages and starting another assault. E.g., if 215x3, 220x2, 225x1 has almost crushed you, back off to 185x3, 190x2, 195x1 and build up again. Power to you!

WAVE THE WEIGHTS FOR POWER

Question: My training partner took your seminar and told me that you recommend waving the weight up and down from set to set. Why?

First of all, you shall get stronger faster. Eastern Europeans' weightlifting sessions are variable. When Russians hit heavy doubles or triples, they often alternate them with singles or doubles with a weight reduced by 5-10%. Another set and rep scheme popular in the former Soviet Union, by Robert Roman, calls for three sets of three reps with a 70% weight and 3x3 @ 75% 1RM. The weights are alternated from set to set.

Your strength depends on your skill to contract your muscles hard – even more than on their size. Since World War II, motor learning, the fine discipline about shortcuts to skill mastery, has made many breakthroughs that are waiting to be recruited in your quest for strength. One such breakthrough is *variable* practice, the powerful alternative to conventional *constant practice*.

Constant practice refers to doing the same thing in every consecutive trial. Multiple sets with the same weight, 455x5x5 or 200x10x3, are examples of constant practice. This method works but it can be improved on. *Variable practice*, or waving the load up and down every set, is a superior alternative. Many motor learning studies (e.g., Kerr & Booth, 1978) show that subjects practicing under variable conditions perform at least as well as the constant practice group – and frequently do better!

In addition to the strength learning benefits, varying your weight from set to set offers other advantages. Lighter sets facilitate recovery for the next heavy set and painlessly increase the tonnage. Recall how critical volume of loading is to strength and muscle gains. A wavy workout is a lot less monotonous and more enjoyable than one with a static weight. Instead of grinding out 200x5x5 sets try something like 185x5, 205x5, 195x5, 210x5, 190x5, 200x5, 185x5. You will manage a couple of extra sets and will not even notice it.

'INTERVAL CIRCUIT TRAINING' FOR POWER ON A TIGHT TIME BUDGET

Question: Watching my friend turn into a powerhouse on a routine of high sets of low reps with plenty of rest in between has convinced me that it is the way to train for raw power. Unfortunately, I can barely spare forty-five minutes for a workout twice a week. Am I doomed to remain a pencilneck?

Not if you try interval or 'slow' circuit training.

Lee (1988) found that the already awesome gains reaped from variable practice, or mixing up the poundage from set to set, explained in the piece above, can be far greater if it is combined with *random practice*. RP is the opposite of blocked practice, or completing all the trials of a drill before moving on to the next one. Doing all your sets of squats before moving on to the bench press is an example of *blocked practice*. *Random practice* involves alternating between various tasks within a practice period. It is kind of like circuit training, except adequate rest is provided between the drills.

Random practice delivers predictably great results. The idea of switching between squats, benches, and deads every set may strike you as a bizarre way to annoy the gym owner by tying up three bars and most of the plates on the floor. Yet a breakthrough study by Shea & Morgan

(1979) determined that random practice is the way to train. Although it results in poorer performance in practice – you don't get a chance to gradually work up to your meat set and simply do not have the luxury of focusing on one lift and getting in the groove – it delivers better numbers when you go for a PR.

Ideally alternate between harder and easier exercises, something old time professional strongmen used to do (Liederman, 1925) and the Soviets took up later (Roman, 1962). For example, if you powerlift, separate your squats and deads with a set of benches: SQ-BP-DL-BP-SQ-BP. This arrangement offers another advantage, namely enhanced recovery due to the *Setchinov principle* formulated in Russia in the early 1900s. According to this principle, heavy use of a bodypart promotes a reflexive relaxation of bodyparts distant from the first one. As a result, a busy person will be able to handle a greater workload within his or her limited training time without sacrificing quality. Linda Crawford who broke four Minnesota State Masters Powerlifting Records routinely knocked off ten sets per each powerlift within a forty-five minute training session – all with at least 80% of her 1RM!

Provided you rest for a couple of minutes between your stations, alternate between tougher and easier exercises and between your legs and upper body, you can build great strength on a very tight schedule. That is if you train at home or are big enough to tie up a few pieces of equipment at a club without consequences.

A SIMPLE POWER CYCLE

Question: I finally understand the reasoning behind powerlifting style cycling. But some of these cycles are so complex, my eyes glaze over! Is there a simpler way to cycle?

Cycles do not need to be fancy to be effective. Fifteen-year-old Armenian immigrant Sarkis Karapetyan recently set a world record at the WABDL Utah State Championship by deadlifting 3.14 times his body weight. He did it by following the as-simple-as-can-be cycle from my book *Power to the People!*

Here is another simple and effective cycle; it was published a few years back in the highly recommended *Powerlifting USA* magazine.

Let us assume that your two best sets of five in a powerlift are 300 pounds. Add five pounds to this number and work back five pounds a week for five weeks:

Week	Weight x reps / sets
1	285x5/2
2	290x5/2
3	295x5/2
4	300x5/2
5	305x5/2

Not fancy, but the job is done. Start another cycle five pounds heavier:

Week	Weight x reps / sets
1	290x5/2
2	295x5/2
3	300x5/2
4	305x5/2
5	310x5/2

Some lifters tend to burn out training so close to their PR all the time. Ten pound jumps will work better giving them a few easier weeks to recover from the last cycle:

Week	Weight x reps / sets
1	265x5/2
2	275x5/2
3	285x5/2
4	295x5/2
5	305x5/2

Keep recycling and a year down the road you will be moving 350x5/2, another year, and it is 400x5/2...

If you occasionally hit a snag and cannot make the projected weights, take a week off and start the cycle over:

Week	Weight x reps / sets	Week	Weight x reps / sets
1	265x5/2	7	265x5/2
2	275x5/2	8	275x5/2
3	285x5/2	9	285x5/2
4	295x5/2	10	295x5/2
5	305x5/1, 4/1	11	305x5/2
6	off		

When there is no contest in sight, just keep repeating the five-week cycle. When training for a meet, schedule your training so it falls on week seven, and work up to a heavy double on week six:

Week	Weight x reps / sets
1	285x5/2
2	290x5/2
3	295x5/2
4	300x5/2
5	305x5/2
6	330x2/1
7	340x1/1 (contest)

'THE RKC LADDER': A SHOCK PROGRAM FOR SHOULDER STRENGTH AND MASS

Question: My bench is not too bad but I just cannot make any progress in my military press. Help!

In the good ole' days when the clean-and-press was the measure of a man and the bench was unheard of, Russian weightlifters had an expression: "To press a lot you must press a lot." The shoulders, unlike the legs, back, and, to a lesser degree, the chest will not budge until you blast them with a high volume of heavy iron.

The following RKC routine is almost guaranteed to ram you through your shoulder strength and size plateau. Pick a kettlebell you can clean and press – a clean before each press that is – roughly six to eight times. C&P it once with your weaker arm and switch hands. Rest briefly. Ideally your training partner will do his set while you chill. Two reps. Another short break. Three reps. Then start over at one… Feel free to rest longer between each series.

Repeat the 1, 2, 3 series five times, which will total you 30 quality reps. Follow this program three to four times a week. Do a skeleton chest and triceps regimen while you are on it.

Add a series per workout until you are up to (1, 2, 3) x 10 = 60 repetitions. Sixty reps with a seven-rep max is a very powerful muscle-building stimulus!

Now start doing 1, 2, 3, 4 reps, starting out with three series which totals 30 reps. As before, build up to 60 total reps, or (1, 2, 3, 4) x 6.

Move up to (1, 2, 3, 4, 5) x 2. Work up to (1, 2, 3, 4, 5) x 4. By now your shoulders will be swelling with dense and powerful muscle. Take a couple of days off and test yourself on the one-arm military press. You will blow your old PR out of the water!

SLOW GEAR FOR STRENGTH

Question: My friend who read your Power to the People! book told me that you are against explosive lifting. Why?

I am not against explosive lifting, but its indiscriminate application.

First, it is not appropriate for beginners. Dremach (1998), from the former Soviet republic of Belarus – famous for its iron athletes of all persuasions – concluded that introducing an explosive deadlift start increased the max of the advanced lifters who participated in the study by 15% – and enabled them to lift the old 1RM for a few repetitions! However, the researcher concluded that this was only appropriate for intermediate and advanced lifters, the cutoff being around a double bodyweight deadlift. V. Dremach warns that a beginner who takes on the explosive DL is likely to get injured and/or fail to develop good technique.

One of the most crucial skills any iron athlete must develop is that of 'staying tight'. And only the elite can stay tight while exploding like a bat out of hell. Even the Westside Barbell Club powerlifters famous for their explosive training dedicate a special day in their schedule to 'grinding'. So forget pyrotechnic displays until you master full body tension and put up some respectable poundages.

Second, explosion may or may not be appropriate for a PR lift. Powerlifting guru Louie Simmons' statement that if you "have so much explosion out of the hole, you do not have sticking points!" sums up the argument for being explosive when going for the max. But there is an opposing point of view. 900-pound deadlifter Mark Henry said that "what makes a good powerlifter is a slow gear." In other words, when you need to pull a car out of a ditch you call a tow truck rather than a Ferrari. Both camps have valid points and have champions to back them up.

Third, when going for a record, even the opponents of being fast recognize the training value of explosive lifting. Legendary Russian coach S.Y. Smolov, Master of Sports advocates *Power to the People!* style 'grinding' on max lifts yet dedicates two weeks of exclusively explosive training for his famous squat cycle.

The last word on lifting explosively (it does not apply to the 'quick lifts': snatches, cleans, etc.). Don't even think about exploding until you have built a respectable level of strength and learned to get and stay tight. Find out whether maxing explosively works for you through trial and error. Periodically introduce acceleration training with moderate weights into your routine. A great set of guidelines can be found in Dr. Fred Hatfield's book *Power: the Scientific Approach*.

TO PAUSE OR NOT TO PAUSE THE DEADLIFTS, THAT IS THE QUESTION

Question: Should I pause on the platform between deadlift reps or touch and go?

As a rule of thumb, pause. First, you need to develop starting strength for a big pull and you will never do that unless you pull a dead weight. FYI, in the olden days the exercise was known as 'the dead weight lift'.

Second, to do a touch and go rep you must lower the barbell in perfect form to set yourself up for a clean next rep and to protect your back. Doing a negative in the deadlift takes experience. Otherwise it is plain dangerous; the bar tends to pull the deadlifter forward on his toes and round his back.

Even if you have succeeded in not letting the bar run forward and bend you over, do not think your troubles are over. You probably have assumed an exaggeratedly upright stance. Your knees have slipped forward and got banged up while your hamstrings have lost tension. You have got yourself into a hideous position for the next rep. Which is why I recommend quickly pushing your hips back, dropping down with the barbell after each repetition, and resetting for each rep as if it is the first one in *Power to the People!*

Nevertheless, experienced lifters have legit reasons to periodically do touch and go deadlifts with controlled negatives. First, it is well known that eccentric contractions are important for stimulating muscle growth. Second, touch and go reps are good for cleaning up one's technique. Prominent Russian powerlifting coach Askold Surovetsky recommends just that. An interesting wrinkle in his program is alternating two types of deadlift workouts: heavy ones with full stops and dead weight starts, and lighter, high volume ones with touch and go reps. Pay attention: do touch and go deads only with lighter weights and make sure to practice deadlifts with full stops between reps as well! For instance, if you follow the *Power to the People!* program, pull the first set with dead stops and the second, lighter, set in the touch and go manner.

In order to do a safe deadlift negative for a touch and go rep the lifter must know how to keep the pressure in his abdomen, pull himself down with his hip flexors, and keep his hamstrings loaded. I have explained all three techniques elsewhere in detail; ignore them at your own risk.

A word on breathing. Breathe shallow and stay tight; letting out too much air at any time is putting your lower back in danger. Inhale on the way down into your tight stomach (it will not be easy), grunt slightly half way up. Don't bounce the bar on the platform, just gently touch it and go up without losing tension or air.

"If done intensely and correctly," promises drug free 800-pound deadlifter Steve Scialpi, who favors touch and go reps with thirty-five pound plates, "your lower back, glutes and hips should be extremely pumped."

LIGHT WEIGHTS, HARD DEADLIFTS

Question: I have made great gains with your deadlift program from "Power to the People!" Unfortunately, I have run out of my 300 pounds and I am afraid to buy more iron as I live in an apartment. What is a good deadlift alternative for someone in my circumstances?

Try the one legged deadlift described by Harry L. Good in his 1940 course *The Keynote to Great Strength*. Even if nothing prevents you from pulling conventional, you will find the one legged dead a worthwhile addition to your routine.

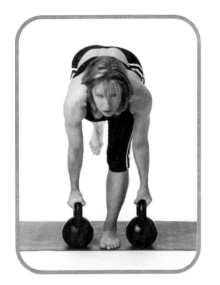

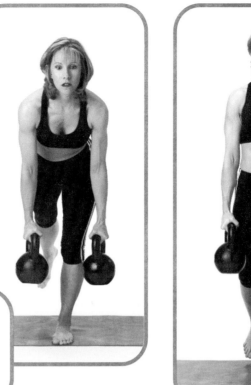

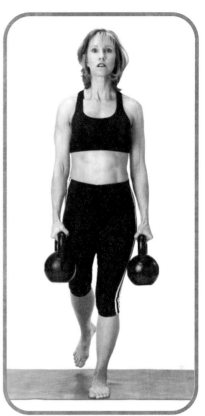

The one-legged deadlift is demonstrated by Brazilian Jiu Jutsu World Champion DC Maxwell of Maxercise.com.

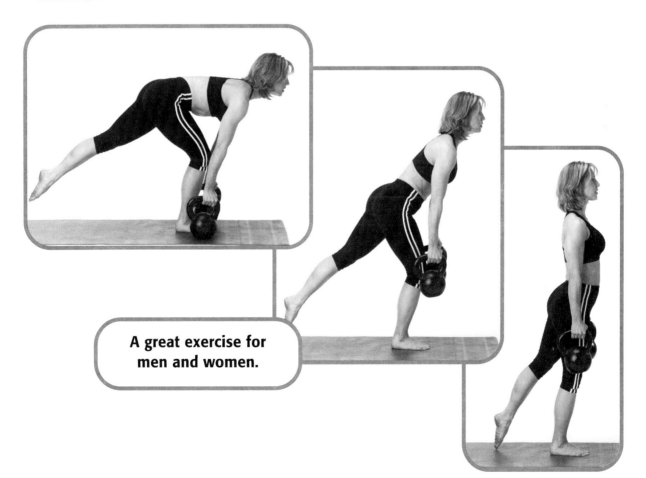

A great exercise for men and women.

Face the bar with one foot centered and the other elevated behind you. Your shin should be an inch or so behind the bar. If you wish, you may extend the pull by standing on an elevation of up to four inches – or by using small plates. You may also do the drill with kettlebells.

Fold forward and semi-squat. Do not let your knee extend over your toes or buckle in. Stick your butt out and grab the bar with the clean or palms down grip. Take a normal breath, tighten up, and lift.

Keep your weight evenly distributed on your foot and your back reasonably straight – the one legged pull is more forgiving than the conventional DL. You will find that you have to contract the glute on the working side very intensely to maintain your balance. Flex it to break the bar off the floor and cramp it even harder at the lockout. It will not take you long to realize that you have discovered one of the most effective glute exercises in existence.

If you start losing balance catch yourself by landing your airborne foot. Carry on once you have got your equilibrium back. Unlike the regular deadlift, the one legged version enables you to lower the weight slowly safely so your neighbors will stop calling the police.

The one legged DL does a fine job of strengthening your ankles, at least if you lift barefoot. An average weak ankle tends to buckle in when the person is standing on one foot, especially with extra weight. The movement of the sole of the foot outward is called 'eversion'. Under the circumstances it is bad news for your leg. A barefoot Good deadlift will strengthen the muscles on the inside of the lower leg responsible for inversion or drawing of the sole inward. Just grip the ground hard with your toes, keep the muscles around your ankle and on the bottom of your foot tight, and make sure that the inside of your foot does not come down to the floor.

Your 300-pound set will serve you for a while now. If you can pull a 300 regular dead, good luck in breaking 135 off the floor.

JURASSIC TRAINING REVISITED: BUILDING TENDON AND LIGAMENT STRENGTH

Question: I hear about 'tendon training' from my strongman competitor friends. What is it? Should I do it?

Although a regular Joe' or Jane's maximal voluntary contraction equals only around 30% of the maximal tensile strength of their tendons (Hirch, 1974), more recent studies reported by Verkhoshansky & Siff (1996) proved what old timers knew all along: increases in quality and quantity of connective tissues may improve the transmission of force from the muscles to the bones! Professor Verkhoshansky explains that a weak or not sufficiently extensive tendon sheath allows the muscle to dissipate some of its force in the wrong direction.

I am convinced that tendon training is a must for experienced iron athletes of all persuasions. Elite muscles generate such high levels of tension that they become stiffer than their tendons for the moment (Zatsiorsky, 1995). Since a muscle with its tendons can be compared to springs in series, it is obvious why tendon strength is so important. The muscles, rigor mortis hard, leave the tendons as the weak link in the chain. That not only predisposes the tendons to injury, but increases the likelihood of your muscle shaking and failing for neural reasons.

Ligament strength is up there with tendon strength on an iron man' or woman's list of priorities. Verkhoshansky & Siff (1996) speculate that the 'muscle fatigue' in exercises with heavy limb loading, often turns out to be ligament fatigue. As they say about a boxer who is due to go out to pasture, 'he has gotten weak in the knees'. According to the *Supertraining* authors, even the fatigue in the legs, back and feet from standing seems to be not muscular in nature!

Spine journal reported that ligaments and spinal disks possess so-called *mechanoreceptors*. When overloaded, they tell the muscle to shut down. Clearly, old salts knew their stuff when they talked about 'ligament strength'. "The best way to get strength is to support a lot of weight in certain positions," Canadian strength pioneer George Jowett was teaching young John Grimek. "More than you can lift normally... this will strengthen your ligaments, your tendons and you'll get more strength out of that than you would if you were just doing flexing exercises."

Although heavy supports in the tradition of Jowett, Anderson, and Grimek are a must for a serious iron athlete, they are only half the connective tissue training equation. Full amplitude high rep work is recommended by Eastern European specialists to stimulate tendon and ligament development. Calisthenics such as the full squats from my book *Super Joints* fit the bill. Kurz (1994) prescribes 3x30 or 1x100-200 after your heavy iron, which should be followed by some stretches. Full stops at the top and the bottom of each rep are a good idea as they shift the load from the muscles to the connective tissues. Clarification: we are not talking about blood and guts high rep sets here; slowly build up your reps until you can handle the required volume with ease.

WHAT ARE THE 'HIGH-TENSION TECHNIQUES'?

Question: You mention 'high tension techniques' in your books and articles. Do you mean 'high <u>intensity</u> techniques'?

No. 'High intensity techniques' such as forced negatives, pre-exhaustion, etc. were devised by HIT Jedis. The idea was to maximize muscular fatigue or 'inroad' within one set. 'Go beyond failure' and similar histrionics.

I use the term 'high-tension techniques' to refer to any maneuvers that amplify the intensity of a muscular contraction via various reflexes and neurological phenomena. Squeezing the barbell to irradiate extra power from the gripping muscles into the arms and shoulders – or tensing the hip adductors to facilitate a stronger contraction of the midsection musculature – are examples of high-tension techniques.

An iron rat named Cliff reported a very typical high tension technique experience on the dragondoor.com training forum: "Anyone who is doubting the effectiveness of these techniques, I can attest they work!.. I haven't done the DL for two years... At that point my 1RM DL was a pathetic looking 455 that left my back aching for a week, despite the belt. Since using... [the high-tension techniques] FOR ONE WEEK ... last night I pulled the same amount for a triple! The kicker is, besides having not touched a weight in 2 years, I'm 65 lbs. lighter, and I did it belt-less... the back feels fine today!"

Where 'high intensity techniques' weaken you and set you up for an injury, 'high tension techniques' protect you and make you strong.

HIGH-TENSION TECHNIQUES: NOT JUST FOR THE GYM

Question: Can the 'high-tension techniques' you teach be applied to sports and work – or are they strictly for the gym?

These techniques can and should be applied whenever you are exerting or absorbing high forces. Following are two unlikely examples that will show you just how versatile the HTTs are.

One of the sharpest physical training instructors in the special operations community, SSgt. Nate Morrison, RKC Sr. of the USAF Pararescue, posted a brief note titled 'High Tension Techniques for Small Boat Ops' on the dragondoor.com forum. "For those who have ever spent days on a Zodiac F450, you know that after about an hour of bouncing around you are slowly reduced to mush and the pain is constant. Well, I am always surprised where High-Tension Techniques (HTT) come in handy. After about three hours of pounding in heavy chop I started squeezing my glutes and pressurizing my abs every time the boat slammed into the water. Low and behold, no more pain!

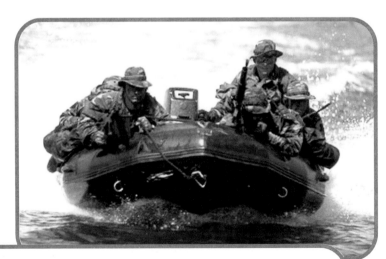

Behold the power of tension in small boat ops!
Photo courtesy MilitaryFitness.org.

As a result, after three days of this I am still pain free while my comrades are in a serious bit of hurt." Behold the power of tension!

And another post by this special operator, titled 'Jumpmaster Notes'. "For those of you who have ever spent hours in a static line parachute harness, you know the back takes a heck of a pounding. While I can't promise you elimination of pain, you will definitely experience some relief if you squeeze your glutes and pressurize your abs. Yes, it still hurts like hell, but at least you won't feel your lumbar and thoracic discs compressing at strange angles. Food for thought." Make sure to read SSgt. Morrison's excellent articles on MilitaryFitness.org.

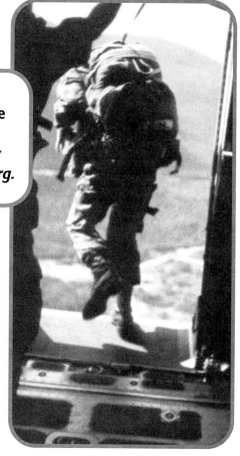

The HTT ease the shock of the static line. *Photo courtesy MilitaryFitness.org.*

'LIFTING THE WEIGHT', 'FEELING THE MUSCLE', OR...?

Question: Can you solve the age-old argument: should one focus on the target muscle or on lifting the weight?

There are two types of focus in strength training: external and internal. The external focus implies thinking of little but lifting the weight somehow, anyhow. When a teenage boy is trying to impress girls with his bench press and elevates the barbell with atrocious form – he will miss his shoulders when they are gone – he is externally focusing. No comment is necessary; you will reap only an illusion of strength and a lifetime of pain.

In a conversation with the Super Slow™ guru Ken Hutchins, his associate Keith Johnson, M.D., coined the word 'internalization' for concentrating on the process of lifting the weight instead of the results: "They urge you to beat the equipment, as… a competitor you must defeat. They teach you to externalize a feigned aggression. You do the opposite. You seem to advocate reaching inside your body. When exercising he [Hutchins' subject] seems to turn off his surrounding environment and concentrate into an internalized trance. That's the fitting word: 'internalize'."

Do not interpret the above as an endorsement of the Super Slow™ but do yourself a favor and learn from the above. And then go a step beyond. 'Feeling the muscle' traditionally implies trying to 'isolate' the primary working muscle while trying to maximally relax the rest of the body. A bad idea. Strength training authority Dr. Ken Leistner once quipped that a body molded with a number of isolation exercises – like leg extensions or triceps kickbacks – looked like 'a collection of body parts'. It just lacks grace, power, and flow. A gymnast or a martial artist whose panther like moves you admire, NEVER isolates. He integrates.

Watch the amazing stunts of the acrobats of the Cirque Du Soleil. You will not see sagging bodies with 'isolated' muscles but long and taught entities. Expert performers **use full body tension as a lens to focus their energy into the primary muscles responsible for the job. So feel all your muscles,** not just one.

KNOW YOUR MAX WITHOUT TESTING IT?

Question: My training partner tells me that I am wasting my time testing my bench max. He showed me a chart that is supposed to calculate it based on an all out multiple rep set. I do not believe him. Who is right?

Your training partner is right about one thing. Unless you compete in powerlifting meets, there is no convincing reason for you to do max attempts. As for the chart, it is a waste of trees. The ratio between an iron athlete's 1RM and, say, 10RM depends on the predominant fiber type, the nervous system organization, recent training, and a host of other factors. In other words, everyone is different. Both you and your buddy might be able to bench 225x10RM, yet you could put up 300x1RM while he might stall at 275x1RM.

Do not give up hope; you might be able to figure out your own PR formula by studying your training log, something powerlifters swear by. A lifter might notice that whenever he can deadlift a certain poundage for three gut busting reps he is good for a max single with fifty pounds more a week later. Needless to say, it will take you months of training and observation to nail down your reps to max ratio. And it is likely to change over time.

USE YOUR HEAD FOR MAX POWER, MUSCLE, AND SAFETY

Question: How should I align my head when lifting?

It depends on the exercise. The following rundown of the so-called 'pose reflexes' by Smirnov & Dubrovsky (2002) will help you figure it out.

Tipping your head down or forward increases the tonus of the arm flexors and leg extensors.

Translation: it is good for curls and leg extensions. But don't try it with squats! Yes, it is easier to come out of the hole with your face down and your butt up. But it is also dangerous for your back and the second half of the lift is likely to get ugly.

Tilting your melon up or back has the opposite effect. The extensors upstairs and the flexors downstairs get a strength boost. Applications. Look up at the bar when military pressing or at the floor when doing handstand pushups (but only if you have the discipline not to arch your back). Press your head down into the bench when benching, especially at the sticking point.

Russian scientists explain the curious reason for the above reflexes' existence: improving the animal's chances of reaching food below or above.

The second group of pose reflexes is fired off by turning the head or tilting it to one side. The extensors on the side the head is facing – and the flexors on the opposite side – get a strength boost. Both the lower and the upper body are affected. Professors Victor Smirnov and Vladimir Dubrovsky explain that these reflexes' job is to maintain your equilibrium. When you turned your head you probably shifted your center of gravity and got off balance. Note how your right quad automatically gets loaded if you lean your head to the right.

Sample applications. Look up and to the right when doing a right arm kettlebell military press. Look down and to the left when curling with the right.

Advanced iron men and women often instinctively come up with more sophisticated 'for professionals only' neck maneuvers. For instance, drug free master powerlifter Fred Peterson starts his deadlift with his head down – don't try it at home! This, as you know, boosts the quads' strength for the start. As the nearly 700 pound barbell passes his knees, Peterson looks up. This fortifies the hamstrings and back and helps the lockout.

'ACTIVE NEGATIVES' FOR POWER, MUSCLE, AND SAFETY

Question: I don't understand what you mean when you say 'pull yourself down into the squat'. How am I supposed to do it and what is the point?

There are two ways you can descend into the low position of the squat or any other exercise. Passively, by yielding to gravity. Which is what most people who have no poundages to brag about do. Or actively, by pulling yourself down against the resistance of your own muscles. Which is what strong people – whose barbells bend under the burden of many wheels – do, consciously or not. An active negative does three things. First, it loads elastic energy into your muscles and tendons, for a more powerful return. Second, it amplifies your strength through the Law of Successive Induction. This law states that a muscle will be stronger immediately after its antagonist's contraction. And third, it dramatically increases your control of the iron and therefore cuts your odds of injuries. Imagine two opposing pulleys controlling a crane, rather than one.

Armed Forces Powerlifting Champion, Jack Reape suggested an excellent drill to teach you how to pull yourself into the squat on the dragondoor.com forum: 'the reverse squat'. "Hold a pull-down rope around the back of your neck, then squat down and bend over. Good for your abs and great for your stabilizers."

The same drill works for the deadlift. For the bench press try the reverse bench row. Set up a barbell for benching, then lie down on the bench with your head facing away from the bar. Scoot under the bar until it is over your sternum and your hips are hanging off the edge of the bench. Grip the bar with your usual BP grip. Force your chest out, and pull it towards the bar in a rowing motion. Try to follow the exact groove of your bench press, hence 'the reverse bench'. Note what it feels like and try to recreate the same pulling sensation when you are lowering your benches.

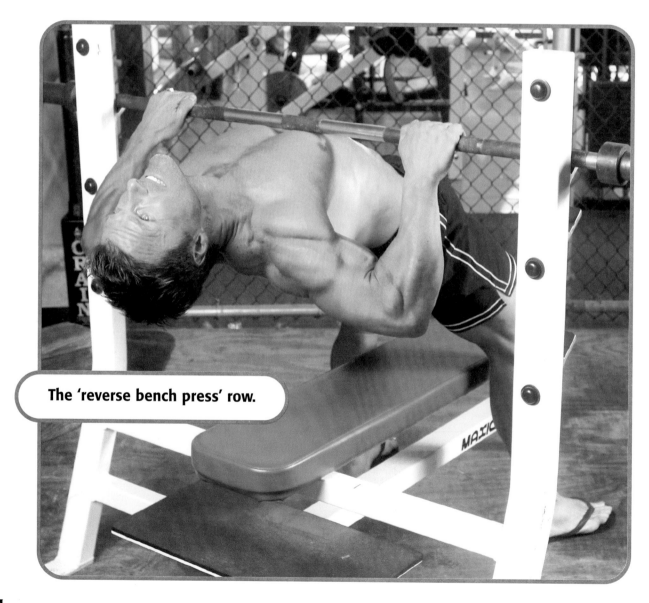

The 'reverse bench press' row.

HEAVYWEIGHT STRENGTH ADVANTAGE FOR THE LEAN

Question: Is it true that fat helps you lift more?

Yes, any tissue, including fat, helps by providing elastic rebound, sort of like powerlifting knee wraps and suit. Watch a super heavyweight lifter squat: his gut gets squished against his knees and his monstrous thighs push against the thick calves.

Of course, gaining fat to get stronger is not a wise choice for anyone but a SHW Pler, but you can fake some of the big guy's leverage and come out with bigger and safer lifts.

The two exercises that lend themselves well to this 'virtual size' leverage are military presses and rock bottom Olympic squats. Watch a big dude military press. His torso and arms are so thick with muscles and fat that his tris get propped up on a cushion and the lift starts almost at the ear level. A skinny guy or gal has to start way down, below the collarbones, because thin arms naturally tuck into the sides.

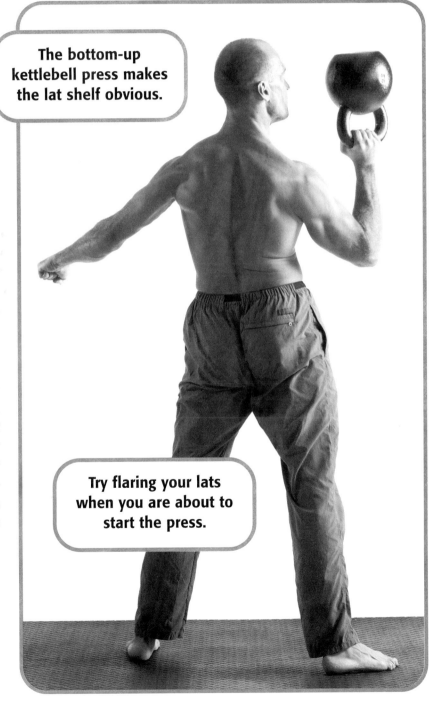

The bottom-up kettlebell press makes the lat shelf obvious.

Try flaring your lats when you are about to start the press.

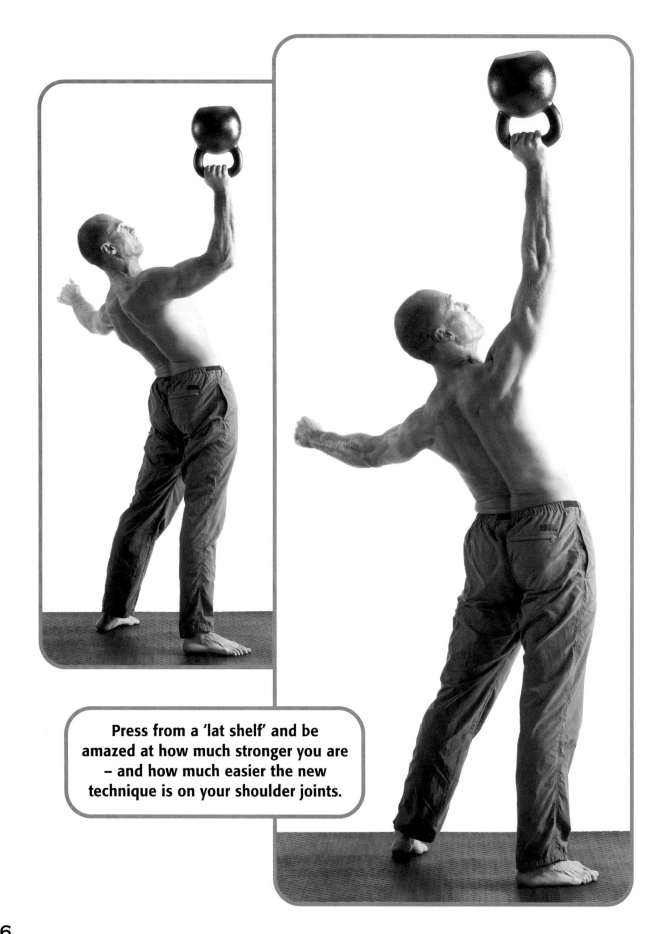

Press from a 'lat shelf' and be amazed at how much stronger you are – and how much easier the new technique is on your shoulder joints.

Try flaring your lats when you are about to start the press. Literally spread them, as if you are trying to impress the gym with your V-shape. A special, partial lateral raise will help you to get the hang of this move. Grab a couple of dumbbells that are way too heavy for lateral raises. Now, without shrugging your shoulders, try to lift them an inch or so, just by tensing your squished lats. The latissimus will flare and push up on your upper arms. Try to recreate the same feeling at the beginning of a military press. Press from a 'lat shelf' and be amazed at how much stronger you are – and how much easier the new technique is on your shoulder joints. But remember to resist the temptation to shrug your shoulders!

When you have mastered the lat shelf for your military presses you can start practicing to apply it to your benches, something record-breaking powerlifters swear by. It is not easy to master but well worth it.

Now apply the 'virtual tissue leverage' technique to rock bottom back or front squats. Start by going rock bottom without any weight and practice getting up an inch or so just by 'thickening' your hamstrings. Once you have it down pat, try it with a weight.

Do it! The 'virtual tissue leverage' technique is not just a gimmick that artificially raises your poundage; it is an effective way to protect your joints.

BOOST YOUR BENCH... WITH SHRUGS!

Question: Is it true that there are dozens of shrug variations? Are they of any use?

Yes and yes. Your shoulder girdle has many degrees of freedom and it stands to reason that working it through many planes will fire up some new muscles and fibers and slap a few pounds on your frame. Besides, according to the shrug expert Paul Kelso, they will make your shoulders more resistant to injuries and up your poundages in other lifts. Here is one such shrug from the highly recommended *Kelso's Shrug Book*. It will boost your ego lift – the bench press.

Stand inside a cable crossover machine – at last, a hardcore application for this sissified contraption! – and stretch your arms out to grab the handles of the high pulleys. Lean back slightly as if you are lying down to bench. If you are not using enough weight to counterbalance yourself, a spot from behind is a good idea.

Inhale and retract your straight arms into the shoulder sockets while forcing your chest out and pinching your shoulder blades together. "There is an odd result with wide grips," comments Paul Kelso, "the direction of pull is not back or up... There is a triangulation from the hands to the focal point of contraction." As if you are sucking your straight arms in your body. Pause in the retracted position for a few seconds, and release the stacks slowly. Do three sets of eight reps with pauses, either after your bench workout or on your back day.

67

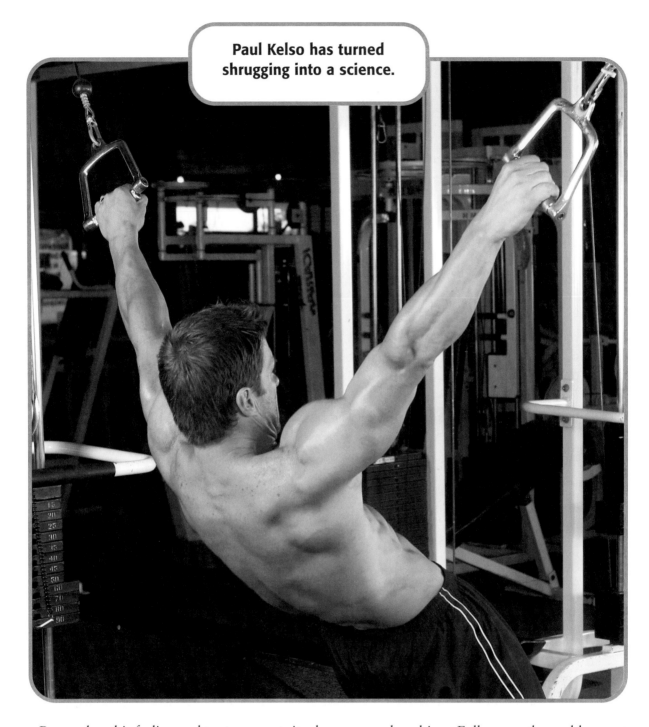

Paul Kelso has turned shrugging into a science.

Remember this feeling and try to recreate it when you are benching. Follow another gold nugget from Kelso's book: 'pull the bar apart' as you are lowering it to your chest. "The tension created is translated through the arms to the upper back and provides... stored "extra energy"..." This subtle championship tip will make your bench go up. Guaranteed.

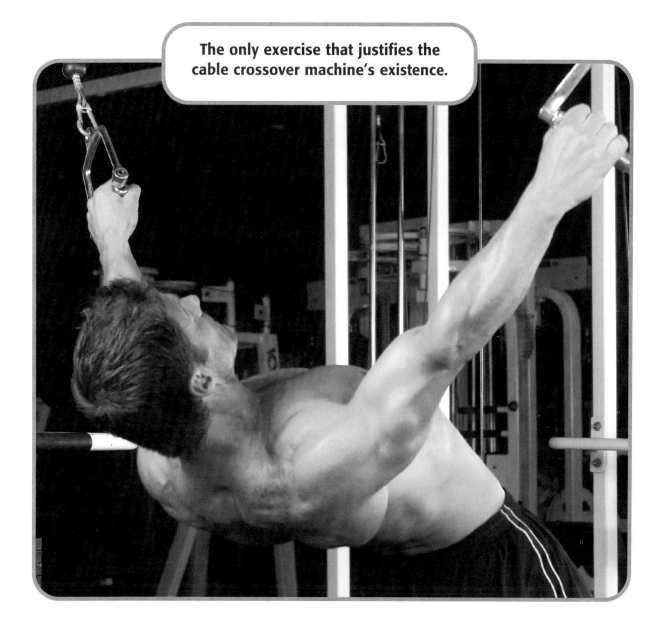

The only exercise that justifies the cable crossover machine's existence.

DUMBBELL BENCH POWER

Question: Could you give me a program to improve my dumbbell bench press? I can do a pair of 90s.

You bet. On Monday work up to a comfortably heavy triple, e.g. 50sx3, 60sx3, 65sx3, 70sx3, 75sx3, 80sx3. On Tuesday do many sets of five with little rest, e.g. 60sx5x10. On Thursday work up to a heavy five of incline bench dumbbell presses, then declines. You might be able to do 45x5, 50x5, 55x5, 60x5, 65x5 on inclines and 65x5, 70x5, 75x5, 80x5 on declines. Understand that these are just examples. The idea is to start light and work up to comfortably heavy, while keeping the reps the same.

Keep your rest between sets brief on Monday, Tuesday, and Thursday. On Saturday do many triples with plenty of rest, e.g. 70s-75sx3x8-12. Do the above program for three weeks. Peak in week four. Work up to a comfortable triple, perhaps 85sx3 by now, on Monday. A double, probably 90sx2, on Tuesday. It should be heavy but do not kill yourself. Do a very easy low rep workout on Thursday just to grease your groove, e.g. 70sx3x3. Test your max on Saturday. Your test might look like this. 50sx3, 60sx3, 70sx2, 80sx1, 90sx1, 95sx1,100sx1. Feel free to apply this pattern to other exercises.

SQUAT BIG WITH BAD KNEES?

Question: I have bad knees and I cannot squat regularly. Is there a way for me to build up my squat without squatting? And to replace the muscle building benefits of this king of exercises?

If your doctor is cool with you squatting at least once in a blue moon, there is a solution. Do what 1959 Mr. Universe Bruce Randall did. A young Marine, Randall wanted to play football for the base team and started lifting and eating. But as his size and strength grew, he lost interest in the ball game and focused on the iron. Bruce had one problem: he had suffered seven leg fractures in a bicycle accident and squatting was very hard on him. He got buried by 190, the first time he tried it!

But the jarhead did not give up. He eventually worked up to a 680-pound squat – without practicing it! But in case you got excited in anticipation of a secret routine that will mix leg presses, extensions, and other easy moves into a big squat, you have another thing coming. Mr. Universe's substitute was at least as hard as the squat; some people would say it is even harder. It was the good morning, the exercise I am yet to see done in an average gym. Because the good morning is so similar to the power squat, the former automatically pushes up the latter.

Now run over to the squat rack before you get cold feet and give this tough exercise a shot. With the bar low on your back set up in your usual squat stance. Take a breath into your stomach, tighten up, and push your hips back. This is very important: don't lean forward but stick your butt out as far as possible. The latter intent is much safer for your back and enables you to put up much heavier weights.

Keep your stomach braced at all times and don't lose your air! You can breathe, but shallow – 'sip' air as the late Dr. Siff would put it –- and without losing tension in your abs. Look straight ahead at all times and keep your spine straight (not to be confused with 'vertical'). Keep your weight on your heels, your knees slightly bent, and your shins vertical, something your knees will appreciate. Keep folding until your torso is parallel to the deck or you cannot go any deeper without rounding your back. Press your feet into the floor and your traps up into the bar, and steadily straighten out.

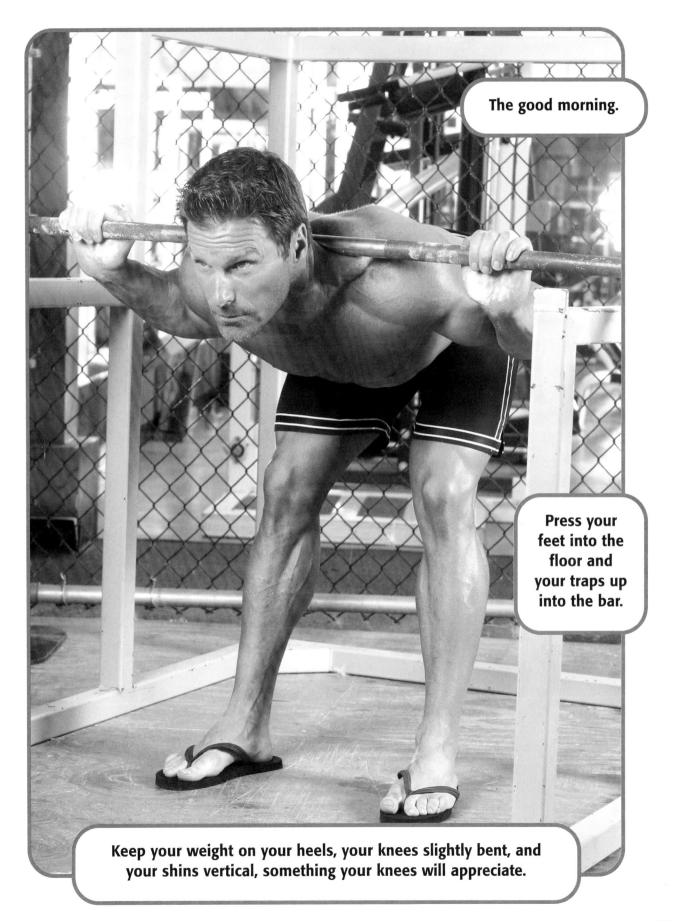

The good morning.

Press your feet into the floor and your traps up into the bar.

Keep your weight on your heels, your knees slightly bent, and your shins vertical, something your knees will appreciate.

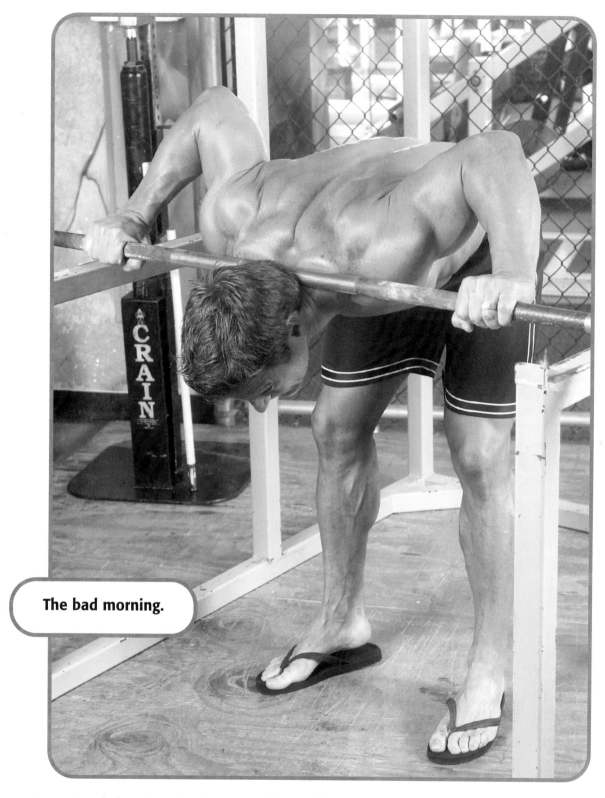

The bad morning.

Bruce Randall used to do three sets. He would pick a weight he could do for sets of five and gradually work them into eights. Then he would add ten to fifteen pounds and start over with sets of five. Do this twice a week and try a comfortably heavy squat once a month. Unlike other squat avoidance schemes, this one will work.

'DEAD SQUATS' FOR POWER

Question: I saw a big dude in my gym squatting from the bottom up from the power rack pins. What is the purpose of this type of training?

I will start with the benefits of 'dead squatting'. First and foremost, it keeps you honest. While you can get cute in the traditional back squat by cutting your depth for instance, the dead weight sitting welded to the pins will accept nothing less than real strength. Second, it is a very safe way to squat. And fun too. The dead squat is the ultimate in muscle tension.

The drawbacks. First, because it de-emphasizes the negative, the dead squat does not build as much muscle as the down-and-up squat. It can be an advantage though, if you are satisfied with your thigh size and just want to get stronger. Second, the dead squat does not teach you to 'store tension' on the way down. It means that you will not improve your regular up-and-down SQ without specific practice in addition to your power rack squats.

Set a light barbell inside a power rack at a level that places your thighs at parallel once you crawl under the bar. Get under – quickly, before your cramp! – take a breath, tighten up, and stand up.

De-emphasize the negative. Do singles. Add small amounts of weight until you work up to a near max, then take off some weight and do one or two back-off sets of five to ten reps. Let the bar rest completely on the pins between each rep. The whole workout might look like this: 185x1, 225x1, 275x1, 295x1, 305x1, 310x1, 225x10. Ease into it as you are likely to get very sore, especially in your hip flexors.

Follow the above routine one to three times a week. You will not need any other hip and thigh work. A few years ago I put two friends of mine, everyday guys in their forties, on this program. They kept improving at least five pounds a week for almost a year without back cycling of any sort.

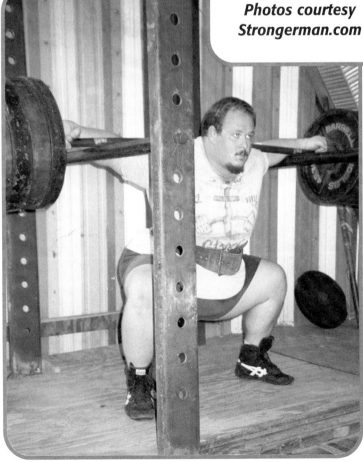

Bud Jeffries dead squatting 900 pounds! His PR is a grand!

Photos courtesy Strongerman.com

73

The definitive text on the dead squat is *How to Squat 900lbs Without Drugs, Powersuits, or Knee Wraps* by Bud Jeffries (Strongerman.com). In the know people consider Jeffries the successor of Anderson. The man parallel dead squatted a grand!

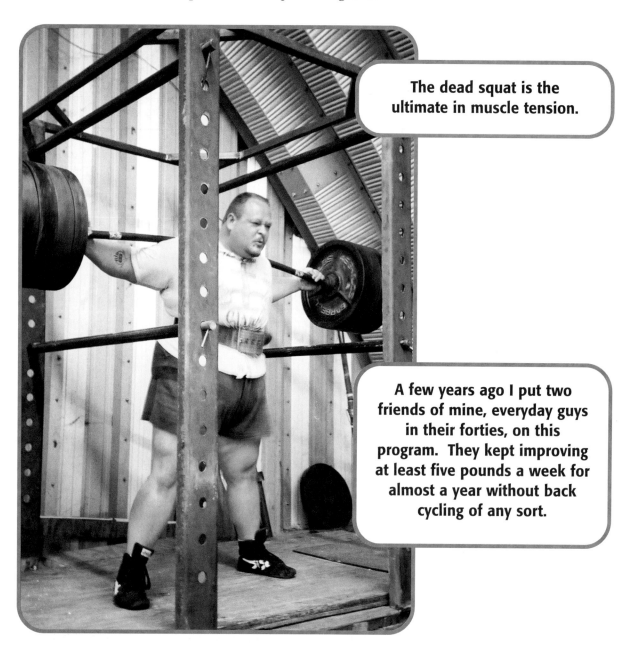

The dead squat is the ultimate in muscle tension.

A few years ago I put two friends of mine, everyday guys in their forties, on this program. They kept improving at least five pounds a week for almost a year without back cycling of any sort.

PROTECT YOUR BACK WITH A 'VIRTUAL BELT'

Question: Should I Power Breathe when I squat and deadlift?

When your spine is compressed by a heavy poundage you cannot afford losing any air, for it protects your back like a pneumatic cushion. So instead of forcefully expelling your breath just pretend that you are – a technique I call 'Virtual Power Breathing'. Obviously, it is not for comrades with heart or blood pressure issues.

Practice a couple of regular Power Breaths as I described elsewhere. Then do the same – but 'catch your breath' in your stomach instead of letting it escape. You will experience comfortable tightness in your waist as your abdomen gets pressurized. Your belly should not stick out or suck in; it will just get rock hard and you will feel very solid inside. Make sure not to flex your spine, try to maintain its normal curve.

Here is how to apply the 'virtual belt' to your powerlifts. Take three quarters of your maximal breath and pressurize your abdomen – as explained before – pulling your dead off the platform. Hold it as the bar is inching up. Power Breathe a little air out at the lockout and park the weight without losing your tightness. Follow a slightly different sequence in the squat: inhale and pressurize at the top, go down and come up while holding your breath, release some air at the top.

Do not forget to employ this technique when you are hauling heavy stuff outside the gym and remember to religiously practice plain vanilla or water Power Breathing to hone your skill of pressurizing your abdomen.

The effects of Virtual Power Breathing are nothing short of miraculous. The usually heavy weight will feel whimsically light and your back is not likely to feel a thing.

"IRON FUNDAMENTALISM"?

Question: Why are you so fundamentalist in your training philosophy? 'Never do more than five reps', 'never go to failure', etc. There are people who got big and strong without following them, aren't there?

I will restate my 'iron communist' views:

1. You must lift heavy.

2. You must limit your reps to five.

3. You must avoid muscle failure.

4. You must cycle your loads.

5. You must stay tight. Tension is power.

6. You must treat your strength as a skill and 'practice' with iron rather than 'work out'.

7. You must strive to do fewer things better.

My 'fundamentalism' is meant to give you the safest and most foolproof path to your goals – size and strength. Why overcomplicate your life with multiple choices if you can get the job done simply?

At a recent RKC seminar one of my senior instructors Rob Lawrence made an excellent point that all training 'laws' are reversible under the right circumstances. Take 'the law of staying tight' as an example. Extreme full body tension is an absolute must for one-rep strength that impresses; I dare you to find a good powerlifter who does not practice it! Yet *gireviks*, athletes who compete in kettlebell lifting, stay as loose as they can when pressing. Tension accelerates fatigue, which is unacceptable in the brutal Russian strength-endurance sport.

All training laws and guidelines are reversible in the right context. The caveat: it takes knowledge and experience to reverse them properly and sometimes you must be willing to pay the price. Until you have been in the iron game for a decade and accomplished something, break these 'laws' at your risk.

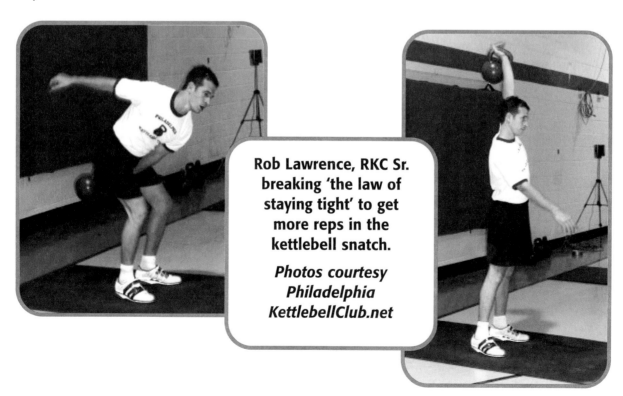

Rob Lawrence, RKC Sr. breaking 'the law of staying tight' to get more reps in the kettlebell snatch.

Photos courtesy Philadelphia KettlebellClub.net

OLD-TIMER TRAINING Q & A

Question: Many old-timers combined weight lifting, gymnastics, and strongman training. Is that necessary today?

Dr. Ken Leistner, one very strong hombre and an influential name in the iron game, once quipped that bodies built with isolation exercises looked like 'a collection of body parts'. That never happens to those who apply their muscles to a variety of natural tasks: lifting awkward objects, acrobatics, heavy manual labor, etc.

One way of combining such training with traditional bodybuilding is starting every workout with the former and wrapping up with the latter. Another approach, more fitting for someone who trains at a public gym, but keeps his logs and tires in the garage, is to emulate Russian strength icon Valentin Dikul. This sixty some year old juggles 180-pound kettlebells and squats a grand! He lifts daily, alternating powerlifting/kettlebell/strongman days and bodybuilding days. Note that although Dikul does isolation exercises like straight-arm pulldowns, he always goes heavy, typically five sets of six.

Question: How could old-timers train each muscle daily and why can't we?

Our great-grandfathers treated their iron time as a *practice* rather than a *workout*. They lifted heavy and often but never to failure or exhaustion. According to *The Strong Men of Old* by Bob Hoffman, Arthur Saxon "would do each stunt only a few times and alternate with brief periods of rest so as to prevent himself from tiring." That explains how Saxon could train daily.

Although frequent, heavy, and non-exhaustive training builds unreal strength, it is not a good full time method for a bodybuilder. Saxon was a strong man but not a muscle man. In 1879 William Blaikie explained in *How to Get Strong and How to Stay So* that "...occasional heavy lifting tends rather to harden the muscle than to rapidly increase its size, protracted effort at lighter but good-sized weights doing the latter to better advantage." An occasional six to eight week gig of daily pure power training will do you a world of good though. Greater strength later applied to high volume bodybuilding will deliver tremendous mass gains.

Question: Are there any "lost" retro exercises that should be resurrected?

Plenty of them. The bent press gets my first vote. This drill is not really a press but a unique flexibility and support feat. Get a weight to your shoulder: a barbell, dumbbell, or kettlebell. Set up so your elbow is resting on your pelvic bone, on the side and even slightly behind you. This calls for some serious shoulder flexibility; chances are it will take you months of partial reps to work into a full bent press.

Slowly lean to the side away from the weight and slightly forward – never back! Keep your eye on the bell at all times and be ready to drop it. Your elbow must rest against your side at all times and your forearm must remain vertical, absolute necessities with heavy weights. The all time record is Arthur Saxon's 370 pounds!

Eventually you will end up in a semi-squat, your arm finally locked out. Slowly stand up with your arm straight overhead.

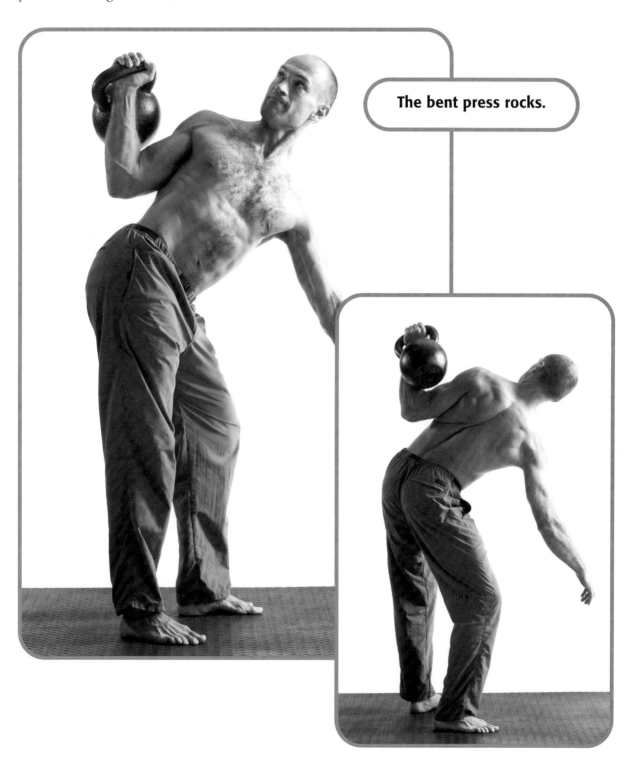

The bent press rocks.

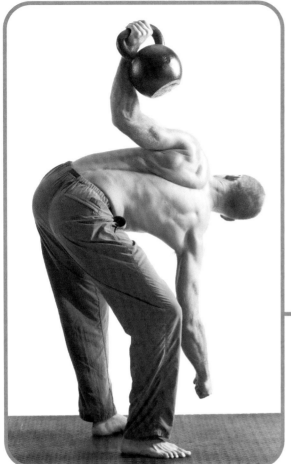

Some tips. Practice where you will have no fear of dropping the weight. Occasionally bent press after your triceps are fried, to discourage you from pressing the bell. At other times practice when your lats are pumped; flaring the lat really helps.

Getting even a marginally passable bent press will take months. Why bother? – Because it is a great lat workout (you would never guess, would you?). Because it develops spectacular shoulder flexibility that will go a long way towards shoulder health. Because it is one of the best moves to work all your core muscles and to make your back injury resistant.

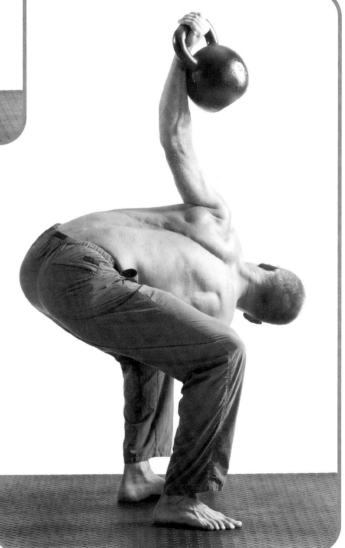

Eugene Sandow, the father of bodybuilding, was a bent press expert and his physique is yet to be topped. There are plenty of bigger guys nowadays but no one comes close to Sandow's total package of superstrength – one-finger pullups, anyone? – muscle density, and symmetry.

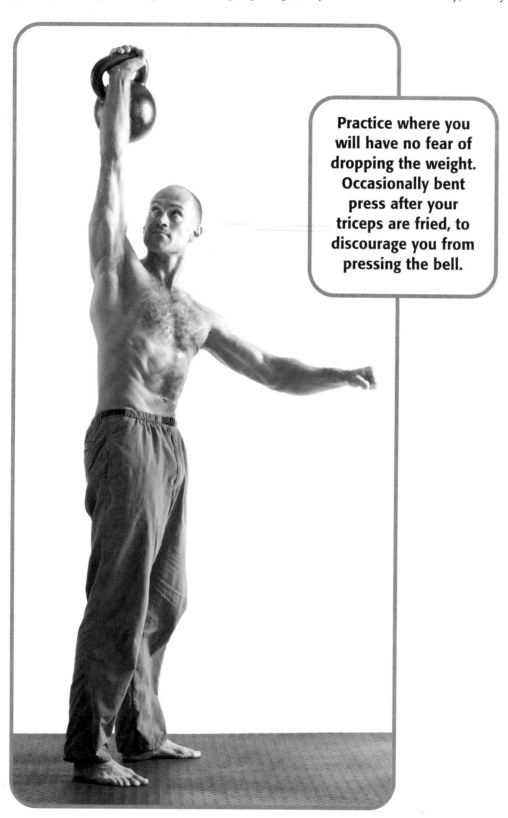

Practice where you will have no fear of dropping the weight. Occasionally bent press after your triceps are fried, to discourage you from pressing the bell.

Question: Why didn't the bodybuilders of the golden age bench and squat?

On the bench press count, it would not occur to our able bodied grandfathers to exercise and test their strength lying down. Besides, in those days 'chest development' meant a huge ribcage, not breast like pecs. The floor pullover was the chest exercise of choice. And yes, contrary to what some modern trainers say, it is possible to expand an adult bodybuilder's rib box. As for the squat, logistics was the problem. Squat stands and power racks did not exist; squat pioneers had to rock a barbell onto their shoulders, a feat in itself.

Is BP and SQ free training worth emulating? – It depends on the look you are after. You will not get truly huge without them. On the other hand, you will not have droopy pecs and chafing thighs either. The retro emphasis on a variety of lifts from the ground and overhead, forge physiques along the lines of antique statues: broad shoulders with just a hint of pecs, back muscles standing out in bold relief, wiry arms, rugged forearms, a cut-up midsection, and strong yet trim legs.

Question: What did the old timers do for cardio and staying lean?

Dig into your family album or go to the library and look up photos of people who lived in the first half of the twentieth century or earlier. I dare you to find an obese person. The lost secret of leanness is simple: hard physical labor every day. Here is some grandfatherly advice: get off your stern and go to work. Real man or woman work, not fifteen minutes on an elliptical trainer every other day. Get a part time job as a mover. Sell your John Deere and get an old-fashioned push mower. Volunteer to clean up a highway. Andrey Dolgov, a Latvian boxing and kickboxing coach extraordinaire, raised a school of fearsome champions whose S&C is old-fashioned labor. These hard and ripped to the bone fighters volunteer to cut and stack firewood for old ladies.

Even an occasional day or two of hard physical work or exercise will do wonders for your body comp. My students always leave a weekend kettlebell course leaner and more muscular. Martial arts seminars are great; recently I took an excellent two and a half day course from Tim Larkin of tftgroup.com and walked away noticeably leaner.

My wife once observed, if you work out for an hour a day and spend twenty-three hours sitting or lying down, do you think your looks will reflect the one hour or the twenty three hours?

Question: What lost bodybuilding secrets can we use today?

There are many – but one stands out: do not train to failure and have patience. Famous Russian strongman Pyotr 'the Kettlebell King' Kryloff said, "The training of amateurs I have been meeting... is driven by records. It is a wrong system and an unhealthy one to top it off... Thanks to my extremely careful and restrained system of training I have kept my strength and muscles, even though, being an old school circus athlete, I had to perform very difficult stunts and sometimes perform shows with very heavy weights a few times a day." As the ancient wisdom goes, "He who understands life does not rush."

DRILLS THAT RULE, DRILLS THAT DROOL

Last week I taught a seminar out of town and hit a gym near my hotel for a workout. What a depressing landscape, Comrades! A dude was doing what he apparently perceived as plyometrics on a Hack squat machine and I almost had to dodge a rocketing kneecap. An intellectual was performing some exotic combo of an internal shoulder rotation and a cable crunch. A lady who could whip both guys was getting a glazed look as she was approaching a trance like state after a hundred crunches...

I cannot fix the whole bodybuilding scene in one day, but putting together an 'A' and a 'Z' list of exercises will be a good start.

ABS

It Drools: the Crunch

I have no clue how such a pathetic exercise has come to dominate the scene. I guess some simple mind came up with a bright idea that not coming up all the way would isolate the abs from the psoas. It does not. But if you have not read my book *Bullet-Proof Abs* you will never know why.

It Rules: the Janda Situp

The crunch brigade is stuck in the industrial age. They treat the body as a simplistic mechanism of pulleys and levers and fail to recognize the vital role of the nervous system in protecting the back – and in making rock hard abs happen.. The Janda situp, a state of the art exercise developed by a top Eastern European back rehab specialist, drags ab fitness into the information age. It 'hacks' into your 'muscle software' to dramatically amplify the intensity of the abdominal contraction while shutting off the potentially back damaging hip flexor muscles.

OBLIQUES

It Drools: the Situp with a Twist

You will miss your back when it is gone.

A broomstick twist is just as dumb as the twisting situp ,but gratefully it has been put to rest by all bodybuilders other than those who have been pumping away in bomb shelters hiding from Soviet ICBMs.

It Rules: the One-Arm Suitcase Style Deadlift

There are a few more goodies on my obliques 'A' list but I chose this one because it will hurt the most, heh-heh. Deadlift a barbell – a dumbbell could be bad news to your toes – as a suitcase. Do not do a side bend; your body should come up evenly as if you have another bar of the same weight in your other hand. Stay tight. You will get a lesson in anatomy the morning after: "I didn't know I had muscles there!"

GLUTES

It Drools: the Fire Hydrant and Anything Else that Happens in a 'Muscle Sculpting' Class

What a pathetic, demeaning exercise. Get off your knees, you are not a dog. Besides, the glutes are very powerful. It takes a lot more than repetitive butt squeezes to get them to shape up.

It Rules: the Hip Pull-through

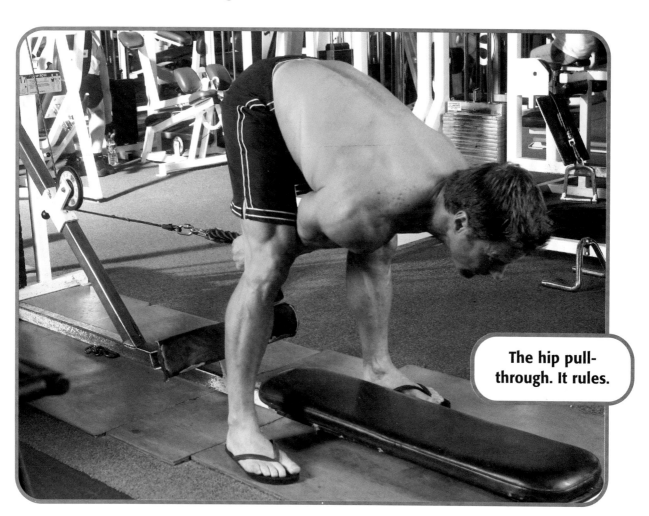

The hip pull-through. It rules.

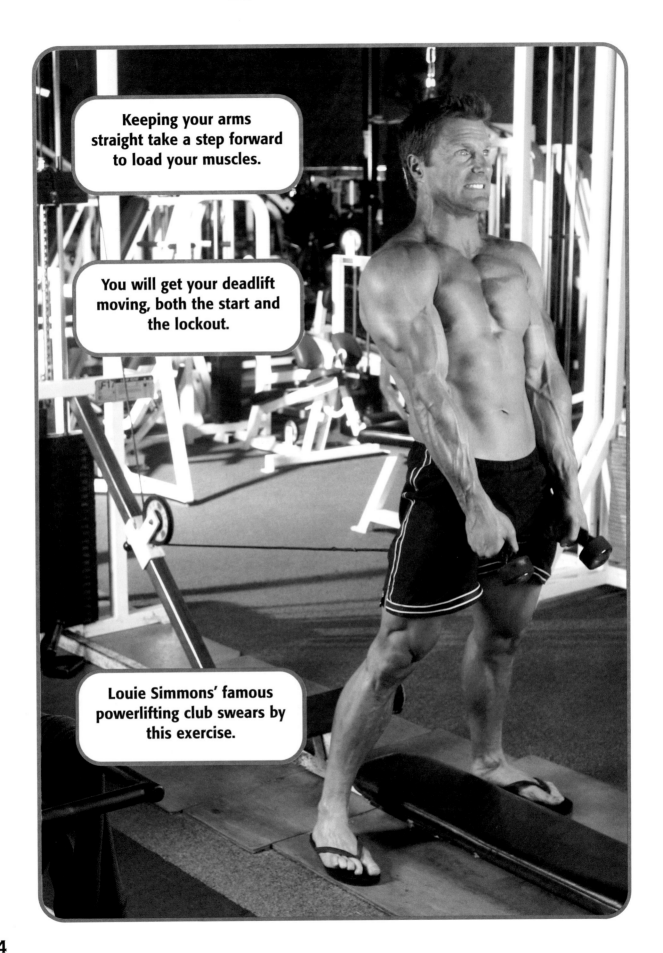

Facing away from a cable machine, stick your arms between your legs and grab a triceps push-down rope attached to the low cable. Keeping your arms straight take a step forward to load your muscles. Now squeeze your glutes and drive your hips forward while locking out your knees. If your knees stay bent, the drill will not work. In addition to a hard butt you will get your deadlift moving, both the start and the lockout. Louie Simmons' famous powerlifting club swears by this exercise.

LOWER BACK
It Drools: the Sissy Deadlift

You have heard of a sissy squat but not a sissy deadlift? – You have seen it, Comrade, trust me. This grotesque deadlift mutation calls for a weight lighter than your top curl and demands that you lock your knees and twist your neck to check out your butt in the mirror. This exercise in vanity will get you nothing but back, neck, and knee problems; your spinal erectors will remain flatter than a road kill.

It Rules: the Deadlift Lockout

Be generous with plates and pull a barbell from your knee level or slightly above. Use a staggered powerlifting grip or straps. Keep your whole body, especially your stomach and butt, tight. Frank Zane digs the partial deadlift for a reason. What reason? — Do the drill and you will not have to ask.

QUADS
It Drools: Any Machine Exercise

Just say no to machines when it comes to leg training! If you cannot, get help. Leg extensions are worthless and can be tough on the knees – as the latter are vulnerable without the backup of contracting hamstrings. Ditto for the Hack squat machine, not to mention additional problems from knee hyperflexion. And the leg press is nothing but an ego lift. Sure, you can impress someone who has never touched a weight with a 1,000 pound leg press. People in the know would be more impressed with a squat with one third of that poundage.

It Rules: the Squat

Nobody does it better. You may opt for any reasonable variation of the squat – the Olympic squat, the powerlifting squat, the front squat, the one-legged squat, the duck style deadlift or the trap bar deadlift – as long as you squat.

HAMSTRINGS

It Drools: the Leg Curl

The most likely 'gain' that you are going to report from this exercise impostor is back pain from trying too hard and getting your hip flexors in the action. Working the hammies as knee flexors just is not productive (unless you are using Dr. Yessis' GHG machine). Treat them as hip extensors and you might eventually come to the gym wearing shorts.

It Rules: the Good Morning

My friend Marty Gallagher, a former coach of the Powerlifting Team USA, laments, "Why does such a manly drill have such a 'hearts and flowers' name?"

I have no idea. But I know that your hamstrings will fill out like a pair of footballs once you put good mornings in your regimen. Make sure to keep your back arched and do not go any deeper than parallel. Do not think of leaning forward, rather keep sticking your butt out while looking straight ahead until you reach the right depth. As a bonus, good mornings will boost your squats into orbit, which is why they are a favorite with most top Russian powerlifters.

CALVES

It Drools: the Standing Machine Calf Raise

When young Arnold trained with Reg Park, the latter used 1,000 pounds for his calf raises, twice Schwarzenegger's training weight. Park explained to the future legend of bodybuilding that the 500 pounds he was toying with "were not making an impression" on his calves at all, because these are very strong muscles (or at least ones with good leverage). Arnold proceeded to work up to a grand. The rest is history.

Superheavy calf training is a must. But great weghts on your shoulders combined with high volume translate into some serious spinal compression, especially if you are not skilled in protecting your back with diaphragmatic pressure against your viscera and your midsection is weak. Regardless of the standing calf raise's effectiveness, you had better ditch it once you work up to big poundages.

It Rules: the Negative Accentuated Foot Extension in a Leg Press Machine

Your calves get worked daily and it takes some unusual stress to spur them into growth. This is where the leg press machine comes in (the only thing it is good for). The sled will enable you to blast your calves with monster weights without back stress – as long as you do not let your butt curl up – and easily lends itself to intense negative accentuated training. Lift the load with two feet, lower it with one. Feel the pain.

LATS

It Drools: the Pulldown Behind the Neck

If you have exceptional active flexibility of the shoulder girdle, can keep your elbows way back and can pull the bar to the nape of your neck without leaning forward and sticking your head out like a chicken about to be beheaded– go ahead and pull behind the neck. Since I do not know anyone except for Olympic weightlifters and gymnasts who can do that, you might as well forget it! The chicken style pulldown behind the neck does little but screw up necks and shoulders.

It Rules: the Pullup/Chinup on Gymnastic Rings

The debate regarding the 'best' pullup grip is as hot as it was half a century ago. Is wide better than narrow? Is the supinated grip better than the pronated one? I have good news for you: you can have it all, just do your pullups or chinups on gymnastic rings. What a stretch! What a contraction! If you do not have the luxury of living next door to the old Santa Monica Muscle Beach go to ringtraining.com and get a set.

TRAPS

It Drools: the Smith Machine Shrug

I have never seen a set of big traps inside a Smith machine. You cannot pull your shoulders back at the top of the movement and your traps will miss all the good stuff. Besides, the machine locks your shoulder girdle in a set track and that could lead to joint problems.

It Rules: the Barbell Shrug with a Hip Thrust

The traps of Soviet weightlifting legend David Rigert stood out like a foreign object, an alien parasite. You can bet that the champion did not get there with uncertain shrugs with little weights. The traps best respond to explosive barbell shrugs assisted by a hip thrust: violently contract your glutes and throw your hips forward as you shrug up and back. Do not bend your arms; it helps to keep your triceps flexed, at least on the bottom of the movement. You may hold the contraction on the last rep for a few seconds followed up by a slow negative. Do not relax under the weight! Breathe shallow.

CHEST

It Drools: the Cable Cross-Over

The pec was designed for power and teasing it with this silly move is a waste of your time. If you want to bring out the 'cuts' you will be much better off etching them in with some old-fashioned iron bending. Go to IronMind.com for nails and instructions. Take a seminar with

Senior RKC Brett Jones of BreakingStrength.com. Brett is the eleventh person to bend Iron Mind's famous Red Nail ™, the second fellow under two hundred pounds.

It Rules: the Legal Powerlifting Bench Press

No need to reinvent the wheel here. You will not find a better chest builder than the barbell bench press. However, to get the most out, of it you had better lose some of your bad bodybuilding habits – such as putting your feet up on the bench and bouncing the bar off your chest. Drive your feet into the floor and pause on your chest for a second without relaxing, as you would in a power meet.

SHOULDERS

It Drools: the Seated Barbell Military Press

Do this one long enough and heavy enough and you can kiss your back goodbye. Get off your butt, you big sissy!

It Rules: the Arnold Press

Let's face it, the big guy knew what he was doing. Even though there are other shoulder drills at least as effective as this one, say the clean-and-press, the Arnold press is a lot more user friendly.

Press two dumbbells from your chest starting with a curl grip. Not straight up though, but back and to the sides in an arc. It helps to bring your elbows as low as possible between reps; you will get a greater deltoid stretch and your shoulder joints will appreciate it.

BICEPS

It Drools: the Zottman Curl

The Z curl calls for curling a dumbbell with a regular palm up grip, then pronating the wrist and doing a reverse curl negative. Unless you are very in tune with your body your smaller flexors on the top of the forearm will be a hurting units for weeks; those negatives creep up without warning.

It Rules: the One-Arm Dumbbell Curl

It is hard to beat this classic provided you curl strict and slow and employ every high-tension technique in the book.

TRICEPS

It Drools: the Triceps Kickback

The long and the lateral heads of the triceps –that is two out of three – just refuse to work until you are handling a respectable weight. Kickbacks? – Forget about 'em!

It Rules: the Close Grip Bench Press

Nothing fancy, but it sure gets the job done. Do not get your hands too close together, almost touching the smooth part of the bar with your index finger is just right.

FOREARMS

It Drools: the Wrist Curl with a Weenie Weight

Most of my arm-wrestling buddies have no trouble slamming a #2 Captains of Crush™ gripper that takes almost 200 pounds to shut. And they have the forearms to show for it. You will never get a spinach endorsement contract, Comrade, if you train your forearms with Malibu Ken and Barbie weights.

It Rules: the Suitcase Barbell Wrist Flexion

Pick up a long bar from the power rack pins set at your hip level, as you would pick up a suitcase. Squeeze the bar and gooseneck your wrist as if you are trying to roll up your fist toward the inside of your elbow. Your elbow will flex somewhat; that is OK. Keep your lat tight and do not shrug your shoulder. It helps to think that you are trying to pull yourself down to the bar.

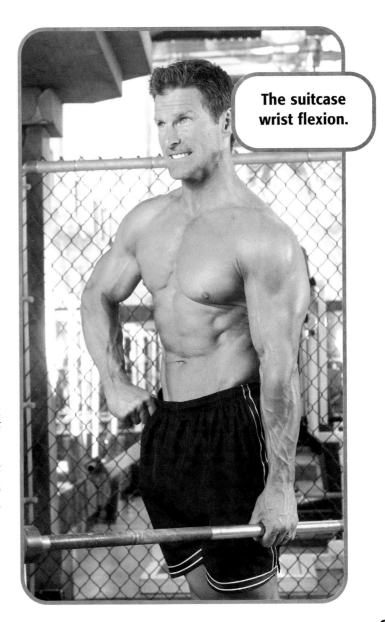

The suitcase wrist flexion.

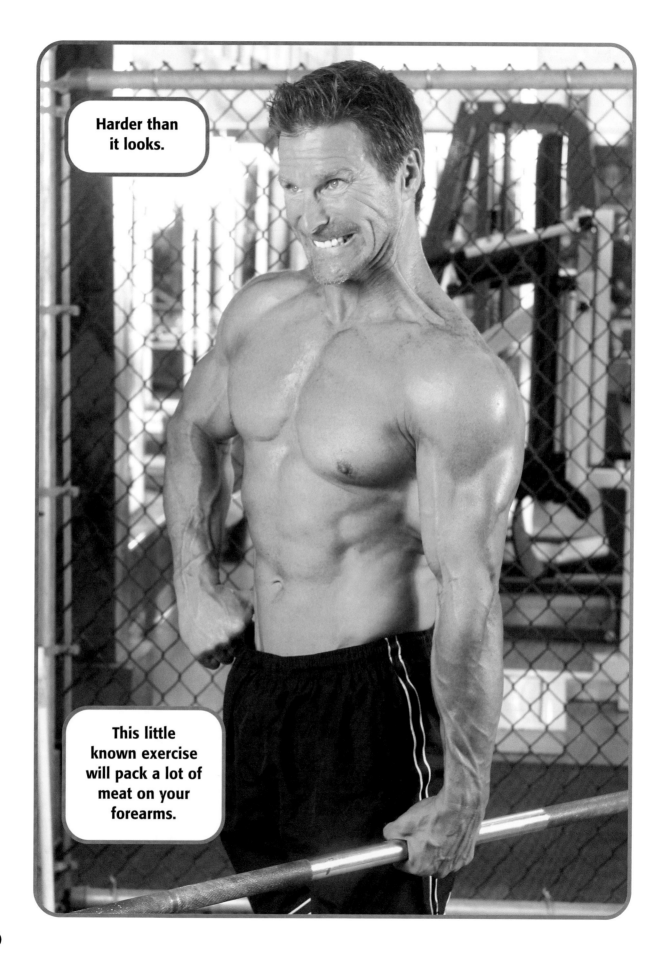

Harder than it looks.

This little known exercise will pack a lot of meat on your forearms.

This little known exercise will pack a lot of meat on your forearms. Still, do not limit your forearm training to wrist flexion. Work other degrees of wrist freedom: extension, abduction, adduction, pronation, and supination. And do not forget your fingers, at least flexion and extension.

Naturally, my 'A' and 'Z' lists are far from being exhaustive. There are many more fine bodybuilding exercises and even more exercises that suck. But it is a start. If I got you to turn your back on a leg curl machine and load up an Olympic bar for good mornings, if you start treating the cable cross-over stack like you would a drug pusher near your kid's school, and if do not let your friends use the leg press machine, except for heavy calf work, I got something accomplished. Now, if I could only get that health club's management to shut off their mall tunes and crank up some AC/DC, I might even go back next time I am in town.

FREE WEIGHTS FOR BEGINNERS?

Question: You indiscriminately push free weights on anyone, including raw beginners like me. Don't you get it that your barbells and kettlebells are very hard to balance and it would be a lot safer to get someone started on machines?

I shall respond with a quote from the authors of Supertraining Prof. Verkhoshansky and Dr. Siff. "Contrary to common belief, the novice must be taught from a base of mobility to progress to stability, just as an infant learns to stand by first moving, staggering and exploring the environment."

Would you like to be 'staggering and exploring' while you are still relatively weak or later, when you have more strength to hurt yourself? I rest my case.

A NO COMPROMISE HOME GYM ON A BUDGET

Question: I am planning to set up a home gym. I have a bare bones budget and very limited space. What should I get?

HOME GYM MINIMUM #1

A barbell set plus a homemade platform. You could get a cheap set made with child labor in the Far East. Or you could spend a few bucks more and get a quality product proudly made in the US, for instance one by the legendary York Barbell Company, YorkBarbell.com.

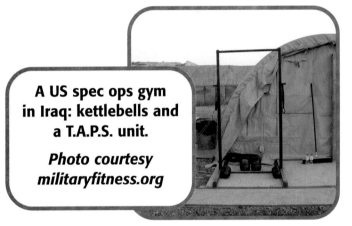

A US spec ops gym in Iraq: kettlebells and a T.A.P.S. unit.

Photo courtesy militaryfitness.org

Throw a 3/4 inch thick sheet of rubber on the floor and you are all set. If you deadlift heavy or drop your overhead lifts you will need a platform. The following home made design that I had learned from former Powerlifting Team USA coach, Marty Gallagher served me well. Cover six old tires of the same size arranged in two tight rows of three with a thick sheet of plywood. Nail a couple of 2x4s on the edges of the platform to prevent the barbell from rolling off. Top off the contraption with a thin sheet of rubber and you are in business.

Where is the exercise bench, you might ask? Isn't it the staple of bodybuilder's arsenal?! – No. Until a few decades ago you could not even find one in any gym. Even in this age of obsession with pecs you can do without one. Do floor presses; it is the same movement as the BP except you are lying on the floor. What about the legs? – Deadlifts, Jefferson, and Hack squats will take care of them. Figure out the rest.

If you have a few bucks left get a power rack. Avoid cages with all the fancy attachments, although a pullup bar would be great.

HOME GYM MINIMUM #2

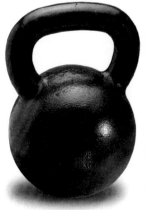

A kettlebell. This classic iron tool available from RussianKettlebell.com enables you to do everything you could do with a dumbbell plus many things you could not: repetition quick lifts, various presses, Turkish get-ups, overhead squats, armwrestling curls... And, what is important when you are on a budget or tight on space, the traditional kettlebell training protocol does not require multiple weights, one or two bells are just dandy.

HOME GYM MINIMUM #3

A pullup bar or a set of gymnastic rings. Or, better yet, both. If you have imagination you can build a powerful upper body with your body-weight alone. Floor exercises take care of themselves; all you need is something to pull yourself up on. Ideally install your bar or rings high enough for you to hang with your legs straight without touching the floor. The Tactical Athlete Pullup System by Jeff Martone, RKC Sr. is an awesome pullup rig. Get one from TacticalAthlete.com. Get your rings from RingTraining.com. You can hook them up to your T.A.P.S. and do a ton of cool stuff, including dips.

Senior RKC Jeff Martone in his home gym: a T.A.P.S. unit + kettlebells + Power Rings.

Photo courtesy TacticalAthlete.com

CAN SINGLE JOINT EXERCISES BUILD STRENGTH?

Question: It seems that everyone praises squats and other compound exercises these days. Do isolation exercises have any future?

Canadian researcher Digby Sale discovered that individual muscles within muscle groups and even motor units within individual muscles have activation patterns that are highly movement specific. In other words, you will not be using the same part of your quads during squats and leg extensions. Depending on your goals, it can mean different things to you. If you are an athlete or a power bodybuilder, forget exercises like leg extensions that do not resemble any sport or real life efforts! "It would be most efficient to induce hypertrophy only in the muscle fibers of the motor units that are activated in the sports movement," explains Sale. "Hypertrophy of irrelevant muscles and motor units might even be counterproductive, particularly in sports which require a high strength to body mass ratio."

At first glance it appears that single joint exercises are a waste of time to anyone but purely cosmetic bodybuilders a.k.a. the Big Sissies. But wait! What if there is a way to circumvent the 'Sale Law' and activate the 'leg extension muscles' during squats?!

Here is the theory based on a long lost secret of Paul Anderson. 'The Wonder of Nature', as the Russians nicknamed him, used to perform his powerlifts and assistance exercises in a circuit. He would do a few squats, rest a bit, do a set of good mornings, then more squats... Big Paul did this to 'coordinate' the strength built with the assistance exercise, with the powerlift. Today we understand what he did and why it worked. The neurons which regularly fire close together tend to get cross-wired and become a part of a single neural network. As a result, the good morning muscles and fibers previously unused in the squat become integrated into it! It might work with single joint exercises too.

On many occasions Paul Anderson devised a training technique decades ahead of his time without knowing neurons from nylons. Russians call this technique *complex training*. It is common among T&F top dogs but somehow failed to catch on with strength athletes. A high jumper may do a heavy triple in the squat followed by some depth jumps, an intense form of plyometrics, and wrap up with a competition style high jump. The result: a transfer of the strength gain in assistance exercises to the primary skill of the sport. So it is conceivable that heavy sets of triceps extensions alternated with benches would strengthen the latter lift. The single-joint exercise would build and neurally strengthen some new fibers – and alternating it with the target compound lift would integrate these fibers into the lift.

If you choose to test this theory, train your 'isolation' exercises as you would the powerlifts – with the high-tension techniques, heavy, and for low reps. Pat Casey, the first man to bench 600 pounds (in a wife beater, not a bench shirt) did insanely heavy one-arm laterals. Try alternating 3x6 of the single joint assistance exercise with 3x3 of the power lift or some other pet lift of yours. It is not clear what rest periods you should use. Start with 2-3 min. No one knows whether uneven intervals, e.g. resting only 1 min after the flies and 3 after the benches, would be of any help. Experiment and drop me a line on the dragondoor.com forum with your results.

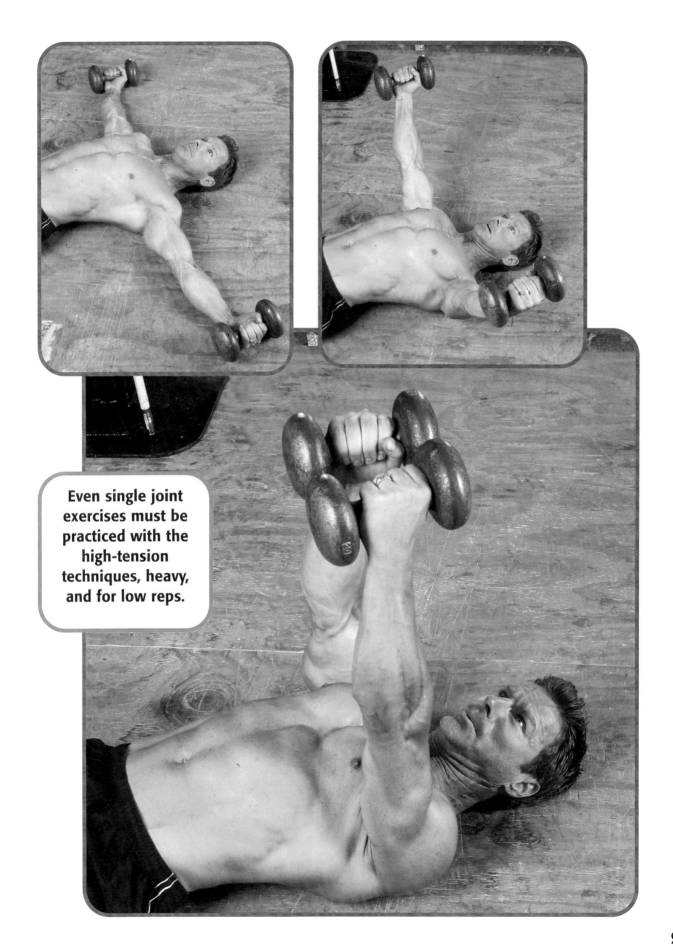

Even single joint exercises must be practiced with the high-tension techniques, heavy, and for low reps.

SECTION TWO
TRAINING PLANNING

CONTENTS

Articles

Questions and Answers

TRAINING PLANNING CONTENTS

Questions and Answers

- *Is varying exercise tempo worth the trouble?*

- *Not satisfied with your rate of progress?*

- *Variety for minimalists*

DIVIDE AND CONQUER: DESIGNING THE PERFECT SPLIT

Comrade, are you having a hard time deciding how many times a week should you lift and how often you should hit each lift or body part? – Not any more. The purpose of this section is to teach you how to customize your iron schedule, split or otherwise.

First, let us consider the pros and cons of full body workouts versus split routines. A full body workout is the most foolproof and harder to overtrain on – clear plusses in a beginner's book. It is time efficient – an asset, unless you dig the gym scene and have no athletic pursuits outside the gym. Finally, a full body session can help you focus on the big bang exercises and reduce the number of flaky, non-productive moves.

On the down side, a full body workout does not allow for specialization training and prevents the trainee from doing a high volume of work. Both are advanced issues. A beginning to intermediate bodybuilder has no business specializing, unless he specializes on the squat. And a high volume of loading does not become a must until you already have some meat on your bones. Which does not imply that a full body routine is for beginners only! Guess how the drug free physical culturalists of the golden age built their strength and physiques?

If you have picked a full body routine, the only decision you have to make is the frequency of training. Here are your choices.

a) Once a week or less. Although hitting each body part once a week works well on a split routine that provides indirect daily stimulation, this frequency – or rather 'infrequency' – will not fly unless all you do is squat and deadlift.

b) Three times in two weeks, e.g. Mon-Fri-next Wed. An appropriate schedule if you are super busy or your lifestyle does not help quick recovery. Be prepared to be sore a lot.

c) Two times a week, e.g. Mon-Thur. Fitting if you are short on time. Also good for advanced comrades who are not good at varying their volume and intensity from workout to workout (cycling).

d) Three times a week. The Mon-Wed-Fri schedule has persevered for decades because it is the most foolproof.

e) Four times a week. One of the best setups for a serious drug free iron man or woman. As gymnastics coach Chris Sommer put it, it "allows maximum work combined with substantial rest." Surprisingly, according to Prof. Arkady Vorobyev, the author of the Russian equivalent of Arnold's *Encyclopedia of Bodybuilding*, Mon-Tue-Thur-Fri is superior to Mon-Wed-Fri-Sat. The reasons are outside the scope of this piece; just remember that the Party is always right.

f) Five times a week or more. Perfect if you have the discipline to follow an ultra abbreviated routine such as *Power to the People*! and strength is more important to you than size.

Onward and upward to split routines. There are two types of splits: by muscle group or body part, and by lift. The latter is the powerlifting approach, but it does not mean it will not work for a bodybuilder. The classic powerlifting split is Monday – the squat, Wednesday – the bench, and Friday – the deadlift with a second, light, BP session often added on Saturday. Start by working the primary lift and wrap up with exercises that would help it, regardless of the body part involved. For instance, on squat days you could do good mornings, usually known as 'a back exercise', to make your squats feel lighter – and presses behind the neck to stretch out your shoulders for a better bar position on your back.

Why bother with the powerlifting split? – to be as strong as you look.

Two more effective power splits. Squat on Mondays and Fridays, deadlift on Wednesdays, and bench on all three days (the great Mike Bridges' schedule). Or lift three days a week, benching every other session and rotating squats and deads: Monday – SQ, Wednesday – BP, Friday – DL, Monday – BP, Wed – SQ, Fri – BP, etc. (Paul Kelso's split). By the way, there is no reason you cannot dedicate your Saturdays to curls and other beach work. The best of both worlds.

If you go the traditional bodybuilding route and split your workouts by body parts, the rule of thumb is to make sure that each muscle group gets to be trained when it is maximally fresh. Pair up body parts that have a minimal negative impact on each other. Legs + arms is better than chest + triceps. Shoulders + biceps rocks and back + biceps sucks. You get the idea.

Dorian Yates' early split teaches you how it is done. Mr. Olympia would work his legs and arms on day one, take a day off, then train his torso: chest, back, and shoulders. The fourth day was a day off. Neat: the arms get blasted once directly and then get a light day when the torso is worked. And the chest, back, and delts cannot help getting an indirect training effect on the arm day, at least if you do real exercises such as dips and cleans rather than weenie triceps kickbacks.

The story of another Mr. Olympia, Lee Haney, will drive home the point of minimal overlap even further. Haney used to follow the push/pull split, that was popular in his day. He would train for three days on, one off: Day 1 – chest, shoulders, triceps, Day 2 – legs, Day 3 – back and biceps. The gains were not great and Mr. O's shoulders were hurting, thanks to the triple assault on this vulnerable joint on day one. As high achievers tend to be, Haney was confident enough to admit that he did not have all the answers. Someone suggested that he switched to this arrangement: Day 1 – chest, biceps, triceps (the tris were worked separate hours later), Day 2 – legs, Day 3 – shoulders and back. Instead of smoking all the 'pushing' muscles on one day and the 'pulling' ones on the other, all were getting heavy days and light days, an essential element of continuous progress. The shoulders healed, the scale needle and the exercise poundages started climbing up again...

Following are two more splits that follow the minimal overlap principle. Plug in the abs and forearms where you think it is best.

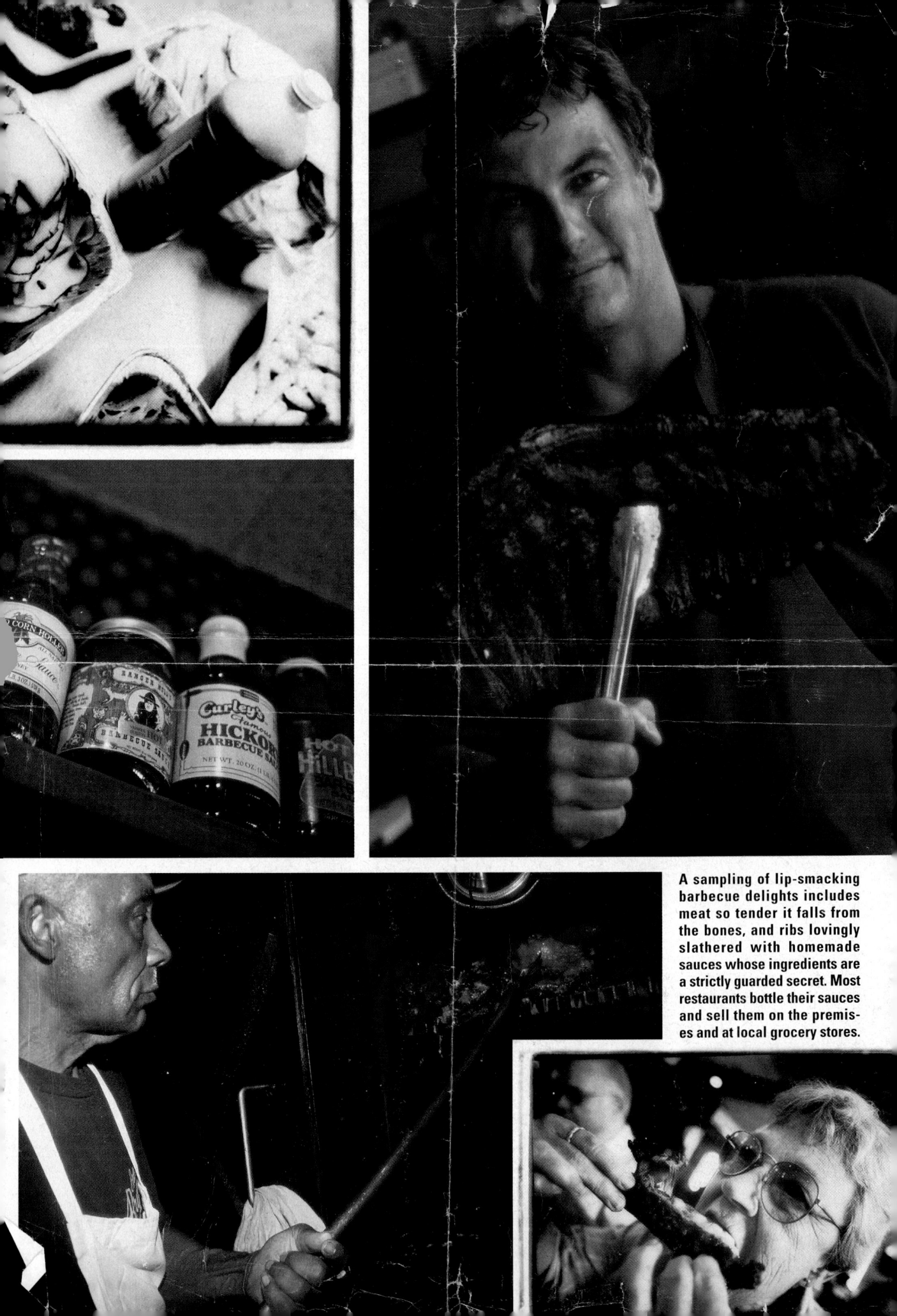

A sampling of lip-smacking barbecue delights includes meat so tender it falls from the bones, and ribs lovingly slathered with homemade sauces whose ingredients are a strictly guarded secret. Most restaurants bottle their sauces and sell them on the premises and at local grocery stores.

A Taste of K.C.

Try these recipes at home for a sample of Kansas City barbecue.

Nuclear Chicken Wings

The Boardroom Bar-B-Q won the 1990 Coors Buffalo Wings round at the American Royal BBQ Contest with this recipe.

5 lbs. chicken wings, tips removed
1 cup dry barbeque spice mixture
2 T. crushed red pepper flakes
1 T. Cajun spice
1 T. cayenne pepper
1 (to 2) cups spicy barbeque sauce

Rinse chicken, pat dry. Sprinkle mixture of barbeque spice, red pepper flakes, Cajun spice and cayenne over chicken in nonreactive dish, stirring to coat. Let sit, covered, in refrigerator for 8 hours or longer. Smoke chicken over indirect heat for 30 minutes, turning once. Baste both sides of wings with barbeque sauce. Grill over direct heat for 5 minutes per side. Serve immediately with a spicy sauce. Yield: 50 servings.

BBQ Pork Tenderloin

Rich Davis' recipe took first place in the American Royal BBQ Contest.

3 large pork tenderloins
Marinade:
1 cup soy sauce
1/3 cup Oriental sesame oil
3 large garlic cloves, minced
1 T. ground ginger
1 tsp. MSG (optional)
Sauce:
1 bottle (18 oz.) K.C. Masterpiece
1/3 cup soy sauce
1/4 cup Oriental sesame oil
1 garlic clove, minced

In a small bowl, combine marinade ingredients. Place tenderloins in glass or enameled pan, pour marinade over meat, cover with plastic wrap and let sit overnight in the refrigerator. Place meat on a charcoal grill (with moistened hickory chips added to smoke) over indirect low fire. Barbecue with lid closed, turning every 15 minutes and basting with marinade, about 1 1/2 hours. Mix together sauce ingredients and heat. Serve with meat. Six to 8 servings.

Arthur Bryant Barbecue

(1) 1727 Brooklyn, Kansas City, Mo; 816-231-1123.

Proclaimed by native son and The New Yorker columnist Calvin Trillin to be the "best single restaurant in the world," it's short on decor, long on legend. Arthur Bryant is the undisputed "grand-daddy" of Kansas City barbecue, having turned out briskets and ribs for nearly 50 years until his death in 1983. The classic entrée: thinly sliced brisket, lightly sauced with their trademark, almost gritty, sauce, piled jaw-stretching high between two slices of white bread, accompanied by a side of delicious lard-fried French fries.

Boardroom Bar-B-Q

(2) 9600 Antioch, Overland Park, Kan; 913-642-6273.

Grand Champion at the 1985 American Royal Barbecue Contest, Scott O'Mara spent a lot of time planning his Boardroom Bar-B-Q with wife, Ann, before chucking the corporate life in 1991. It's located near a large corporate office park and attracts many business people; hence the name of the restaurant and many of its specials. Second biggest seller, after ribs, are "Burnt Ends" — the ends of the beef brisket too small and irregular to slice. Instead, they're cubed and resmoked until they become very smoky and very tender.

Gates Bar-B-Q

Five locations: 1221 Brooklyn Ave., Kansas City, Mo; 816-483-3880; 1026 State Ave., Kansas City, Kan; 913-621-1134; 1044 E. 40 Hwy, Independence, Mo; 816-353-5880; 2001 W. 103rd Terrace, Leawood, Kan; 913-383-1752; 3201 Main, Kansas City, Mo; 816-753-0828.

Another Kansas City barbecue pioneer was George Gates, whose son, Ollie, now supervises operations of the restaurants, and of Gates' prize-winning barbecue sauce, available bottled in many local supermarkets and by mail order. With locations on both sides of the Kansas/Missouri border, and with all employees graduates of Gates' "Rib Tech" employee training program, expect the same efficient service and good food at any Gates Bar-B-Q. Highlights include the lamb and pork ribs, a tangy potato salad and sweet-potato pie.

K.C. Masterpiece Barbecue & Grill

(4) 4747 Wyandotte, Kansas City, Mo; 816-531-7111; (5) Interstate 435 and Metcalf Ave., Overland Park, Kan; 913-345-1199.

The K.C. Masterpiece Sauce that Dr. Rich Davis developed became so successful, he gave up his psychiatric practice for barbecue endeavors. He eventually sold the sauce business and he and his sons now concentrate on their restaurants. Two appetizer favorites are Doc's Dip, a puréed and seasoned spinach, tomato and cream cheese mixture; and the yummy "Onion Straws," thin onion slices, lightly battered and fried. Be sure to save room for the Chocolate Peanut Butter Ice Cream Pie.

L.C.'s Bar-B-Q

(6) 5800 Blue Parkway, Kansas City, Mo; 816-923-4484.

A local secret until recently, it's now one of the current barbecue "hot spots." What it lacks in decor it more than makes up for in food. The smoker, fired up 24 hours a day, turns out great brisket and ribs, with a not-too-sweet sauce that complements the meat's smoky, sweet flavor. The crisp, thick-cut fries are hard to resist. L.C.'s is a favorite "pit stop" for fans headed to the Kansas City Chiefs games.

Lil' Jake's Eat It & Beat It

(7) 1227 Grand Blvd, Kansas City, Mo; 816-283-0880.

This pint-size lunch spot depends on rapid service — and eating — to handle its brisk business. You can wait your turn for one of 18 counter seats, or place your order in the fast-moving carryout line.

Split One

1 Shoulders, biceps
2 Legs
3 Chest, triceps
4 Back
5 off

Split Two

1 Chest   5 Back
2 Biceps   6 Shoulders
3 Legs   7 off
4 Triceps

More sophisticated splits are an option for experienced bodybuilders. For instance, you could train your legs three times in two weeks, your chest twice a week, and your arms three times a week as suggested by Shawn Phillips. Dr. Fred Hatfield's books will give you plenty of ideas if you want to go the custom split route.

And if you feel like keeping things simple, I will make the choice for you. Train your whole body on Mondays, Wednesdays, and Fridays, each time with a slightly different emphasis. For instance, on Mondays start with many sets for the chest and have an easy workout for your legs. On Wednesdays focus on the squats and do just a couple of light sets of benches. On Fridays prioritize your back and take it easy on everything else. On Saturdays just go and have fun with curls and what have you. To the point, fun, and effective.

Most importantly, keep it simple and do not obsess about getting your recovery 'just right'. Your body is highly adaptable and your schedule needs to be good, but it does not have to be perfect. That 'narrow overcompensation window' you have read so much about is a fairy tale; if it was for real, only PhDs in labs could build muscle. I do not have the time to go on this tangent, so pick up a copy of Prof. Vladimir Zatsiorsky's textbook and read about 'fitness/fatigue' if you want to know why. But first – divide and conquer!

PERIODIZATION DEMYSTIFIED

Comrade, can you tell periodization from perestroika and Leonid Matveyev from Leonid Brezhnev? Da or nyet, it is time to incorporate this Soviet breakthrough into your training!

Why should you? – For gains superior to those possible with any other system of training! These strong words are backed up with gold. Hundreds of world champions speaking my native language are the poster children of periodization. You don't really think that Ivan brings Olympic medals to Mother Russia, after 'realizing his full muscular potential in a year, with HIT', do you?

Periodization is defined as planned – according to certain principles! – variation of the training variables such as intensity and volume within a specified period of time culminating in peak performance. Although its origins can be traced to tsarist Russia, periodization did not come alive until L. P. Matveyev published his milestone *The Problems of Periodization in Sports Training* in 1964. Comrade Matveyev even applied this revolutionary concept to his own quest for a 100 kg, or 222 lb, clean and press. In the process 'the father of periodization' changed the face of athletic training as we know it.

In the West periodization has either been overdone with yawn drawing charts and alien Russian terminology or dumbed down to 'do high reps, then switch to heavy weights'. I'll fix it. Here it is, the real thing, no more complicated than it has to be, yet not watered down.

I am not going to repeat the mistake of charting out Dow Jones looking graphs and prescribing every exercise, sets, weights, etc. "Over-reliance on numerical computations in preparing a periodization chart is a major reason why some coaches tend to dismiss their relevance," lament Drs. Verkhoshansky and Siff. The authors of *Supertraining* proposed 'cybernetic programming', essentially old-fashioned instinctive training plugged into a periodization master plan.

Indeed, many variables, from sunlight to your recent argument with your boss, affect your performance and it is difficult to map out a rigid twenty-week plan and follow it rep for rep. Bulgarian weightlifters, scientific as they are, use their judgment in determining the optimal training weight for every set. You should take this idea a step further. This piece is going to teach you how to strip periodization down to its fundamental principles, namely *cycling, sequential development, the optimal volume/intensity relationship,* and *delayed adaptation,* and then superimpose them into your workout free style.

CYCLING

Gym rats love reciting the legend of Milo of Crotona. As the story goes, this ancient Greek stud started lifting a young calf daily. Milo kept growing stronger and stronger as the animal grew into a bull. From calves to bulls, from bulls to elephants, from elephants to whales.

Sure. Dream on. According to the physiological Law of Accommodation, after a short period of time the body stops responding to a given stimulus. It takes a greater load to get it to improve again. The bummer is, you cannot increase the load indefinitely. It just does not work that way; eventually you will hit the wall.

Why can't you train hard full time and progress till you die as the HIT Jedis claim to do in their galaxy far away? Estonian Dr. Atko Viru and other big brains from the former Soviet Union have offered many esoteric theories. It could be systemic neurological or endocrine exhaustion. Perhaps the hypothalamus, the part of the brain in charge of adaptation, just calls it quits? Or maybe the local genetic apparatus in your muscles has had it for a while? It could be some unknown regulatory mechanism that forbids continuous unidirectional adaptation... Who knows, and who cares! The point is, it happens, and you cannot hide your head in the sand if you expect to keep on getting bigger and stronger!

Russian scientists concluded that periodic gain and loss of sporting form is a law of physiology and it dictates a cyclical organization of the training process. "Human life can be considered one big wave with its climbing, peaking, and declining phase," writes Polish immigrant coach Thomas Kurz, MS, the author of highly recommended *The Science of Sports Training* (stadion.com). "Several smaller waves are superimposed on our life wave. Some last years, some days, some hours, and some even less than a second. Rational athletic training should take this cyclical character of life into an account."

Thus cycling of loads was born. This radical concept is simple: if your muscles have stopped responding to a training stimulus and rebel against a further load increase – just back off to resensitize them! 'Soften them up' for future gains, as English cycling crusader Stuart McRobert put it.

Like a Russian nesting doll, the cycling principle applies to your training months and weeks and repeats itself even within a workout. Multiple sets with a static weight, e.g. 200kgx5x5, are frowned upon by Russian weightlifters. They have the habit of following up a heavy triple or double with a double or a single with a weight reduced by 5-10% before making another heavy lift. Their Bulgarian colleagues follow a similar pattern that they call 'segments': work up to a heavy single, then back off some, then push again, etc. In addition to being more effective for obscure motor learning reasons, such a wavy workout is a lot less monotonous and more enjoyable. More important, according to Matveyev, non-stop variation of volume and intensity reduces the possibility of overtraining and enhances the performance peaks.

Many Western proponents of periodization are under the impression that the load should change ever so gradually. While this may often be true for the overall, months long, pattern, taking baby steps in workouts and microcycles, or training weeks, and playing with quarter pound Malibu Ken and Barbie plates is far from being your best choice. Explains Prof. Vorobyev: "Although not excluding the principle of gradual overload, we propose sudden changes in load - 'jumps' that are tailored to the given athlete's functional abilities. This principle of organizing the training loads allows one to achieve higher results with a smaller loading volume."

Instead of increasing your bench numbers – within one workout or in consecutive sessions – in a linear fashion, e.g. 225-230-235-240-245-250, try something wild, say 225-240-215-235-220-250. The overall pattern of increasing the intensity is still observed, but irregular jumps back and forth will bring you to your goal faster than pussyfooting towards it. Do the same step gig with the volume, or the total number of reps in your muscle building session. If you are one of those sick people who like doing their taxes, apply the 60% Rule to your load planning. According to this experimentally calculated formula, the volume of the lowest load training unit (a workout, a microcycle/week, a mesocycle/month) should equal approximately 60% of the highest load unit, provided they are of the same length.

For illustration purposes let us say that you follow the popular bodybuilding split which requires that you work each muscle group once a week. Say the most total reps you ever do is 100 per muscle group. The volume is calculated by adding all the reps minus the warm-ups, e.g. military press 5x10 = 50, upright rows 5x10 =50; the workout volume for the shoulders is 50+50 =100 reps.

Every fourth week cut your volume to 60% of your peak load – which happens to be a standard practice in the Bulgarian and Chinese weightlifting teams. Your deltoid workout would chill out by 40%: (3x10) + (3x10) =60 reps. Your weekly volume distribution in one month might look like this: 90-70-100-60, 70-85-60-100, 60-80-100-65, etc. The variations are endless, just do not fall for slick sequences like 60-70-80-90 or 95-85-75-65. Dr. Matveyev states point blank: sharp changes in training volume and intensity are more effective than smooth ones!

Cycling implies that the difficulty of your training will vary greatly. Alternating hard and easy workouts used to be a standard practice in bodybuilding. According to Kurz, even ancient Greeks had a moderate load training session in their four-day training cycles. During the golden age of American iron sports many ninety-eight pound weaklings transformed themselves into he-men following the heavy-light-medium principle. Then the vocal HIT Jedis convinced the muscle heads that they have no business lifting a weight unless they go balls to the wall. The pencilneck count in the gyms across the fruited plain has been going up ever since.

Soviet research data is clear: easy workouts restore your strength and brawn much faster than channel surfing! "The best conditions for anabolic processes are when small (2-4 ton) loads with low intensity follow large loads," stated Arkady Vorobyev, a champion, a scientist, a coach.

Another reason to have an easy workout, on days when you feel like hanging up your belt ,is what Russian textbooks refer to as 'the continuity of the training process'. Think of it this way: if you include the squat in your leg workout only once in a blue moon, your squatting gains will be non-existent. Your body does not adapt to a stimulus immediately because it does not want to go to all the trouble if the stressor is a fluke. The more often you squat – the stronger you get. Eastern European weightlifters squat daily – but rarely to their 700-800 pound limit. Constantly exposed to the deep knee bends and unable to get out of touch with their purpose, these athletes' legs transform into super squatting machines. So do not be afraid to have easy workouts or sets here and there. They serve a greater purpose than an excuse to hang out at the gym.

While the simple approach of sticking to the same exercises and only cycling the load works for powerlifters, bodybuilders, at least advanced ones, need more variety in their training. The periodization model takes your needs into account. According to the data from the scientific experiment conducted in Moscow in by V.S. Avanesov, a complex of weight training exercises provides good results for one to one and a half months, then it should be changed. But not more often than that!

Dorian Yates warned against excessive muscle confusion. The bodybuilding legend explained that variety for variety's sake is just a distraction from purposeful intense training. According to Y. Verkhoshansky and M. Siff, when exercises are switched more often than once every four to six weeks, the body goes into what is known as a *transient accumulation process*. In non-geek speak, it does not have the time to catch on to what it is supposed to adapt to and in the end hardly adapts at all! Nature does not tolerate extremes. Either changing your workout too often or never changing it is a raw deal.

THE OPTIMAL VOLUME/INTENSITY RELATIONSHIP

The inverse relationship between the loading volume and intensity ('you can't sprint a marathon') is a myth. All volume/intensity combos serve their purposes.

Medium/medium workouts are the bread and butter of training.

High/high sessions push one into mild overtraining and lead to greater gains once followed by a taper.

Low/low sessions are used for active recovery or when the team is likely to go into combat.

Low/highs set PRs.

High/lows build foundation for stable gains.

Then there are medium/highs, low/mediums... Every combo has its purpose. This is a good time to dispel a myth popular in the West, that the volume and intensity are inversely related – the higher the intensity, the lower the volume and vice versa. Smart men like US Armed Forces Powerlifting Champion Jack Reape and Belorussian kettlebell expert N. V. Galenchik, stress that *volume and intensity must be uncoupled*. "Overall load [sets, reps, proximity to failure, rest between sets, the number and order of the exercises, the degree of recovery from the last workout, the length of the session, etc.] must vary so that some days you barely leave... and others you would love to do more but can't – the plan forbids." (Galenchik, 1999)

I repeat: the volume and intensity are random and not dependent on each other.

Load variation is critically important to strength success, but it must follow one rigid rule: concentrate on volume and do not abuse high intensity training! Whether you interpret intensity as a percentage of one rep max (the Russian definition) or of momentary ability (the American definition), you will not build much beef if you HIT regularly! Short-lived strength gains are all you can hope for. Which is why high intensity should be a rare visitor to your regimen.

"When one is after long term adaptation and aims at significant structural, and not just functional changes" – that is muscle mass versus strength – "the volume of loading is increased first and foremost," states Leonid Matveyev. "When, on the other hand, one aims to realize the acquired ability as a sudden increase in athletic performance, the training intensity gets top importance." In other words, build beef with a lot of sets and reps, then get as strong as you look by occasionally pushing the pedal to the metal.

Bench a mind boggling weight once in awhile, get the whole gym talking– and immediately back off! Doggedly attempting to maintain the strength peak just dooms the iron rat to failure, something powerlifters learned the hard way three decades ago. The volatility of the gains – they can be maintained for five to ten days at best according to Dr. Arkady Vorobyev – and a higher risk of injuries and overtraining, are not the only problems of high intensity training. Russian scientists warn that attempting to maintain top condition is detrimental to future progress! Just one more reason why most of the time volume rules.

The proponents of one-set training should go back to school. Russian scientists uncompromisingly state that lasting muscle growth in elite athletes can only be achieved through high volume of loading! No wonder East German specialists recommended up to 150 total reps per muscle group in one muscle building workout. Hey, if 'low volume/high intensity training' was all its proponents claim it is, don't you think there would have been a lot more muscular studs walking around?

105

SEQUENTIAL DEVELOPMENT

If you have read Prof. Vladimir Zatsiorsky's *Science and Practice of Strength Training,* you may have noticed that Russians said goodbye to the pyramid in 1964, which happens to be the year periodization was born. Coincidence? Do not be naïve, Comrade.

Soviet scientists such as Y. V. Verkhoshansky observed that the athlete's body adapts much better if it is presented with a focused and limited training objective, rather than a host of often conflicting demands – get big and strong, and fast, and run a marathon… Since different rep ranges have a specific effect on the muscles – low power reps increase the muscle density, medium reps build the contractile proteins, and high reps develop mitochondria, sarcoplasm, and capillaries – the obvious implication of this discovery on bodybuilding is not to spread your workout over a large rep range. Top strength coaches like Charles Poliquin feel strongly about it.

Just to clarify, narrow rep range pyramids like 5-4-3-2-1-2-3-4-5, 6-4-2-2-4-6, or 12-10-8-10-12 are cool. I am not going to put my foot in my mouth and state that pyramids with a wider rep spread, say 12-10-8-6-4-2-2-4-6-8-10-12, don't work at all. As we all know from experience, they do. Just loading schedules with a narrower focus work better.

The idea of a 'finisher' does not sit well with the periodization model either. The 'finisher' is an endurance smoker done at the end of a strength workout, for example, a farmer's walk after deadlift singles, a sprint after squat fives, or fifty pushups after heavy benches. Unless circumstances force you to train all aspects of strength and conditioning (e.g. 'complex PT sessions' in the Russian military) or all muscle tissues at once, don't. Train different goals in different cycles, or at least on different days.

Do not interpret the above as an admonition not to do back-off sets! Do them by all means, just keep them in the ballpark of the top sets. Examples of 'Party approved' programs with back-off sets are old powerlifting routines by Hugh Cassidy, Dr. Ken Leistner, and John Inzer. Inzer would work up to a heavy, occasionally maximal, deadlift single and chase it down with 3-5x3-10, still heavy. Cassidy might do a heavy fiver followed by three sets of ten. Dr. Ken would put up something like a heavy double followed by a hard set of six. Note that I am referring to Dr, Leistner's powerlifting peaking routines, not his off-season high rep HIT.

So pump up your sarcoplasm, the muscle cell filler, with burning hundred rep sets in one workout (you big sissy!). Up your power and muscle density with singles, doubles, and triples in your next session for the given body part. Build the myofibrils with sets of four to twelve repetitions on your third trip to your iron pit. If you follow a four on/one off split, the whole sequence will take you fifteen days. This approach is known as *sequential development* in contrast with the antiquated *parallel development* with pyramids.

Although, unlike a track and field athlete, a bodybuilder does not need to sequence different workouts in a particular order, he should follow one rule. Namely, spend most of his training time in the four to twelve rep range. Allow me to explain.

When the Beatles were busy recording *Sergeant Pepper* German scientist T. Hettinger discovered that strength built quickly, is lost quickly and vice versa. Soviet scientists such as V. Platonov added that different training benefits are acquired and lost at various rates. For instance, myofibrilllar hypertrophy (4-12 reps) is developed and lost slower than sarcoplasmic hypertrophy (up to 100 reps) or pure strength (1-3 reps). That means two things. First, your hard earned beef will not shrink away if you switch your focus to power or endurance training for a session or two. Second, because gains in max strength and muscular endurance come about so quick, all you need is an occasional session or two to bring them up to a respectable level.

The bottom line. Roughly two out of three workouts should be dedicated to building mass with medium reps. Other workouts can zero in on ultra high or ultra low repetitions. Let your instinct determine the optimal order of these sessions. *

* This piece was originally meant to be the one-stop shop for any bodybuilder, including the 'holistic' types and other misguided characters who do higher reps. I reluctantly give recommendations for such training but I would be much happier if you stopped fooling around with pump and burn and kept your reps in the three to five range. I drive this point home in the piece titled *Holistic bodybuilding'? – No! Power bodybuilding.*

DELAYED ADAPTATION

There is a Russian anecdote about a giraffe who laughs at a joke three times: the first time because everyone laughs, the second time when he gets it, and the third time he laughs at himself for not getting it in the first place. Every living organism is a proverbial giraffe; it responds to any stressor with a lag. For example, the once popular rotation diet did its job by reducing the calories for a day or two and then bringing them back up. A couple of pounds were conquered before the BMR had the time to downregulate.

Renegade Russian scientist Prof. Zatsiorsky explains the *delayed training effect,* "In general, during periods of strenuous training, athletes cannot achieve the best performance results for two main reasons. First, it takes time to adapt to the training stimulus. Second, hard training work induces fatigue that accumulates over time. So a period of relatively easy exercise is needed to realize the effect of the previous hard sessions – to reveal the delayed training effect. Adaptation occurs mainly when a retaining or detraining load is used after a stimulating load."

The adaptation lag has a tremendous impact on strength and muscle training. Once you appreciate its power, you will be freed of the fear of overtraining, which plagues the gyms. Indeed, intelligent short term overtraining is one of the most powerful tools in the bodybuilding arsenal! While a novice or intermediate bodybuilder should allow for complete recovery between his workouts, for an advanced athlete such *distributed loading* is what Estonian sports science mastermind Dr. Atko Viru called 'a waste of time'.

Concentrated loading, Prof. Verkhoshansky's baby, is an advanced alternative. In essence, it is short term overtraining, which is followed by an unusually high supercompensation peak, if the athlete is smart enough to back off before acute overtraining sets in. "A river with a dam has

107

more power," as the Lithuanian saying goes. Aaron Baker, David Dearth, and other bodybuilders reported sensational gains when they gave Mike Mentzer's workout a shot, after doing high volume training for a while. They are the poster children of concentrated loading – or 'overreaching' as it is usually called on this side of the late Berlin Wall – followed by a taper.

"...the more extensive and longer the exhaustion of the body's energy resources by concentrated loading... (obviously within reasonable limits), the higher their subsequent super-restoration and the longer the new functional level is maintained," explain Prof. Verkhoshansky and his colleague Dr. Siff. The scientists warn to keep against going overboard on training intensity when employing concentrated loading; the means are already very powerful and court excessive overtraining. I must add that you should save this thermonuclear weapon until your physique gets startled looks, instead of stupid 'been working out?' comments.

THE TEN COMMANDMENTS OF FREE STYLE PERIODIZATION

1. The volume and intensity are not dependent on each other. All volume/intensity combos serve their purposes.

2. Vary your volume and intensity every workout. Make sudden jumps rather than gradual changes. If you do not mind the math, employ the 60% Rule to your volume planning.

3. Change your exercises every four to six weeks.

4. High intensity training should be employed infrequently. It is only marginally effective for hypertrophy and primarily causes short-lived strength gains. Frequent use of heavy weights and training to failure are also detrimental to future gains.

5. High volume is the key to bodybuilding success. An advanced bodybuilder's high load workout should include up to 150 repetitions per body part.

6. Limit each workout to a narrow rep range: 1-3, 4-7, 8-12, and 12+. Do not employ pyramids.

7. Vary the intensity (both the poundage and the proximity to muscle failure) within each workout while staying in the specified rep range. For example 275x3, 300x3RM, 285x2, 250x3, 295x2, 315x1RM instead of 285x5x3.

8. 4-12 repetitions are the meat of a scientific bodybuilding regimen. No more than one out of three workouts should be dedicated to very low, 1-3, or high, 12 and over, reps.

Chart continued next page

THE TEN COMMANDMENTS OF FREE STYLE PERIODIZATION CONTINUED

9. Relatively easy sessions are more effective than complete rest. Active recovery workouts may be planned or taken instinctively.

10. Controlled short term volume overtraining followed by a low volume/low intensity taper is a very powerful training anabolic. You may plan for concentrated loading or simply take advantage of the accidental overtraining every ambitious trainee is prone to.

Here you have it, the blueprints of a secret Russian weapon that will bomb your competition back to the stone age! Do not even dare to think that because periodization has been around for decades and volumes have been written about it, Westerners understand it better than alien technology in Area 51! The Russkies constantly make corrections and improvements on the go, which are impossible to keep up with unless you are an insider. It is like the old Russian joke about an American spy who got hold of the blueprints of the newest Soviet missile. When a military contractor built it, it turned out to be a steam engine. The irate intelligence officer went back to his source at the Russian defense installation and confronted him. The traitor slapped himself on the forehead, "You mean I forgot to give you the nineteen volumes of upgrades?!"

Let others ride the steam engine. You have the missile plans and the upgrades. Study them. Use them. Dominate.

QUESTIONS & ANSWERS:

THE UPPER BODY SOLUTION FOR 'HIGH INTENSITY' BODYBUILDERS

Question: I am following a 'HIT' (high intensity/low volume) routine that consists of one or two hard sets of a few compound exercises twice a week. Although I am shot for days after each workout, I am making good gains in my lower body. But my upper body just refuses to grow or get stronger. Help!

Although I am not a fan of 'HIT', I will not argue that one or two all out high rep sets of squats or deadlifts pack muscle on the bodybuilders who survive it without getting hurt. Yet I have met very few talented iron rats who have made gains on this type of training in their upper body. Stop denying the reality! The problem is not that you are not working hard enough; the problem is in your routine, emotion rather than science and experience based.

Up the volume, the poundage, and the frequency. Cut the reps and say no to the failure shtick. Consider the classic 5x5 system; unlike HIT, it has never failed to build strength and muscle. Take a weight that is slightly below your 5RM and try to do 5x5 with five minutes of rest in between. Don't fail on any of your sets! It will not be easy, given your HIT mindset, but if it was easy, everyone would be doing it.

Chances are, you will manage something like 5, 5, 4, 3, 3. Stay with this weight and train two to three times a week. Next time you might do 5, 5, 5, 4, 4. A workout or two later you will put up 5x5. Then add five pounds and repeat the procedure. Six weeks later, fresher, and noticeably meatier, you will start reconsidering your lower body routine, even if you are still making gains.

ARE LAYOFFS ANY GOOD?

Question: Is it a good idea to take a month off training once in awhile?

World champion weightlifter Trofim Lomakin would barely show up at the gym once or twice a week, mostly to check in with his boss. Then, three months before a USSR or a world championship, the square jawed Siberian would kick up his training into high gear – and win. Lomakin remained the king of the hill for ten years, well into his thirties.

Working on his 1997 thesis, Vladlen Voropayev, one of the leading kettlebell lifting experts in the world, observed sixty top gireviks, or kettlebell lifters, members of the Russian National Team and regional teams. A whopping 59.3% of these iron athletes reported taking 1-4 months long layoffs from training!

Weightlifting, kettlebell lifting, or bodybuilding, certain things are the same in all iron sports. An occasional layoff, perhaps a month each year or two weeks every six months, will recharge your batteries and will make you want to go to the gym. More importantly, your muscles and the nervous system will become more responsive to training once you resume training; the gains will be fast and furious. Here is how to make the most of this phenomenon.

Start with very, very easy training. Not just for the sake of safety but to make as much gains in the next couple of months as possible. A detrained body will not need much of a stimulus to make it respond. But eventually, as you adapt, a bigger and bigger dosage is needed. Exercise is not that different from drugs in this sense. If you are disciplined enough to set up a powerlifting style cycle – where you start with easy training and do not pop more 'iron pills' until the old dose stops working – you will have a smoothride with three to four months of size and strength gains.

PLANNED VS. FREE STYLE TRAINING

Question: I know bodybuilders who rigidly stick to a routine and others who just wing it. Which is the better way?

In the aforementioned study of elite kettlebell lifters, 57.7% of the athletes followed a training plan, 23% free styled it, and 11.6% did not answer. The same is true among top athletes from other iron sports: some have plotted their ascent to the top while others just winged it.

Obviously, you can succeed either way, but you had better have some structure, at least until you have learned to listen to your body. US Armed Forces Powerlifting Champion Jack Reape made some interesting observations on the dragondoor.com forum: "…most people have no business free styling their training. It just takes too much experience, discipline, and self-knowledge to go in and continuously go by feel, IMHO. Almost nobody who freestyles ever sufficiently backs off. There are days you feel like hell but you can have a good training day. In training, for me, bad warm-ups are a good sign, and easy warm-ups can be a sign of a not so good day. Most new trainees are not physically or mentally tough enough and consequently back away much too early. Most experienced trainees don't know when to back off… I MIGHT have been guilty of this myself a time or two!

Not that everybody needs a 16 week periodized peaking schedule… Having a basic plan to follow is key to making progress, as you must be able to handle more volume and intensity as you progress, or you won't progress. A simple scientific fact… You don't need to be pedantic although that IS allowed, you just need to have it clear in your mind what you are doing this week, month and year, then balance it with your time constraints and priorities.

"No plan survives contact with the enemy, but no one without a plan survives contact with the enemy either!"

Well said.

TWICE-A-DAY TRAINING: THE EDGE OR OVERTRAINING?

Question: I hear contradictory opinions on training twice a day. Some coaches say that these days you cannot succeed in any iron sport without it and others claim it just leads to overtraining. Who is right?

Twice-a-day training has a fascinating history. Upcoming Russian weightlifter David Rigert met the great coach Rudolph Plukfelder (in case you are wondering about the names, both R. and P. are Russified Germans). Committed to his training, young David moved to Plukfelder's hometown Shakhti. Obsessed with strength, Rigert wanted even more pain than whatever his coach was dealing out to him. He secretly made a copy of the key to the gym and started sneaking in for another workout at night. When Plukfelder's backstabbing enemies learned about Rigert's insane regimen they snitched on the coach to the authorities claiming he was killing the young athlete. But a following medical commission found Rigert in excellent health. Rigert went on to become one of the greatest weightlifters ever. Science validated twice-a-day training. Bulgarian coaches visited Plukfelder to learn his moves. You know the rest of the story: a continuous domination of the Russian weightlifters and an explosive rise of the Bulgarians.

Yet there is an expert opinion that such training has led to the decline of American weightlifting. In his interview to powerathletesmag.com weightlifting legend Tommy Kono said that "The U.S. lifters have to go back to the American system of training and not follow what the Europeans are doing. The lifters must return to basics and not have tonnage or intensity govern their training. Believe it or not, it is the old system of light, medium and heavy training 3 to 4 times a week and each workout lasting no more than 90 minutes. It is a matter of taxing your muscles and giving ample time to recover. Too many of our current lifters are over-trained and getting injuries because they lack the recovery time."

Who is right? Don't be mislead by the weightlifting examples, the same two camps exist in bodybuilding. Lee Haney has successfully lifted twice a day while others burned out.

The bottom line is, twice a day lifting works great, but only if you have a military discipline and a relaxed life style, listen to your body, and keep a detailed training log. Do not suddenly add an hour-long evening workout to your usual hour long morning session. That is a sure recipe for overtraining. Do two thirty minute workouts instead– essentially split your normal session in two. This approach, taking your current workload and fragmenting it, has been documented to be very effective by Russian scientists. Which does not mean that it is right for you. It is a high maintenance, non-forgiving regimen. You are probably better off listening to Mr. Kono.

Go lift now. As Rigert used to say, "No squealing. No whining. No complaining."

THE PERFECT SPLIT FOR THE 'STRONG AS YOU LOOK' SERIES

Question: What split should I use with your 'Strong as You Look' series workouts?

One high volume/high intensity workout a week for each body part will do the job. This arrangement hits all your muscles hard and direct every seven days – and indirect a couple of times a week. It as a unique form of cycling invented by American bodybuilders, rather than borrowed from Russian weightlifters or American powerlifters.

I suggest the following breakdown:

Monday	chest
Tuesday	back
Wednesday	abs
Thursday	arms
Friday	legs
Saturday	shoulders
Sunday	off

After three weeks, reduce the reps by 33-50% for a week. E.g., instead of 4x4 do four sets of two reps. Five sets of three instead of 5x5. Two sets of six instead of three sets. You get the idea. The last week of the month will be very easy. It is supposed to be. The unloading week will rejuvenate you physically and mentally and set you up for great gains in the next month.

After a nine-week growth spurt, switch to an altogether different routine. Since you have been working all your muscles with a variety of exercises, mercilessly cut back to the basics, e.g. the powerlifts plus pullups. Because you have been putting in high volume, cut way back, e.g. 3x6 per lift, a mere twelve sets for the whole body. You have been blasting each body part once a week; now train moderately three times a week. This radically different course of action will once again stir up your muscles to new growth.

WHY CAN THE ABS BE TRAINED DAILY AND OTHER MUSCLES CANNOT?

Question: Why is it that the abs can be trained daily and other muscles need two, three, and even more days to recover?

Any muscle can be trained daily provided there is time and a good reason. The Russian National Powerlifting Team benches up to eight times a week. It has been shown that fragmentation of the training load in many mini workouts boosts strength gains (Zatsiorsky, 1995). The idea is to lift heavy as often as possible without tearing down the muscle. If you are training for strength and are not concerned with mass you will be better off doing 1x5 every day rather than 5x5 every five days. This mother of all splits is not ideal for hypertrophy though; Alexey Sivokon benches almost 500 pounds but weighs only 148. A bodybuilder is better off working his or her muscles harder and less frequently.

Since most physical culturists do not dig abs bigger than their pecs, working your midsection daily, heavy but not to exhaustion, e.g. 3x3, is indeed a good choice. Your waist will get tight and strong – and your lower back will thank you for it when you squat or pull.

TURNING LEMONS INTO LEMONADE: OVERTRAINING FOR GAINS

Question: I read that Russian power athletes purposefully overtrain to make greater gains. Can a bodybuilder do that?

Soviet coaches realized that waiting for complete recovery between workouts could take an athlete only so far. Indeed, controlled overtraining – known in the US as 'overreaching' – followed by a taper, leads to gains far superior to those possible with total recovery training.

Although Russians employ some very sophisticated controlled overtraining models it does not have to be rocket science. Any intermediate to advanced bodybuilder can easily follow the approach suggested in one of the free articles posted on dragondoor.com. Work your whole body for two or three days in a row. Then either take a day or two off or taper with very easy, active recovery training. Push, back off, push, back off…

If you like your training cycle to fit nicely into a week, try training Monday through Thursday and take Friday through Sunday off. A fellow named Uru I corresponded with a few years back used that schedule with great success. But with either plan it is essential that you listen to your body. Overreaching is a powerful tool and if abused it can lead to overuse injuries. So use your head!

As a bodybuilder who favors split training you might not like training like this full time. No problem, you should not anyway. Explains former world weightlifting champion Prof. Arkady Vorobyev, "...constant training on the background of incomplete restoration can have dangerous consequences... chronic fatigue and overtraining. Therefore the organism needs a chance to recover completely."

Overreaching for a week every month is more than adequate for a bodybuilder. You will experience great muscle growth, but surprisingly, the best gains are likely to take place during the first week of going back to conventional full recovery split training.

I urge you not to misinterpret the above as the superiority of full recovery training! This is a delayed adaptation made possible by earlier overreaching. Vorobyev explains that incomplete restoration training stimulates the recovery ability; your body literally has to learn how to recoup faster or else! To give you an analogy, say you signed up as a logger and got very sore after the first day of work. If you persist and keep logging day after day through soreness and fatigue eventually your body will adapt and have no problem handling the daily grind. On the other hand, if you were given the unlikely choice of chopping the wood only when you have totally recovered, you would be working twice a week at the most and always recover slowly and painfully (sounds familiar?).

By taxing your recovery ability through intense daily training, you will be building up your adaptation reserves. When you finally go back to hitting up each muscle every three to five days, your muscles will fill out with power like never before!

MATHEMATICS OF MUSCLE GROWTH

Question: You have stated before that a muscle will grow if "it gets pumped with a heavy weight." I am not an instinctive bodybuilder and I would like a less subjective guideline.

Recall that best size gains call for a high percentage of your max lifted for as many total reps as possible in the shortest time. Naturally, these requirements contradict each other so a bodybuilder needs to find the best compromise between the intensity (the average training weight), volume (the total poundage), and density (work to rest ratio).

If you do not like lifting by the seat of your pants use the 'power index' proposed by John Little and Peter Sisco in their book *Power Factor Training*. Say you have squatted 3x10 with 200 pounds in 12 minutes. Start by adding all the poundage lifted: 3x10x200=6,000. Square that number, or multiply it by itself: 6,000x6,000=36,000,000. Squaring the tonnage was a very smart move on the authors' part as it encourages the bodybuilder to up his volume; even a small increase leads to a noticeable jump in the power index.

The final step is to divide the result by the time it took you to complete all the sets. 36,000,000/12=3,000,000. To keep your life simple get rid of six zeroes. You will get the power index – which should really be called 'the mass index' – of 3.

To quantify your training further, start tracking your intensity in its Russian weightlifting definition (Chernyak, 1978). That means the average weight lifted per set. Just divide your total poundage, 6,000, by the total reps performed or 30 (3x10). The intensity will add up to 200 pounds. It goes without saying that if you employ different weights from set to set, your calculations will be a little more involved. Say you have squatted 200x10, 210x8, 220x6. First add up the tonnage of each individual set. 200x10=2,000. 210x8=1,680. 220x6=1,320. Then add them up to get the total poundage: 2,000+1,680+1,320=5,000. Add all the reps, 10+8+6=24. Finally, divide the poundage by the reps, 5,000/24=208. The average intensity is 208 pounds.

Now all you have to do is strive to improve your power index and your average training weights – and meat will start sticking to your bones, if you eat enough. Very quickly the numbers will teach you to lift moderately heavy, keep your reps low, do a lot of sets without lollygagging too much in between, and terminate them before you reach muscle failure.

Understand that although you should up your power index and absolute intensity over a long haul, striving to do so in every workout is unnecessary and even counterproductive. Your loads should wave up and down to pack the greatest punch.

A recent development: Charles Staley's 'Escalating Density Training™' is the most ingenious and foolproof way to plan your power bodybuilding workouts I have ever seen. EDT takes all the guesswork out of your weights, sets, and reps selection. More importantly, it builds muscles that are as strong as they look. Alternating EDT and neural strength programs such as Power to the People!, "Grease the Groove", or 5x5x5 every six weeks will give you the look and the strength of an old-time physical culturist.

Buy Charles' book from edtsecrets.com. Or else.

IS VARYING THE EXERCISE TEMPO WORTH THE TROUBLE?

Question: Is varying exercise tempo worth the trouble?

Lelikov (1975) investigated the effects of the rate of exercise performance on strength gains. He learned that a fast tempo was inferior, very slow lifting was a little better, and a medium pace was the best. However, when the tempo was varied, the gains were 50% greater than those from the leading medium tempo!

Yes, slowing down or speeding up your reps will help you make greater progress in strength and size. And it does not have to be rocket science.

Most of the time you should train at a moderately slow pace, it is conducive to generating the greatest muscular tension. This patient tempo mimics a grinding max lift. You do not need to purposefully slow down; if you keep your whole body tight and lift with calm confidence, your muscles will naturally find their rhythm.

Once in awhile go on a brief stretch of compensatory acceleration or exaggeratedly slow training. My good friend Marty Gallagher, former Coach Powerlifting Team USA, occasionally does a few weeks of Super Slow™ 'for diversion'. In a squat cycle by S. Y. Smolov, Master of Sports, that is popular among powerlifters, two one month long 'grinding' mesocycles are separated by a two week 'switching' period of explosive training and plyometrics. The idea is to provide a radically different stimulus to the nervous system and the muscles – and to get a break between two gruesome phases.

NOT SATISFIED WITH YOUR RATE OF PROGRESS?

Question: I'm totally unsatisfied with my progress. I train my heart out, yet it seems like I have hit a wall; I haven't gained any muscle and strength in six months. Have I reached my genetic ceiling?

Have you noticed that many bodybuilders, stars and everyday guys and gals alike, burn out or get hurt after just a few years of training and quit? On the other hand, there is the powerlifting community where a career spanning decades is common, forty some year olds set world records, and sixty year olds pull triple bodyweight deadlifts. What is it that your iron brothers and sisters know that you do not?

The answer is cycling, the method of starting out with light weights, not training to failure, and slowly building up to a new peak that is weeks or months away. Lifters do not try to impress the gym with their prowess by pushing up max weights every time. A five hundred pound bencher is content with training with three or four wheels, only to add another five pounds to his ponderous max at a meet that is twelve weeks away. In fact, it is the rare powerlifter who maxes more than three or four times a year – and these PRs are never wasted in the gym but carefully saved up for a competition.

Although structured formal powerlifting cycling is a great idea, there are other ways of implementing this conservative attitude into your training. Learn from the post a comrade named Jake Mueller made on the dragondoor.com forum. "I have come upon a new principle that is certainly not new, but new to my own training: Building Momentum... a good way to go about things is to gently "nudge" or "prod" your progress along. For instance, my practice of the barbell clean and military press involves me varying the load each workout… The last two weeks I did 195x10x3 (sets x reps), 235x8x1, 205x10x2, 225x12x1. Now, I might be able to do 225 for 3 sets of 3, or 205 for sets of 5, but the point of this was to practice the lift with relatively heavy weights (75-90%) and NOT incur excessive fatigue. When I start this over again, I'll only add 5 lbs. to each training weight, using 200, 240, 210, 230 respectively. Like Dan John once wrote years ago, "5 lbs. here, a rep there" is what leads to progress, not going to every sort of limit each time you hit the weight room. Progress steadily, backing off occasionally, and you will keep your momentum and avoid burnout (physical and mental)."

As the ancient wisdom goes, "He who understands life does not rush."

VARIETY FOR MINIMALISTS

Question: On one hand you advocate the minimalist approach to training and on the other you teach all these weird exercises and their variations. How do you reconcile minimalism and variety?

The fewer parts something has, the less likely it is to break down. The success of the famous – or infamous – Russian Kalashnikov assault rifle is a case in point. My routines are maximally simplified. They always consist of a very limited number of exercises, all basics, but sometimes with a twist. Here is the logic behind the 'twists'. On one hand, experience has shown that basic moves like squats and deads deliver maximum strength and size gains. On the other, 'the basic variations of the basics' do not always work around injuries and sometimes fail to target one's weak links, be it in strength or in development. Properly selected mutations of the basics do – and much better than the sissy isolation exercises. A couple of examples are in order.

EXAMPLE #1

Bob's bench press has stalled. He has a sticking point a couple of inches off his chest. His training partner diagnoses the problem as a deltoid weakness and recommends military presses and front raises. Three weeks later Bob's bench is still stuck and his shoulders start hurting.

Bob says no to his non-specific overtraining, heals up, and asks a powerlifting coach for advice. The latter lays a couple of 2x4s or a phone book on the bodybuilder's chest. Bob is told to lower the bar until it touches the boards, which places it exactly at his sticking point. Bob is supposed to pause to kill the bounce (without letting the bar sink in) and push back up (without heaving or getting cute in any other way). The power coach prescribes regular benches once a week moderately heavy plus two days a week of intense board pressing. A month later Bob's sticking point is history and his bench is up 15 pounds to a PR of 335.

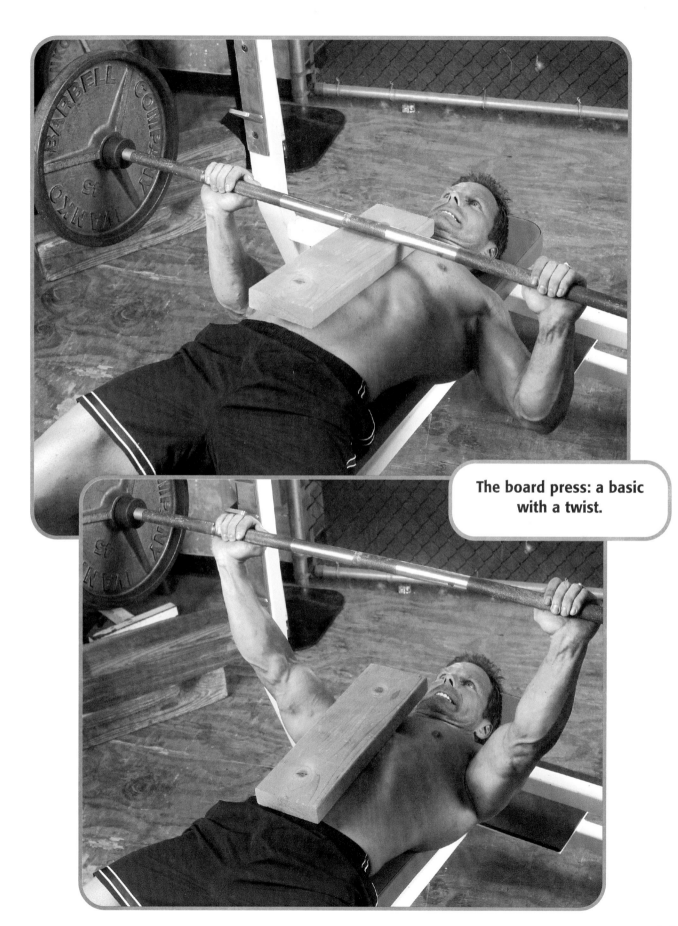

The board press: a basic with a twist.

EXAMPLE #2

Jane wants to cut up her 'lower quads'. She is not happy with the squat-based routine she has been doing as it has bulked up her legs. She follows the gym standard operating procedure and switches to leg extensions. A month later Jane's strength is down; she can tell during her softball games. Her quads have started cutting up but her knees have started aching.

Jane meets a trainer who has been around the block. She explains to Jane that many folks' knees cannot take leg extensions and nothing beats squat type exercises. Jane argues that squats have bulked her up. That is because the loading parameters were wrong for her goals, points out the trainer. To avoid hypertrophy while strengthening and toning the muscles the reps and the sets must be kept low. Furthermore, de-emphasizing the negative will help prevent the unwanted muscle growth.

The trainer tells Jane to do behind the back deadlifts. This cross between the SQ and the DL targets the 'tear drop' vastus medialis muscle and makes it safe to de-emphasize the negative. 3x3 twice a week is the trainer's recommendation. A month later Jane's quads got defined without getting bigger, her knees stopped hurting, and she was faster than ever on the softball diamond.

As you can see from the above examples, a highly abbreviated basic routine can be customized to your individual strength and physique goals, weaknesses, and injuries. Well thought through variations of the basic 'big' exercises is the way to go. Stick with one variation for six weeks or so, then go back to the 'basic-basic' or find another variation to address another weakness. This is the essence of the 'minimalist variety' approach to strength and muscle training.

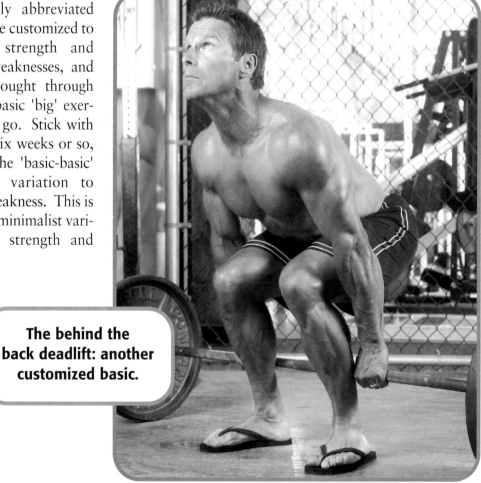

The behind the back deadlift: another customized basic.

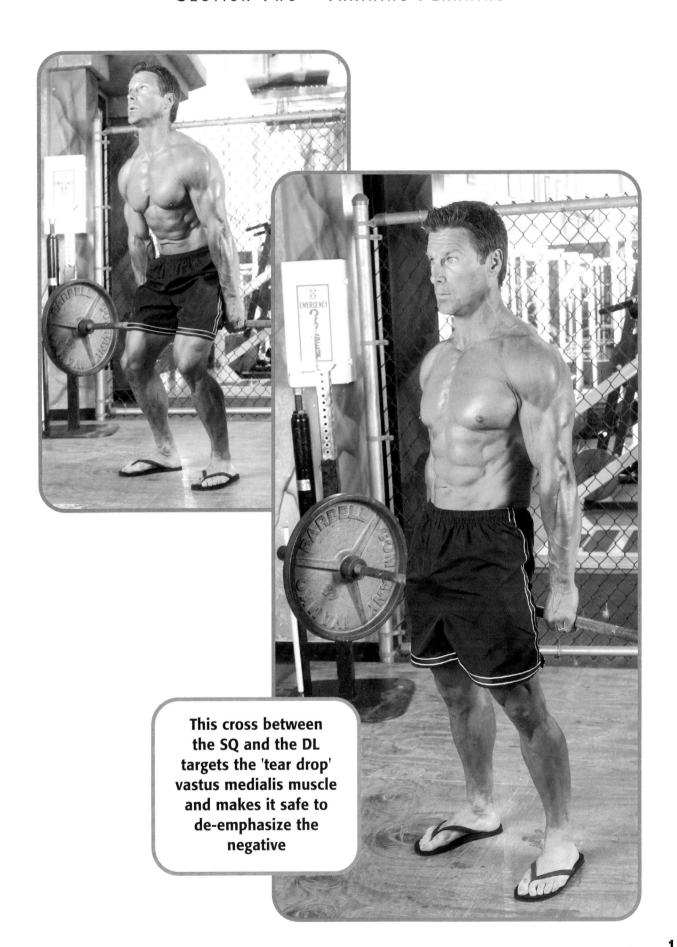

This cross between the SQ and the DL targets the 'tear drop' vastus medialis muscle and makes it safe to de-emphasize the negative

Section Three

Back

Contents

Articles

Questions and Answers

CALLING FOR BACK-UP!
(THE 'STRONG AS YOU LOOK' SERIES)

1. One-arm suitcase deadlift

2. Pullup

3. Hise shrug

4. Dimel deadlift

1. ONE-ARM SUITCASE DEADLIFT

When it comes to all around back development the deadlift rules! The dead has many powerful incarnations and the one-arm DL is way up on the list.

The authentic one arm deadlift is performed with a seven-foot Olympic barbell and is a tremendous feet of grip strength. The dumbbell version is more appropriate for a bodybuilder who wants to blast his back from top to bottom. To make you more miserable, while reducing the poundage required to get a great workout, I shall have you lift the bell on the outside of your hip as a suitcase rather than straddle style.

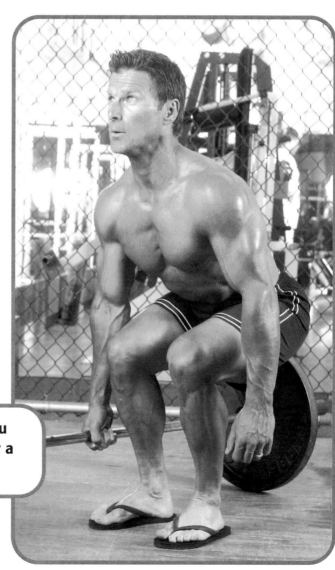

Semi-squat as if you are getting ready for a vertical jump.

Semi-squat as if you are getting ready for a vertical jump and grab a heavy dumbbell outside your foot. Lock your elbow by flexing your triceps. It is imperative for elbow safety and max power. Tense your lat hard so it forms a 'shelf' for your arm.

Inhale, take a breath into your belly, tighten your abs and your whole body, and squeeze the bell off the floor.

Do not let your unloaded side shoot up first! This is not a side bend. Rise evenly, as if you have another dumbbell of the same weight in your free hand. You will notice that you have to flex your glute and obliques on the unloaded side in order to maintain the balance. It will not take you long to painfully realize that the suitcase style dead-lift is more than just a back exercise; it is a full body feat!

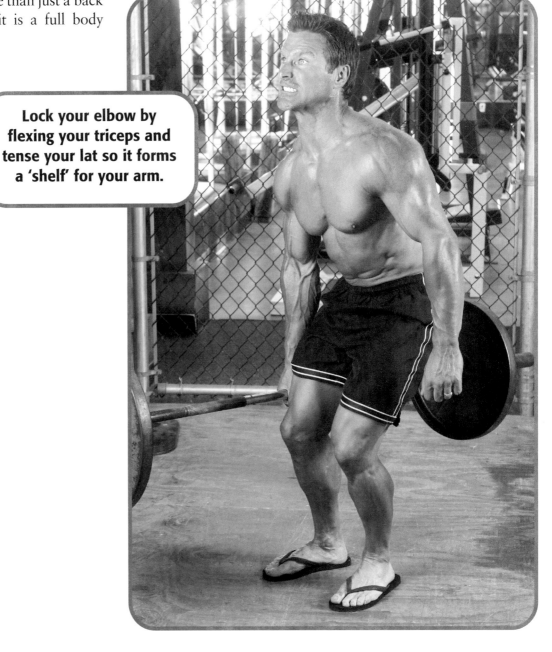

Lock your elbow by flexing your triceps and tense your lat so it forms a 'shelf' for your arm.

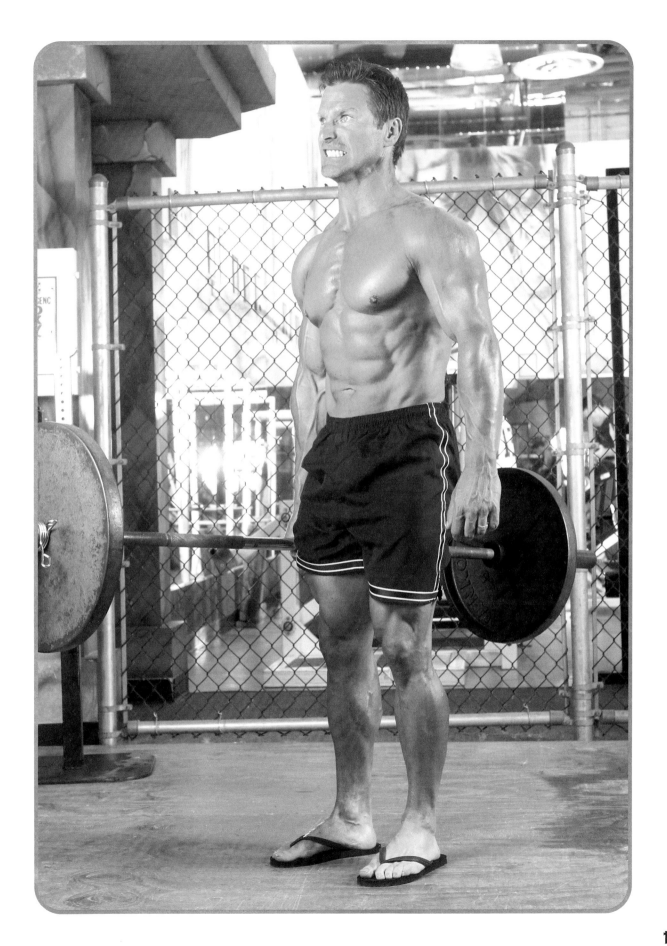

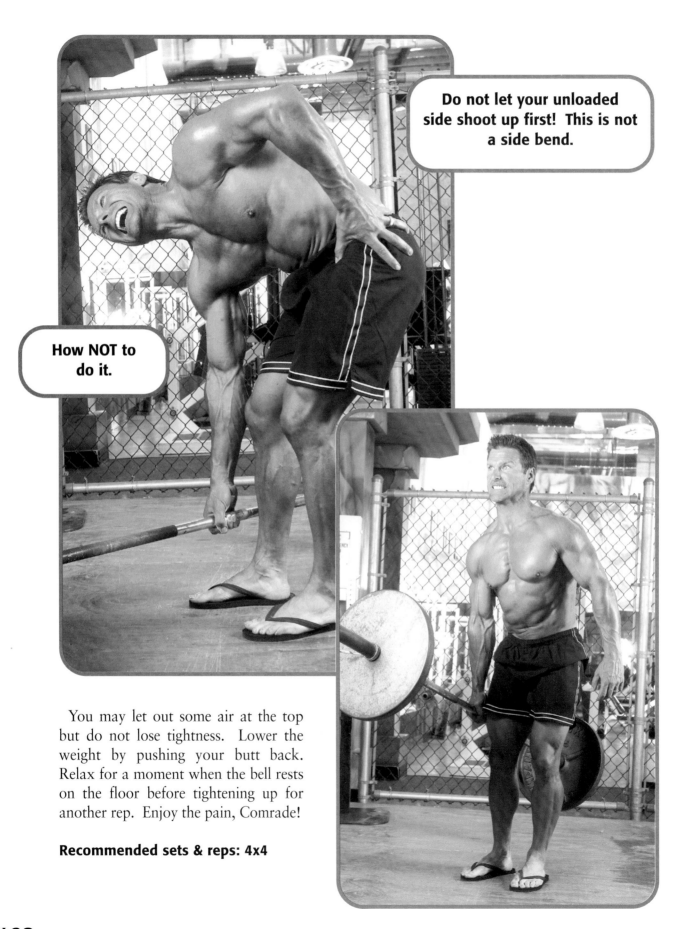

Do not let your unloaded side shoot up first! This is not a side bend.

How NOT to do it.

You may let out some air at the top but do not lose tightness. Lower the weight by pushing your butt back. Relax for a moment when the bell rests on the floor before tightening up for another rep. Enjoy the pain, Comrade!

Recommended sets & reps: 4x4

2. PULLUP

Knock off your silly seated rows and lat pull-downs. Focus all your energy into pullups and your armpits will be chafing in no time flat. Finally you can do 'the walk' without simulating lats.

With a thumbless over-hand grip, from a dead hang, till your neck or chest touches the bar. Anything less is a joke.

Recommended sets & reps: as many sets of 2/3 of your rep max (e.g., sets of 6 if your best is 10RM) as you can manage

With a thumbless overhand grip, from a dead hang till your neck or chest touches the bar. Anything less is a joke.

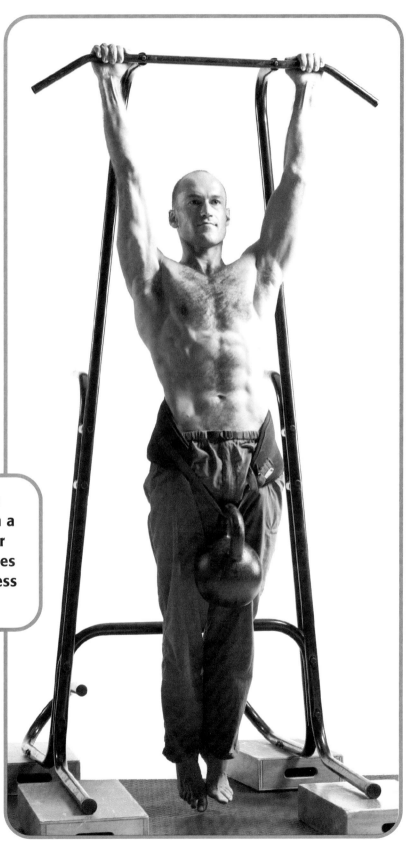

3. HISE SHRUG

This cool shrug, invented by Joseph C. Hise of twenty-rep squat fame, is popular with modern day powerlifters who want their squats to feel ridiculously light. It will do the same for you while adding slabs of beef to your traps and neck.

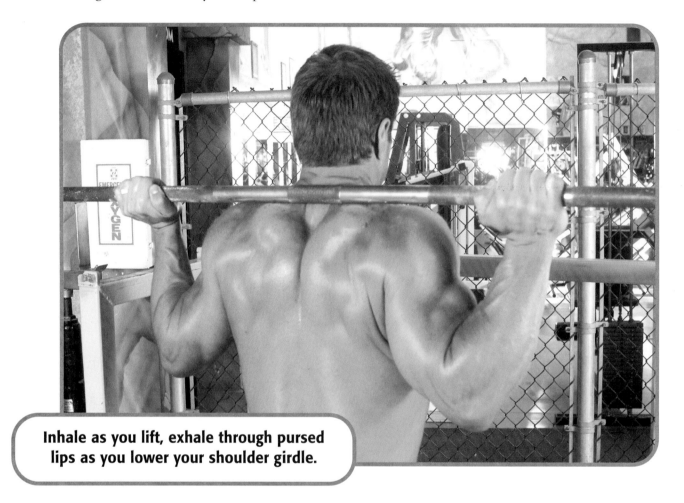

Inhale as you lift, exhale through pursed lips as you lower your shoulder girdle.

Unrack a barbell as you would for a squat, walk out, bend forward slightly to protect your back from hyperextension, and start shrugging. Inhale as you lift, exhale through pursed lips as you lower your shoulder girdle. Keep your waist tight and make sure not to let all the air out.

Do not carry the bar too high or too low on your back. Position your hands in a way that does not put undue stress on your wrists, elbows, or shoulders.

Joseph Hise shrugged with a cambered bar that made the exercise easier on his joints. You can get one from IronMind.com; it is called the Buffalo Bar™. If you do not have one you will be smart to dust off the bent old bar in the corner that no one at the gym wants to touch. And while I would never endorse squatting with a towel across your back you will definitely need some padding for the Hise shrug.

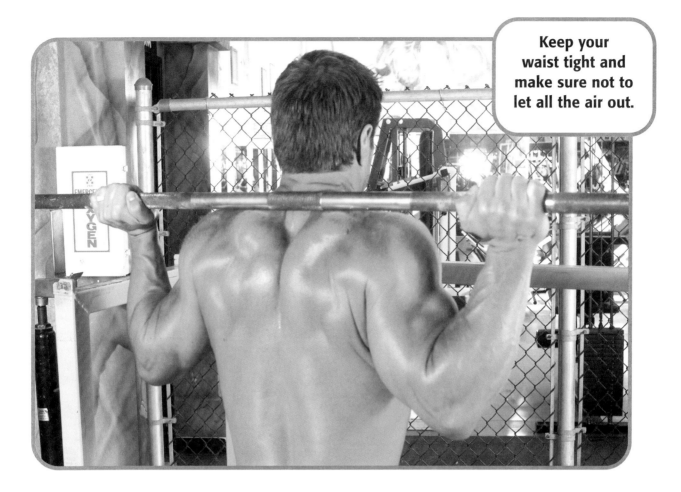

Keep your waist tight and make sure not to let all the air out.

Go get 'em, tiger! The traps to make an Olympic weightlifter take notice.

Recommended sets & reps: 2x20-25

4. DIMEL DEADLIFT

Powerlifting coach Louie Simmons credits this unique drill for him taking the late Matt Dimel's squat to 1,010 and Steve Wilson's deadlift to 865. A bodybuilder will find the Dimel deadlift an exceptional back and hamstring developer.

Deadlift a very light barbell – Wilson used 225-275 pounds, which was a paltry 30% of his max dead – with an overhand grip.   Push your butt back and let the bar drop to slightly below your knee. Your shins should remain vertical. Keep a tight arch in your lower back! Snap your hips through explosively and lock out. Knock off fifteen to twenty reps at a rapid clip.

Dimel deadlifts will be fine while you are at them, but I can assure you that your backside will be barking the morning after.

Recommended sets & reps: 2-3-15-20 two to four times a week

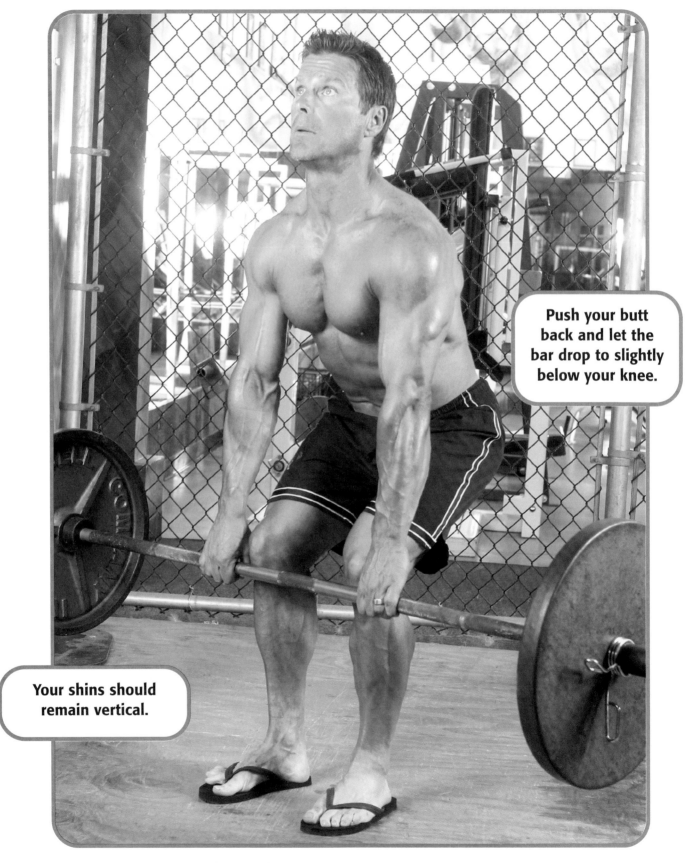

Push your butt back and let the bar drop to slightly below your knee.

Your shins should remain vertical.

Wrap up your back workout by stretching your back and hamstrings and hanging from a pullup bar to decompress your spine.

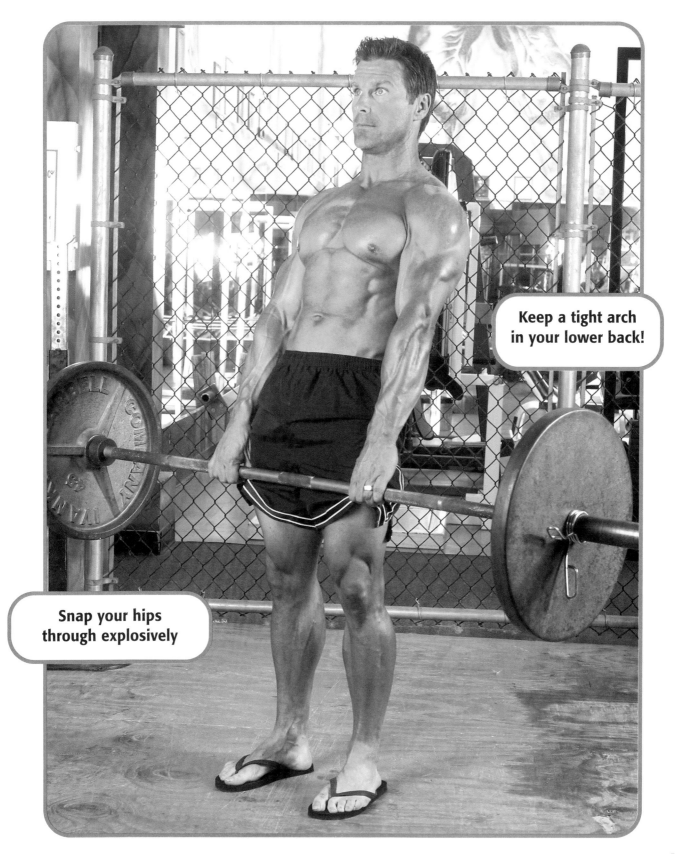

Keep a tight arch in your lower back!

Snap your hips through explosively

BACK TRAINING FAQ

Question: Aren't deadlifts dangerous?

Prominent Russian strength coach S. Y. Smolov, Master of Sports asks, "Which movement skills are vital to a person? Some people will tell you running and jumping, others skiing and biking, and someone else will say swimming. They are all right. Yet no one will list lifting a weight off the floor as one of the most vital skills. Nevertheless in our industrial age the majority of the population does not run, jump, ski, bike, or swim. Yet every one of us, from a school kid to a retired person, lifts and carries something all day long: briefcases, bags, various household items, tools, etc."

Alexey Vorotintsev, Master of Sports, a former USSR record holder in kettlebell lifting, is so determined to teach everyone how to lift things off the ground properly that he has been crusading for introducing deadlifts into the Russian high school Phys. Ed. Curriculum. Myself, I have dedicated a whole book, *Power to the People!*, to the deadlift. You are not going to avoid deads in your day-to-day life so you might as well learn how to do them right, and I do not mean the inadequate and unrealistic OSHA recommendations to stay upright and lift with your legs.

Comrade Smolov goes on, "Haven't you seen a person grab his back and writhe in pain having tried to lift something heavy? I am convinced that everyone has witnessed such a scene, and regretfully more than once. Now try to prove that the deadlift is not a vital skill!"

Case closed.

Question: Is it true that my lats will grow faster if I stretch them?

Yes. To keep in line with Russian muscle research and Arnold's Muscle Beach experience, stretch your lats between the sets. With your hands close together hold on to a sturdy object at your waist level. A power rack is great, but the doorknob of an open door will do, if you are certain that the door will not collapse under your muscular weight. Face the edge of an open door and hold on to the knobs on both sides of it. Your feet should straddle the door under your hands.

Stick your butt out and hang on the door or the squat cage while keeping your arms nearly straight, your head down, and your back rounded. Yes, rounded! Your knees should stay slightly bent throughout the drill.

Spread your shoulder blades if you can. By humping your back and imagining that you are pushing away from the doorknob you should make them kick out in a short time. If you have done it right, you should feel a pleasant stretch between your scapulae. Do not get bummed out if it takes a few workouts to get it right.

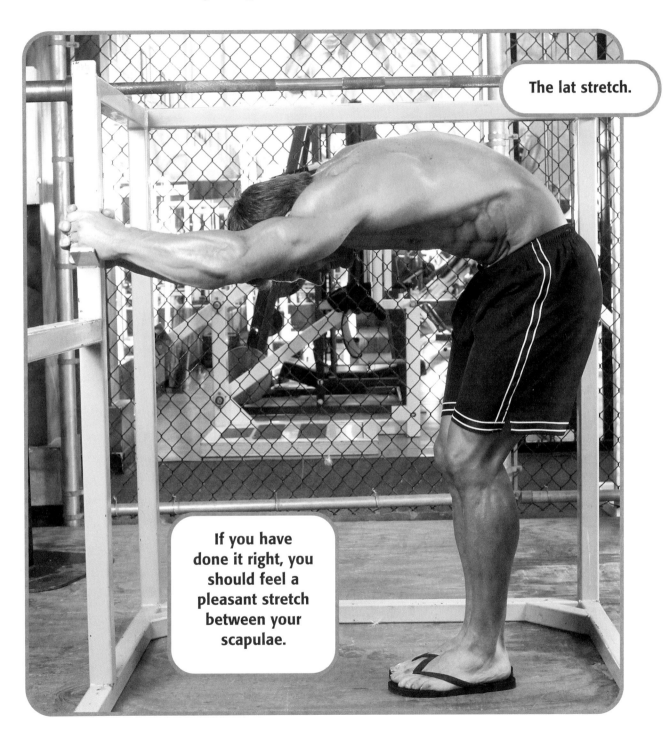

The lat stretch.

If you have done it right, you should feel a pleasant stretch between your scapulae.

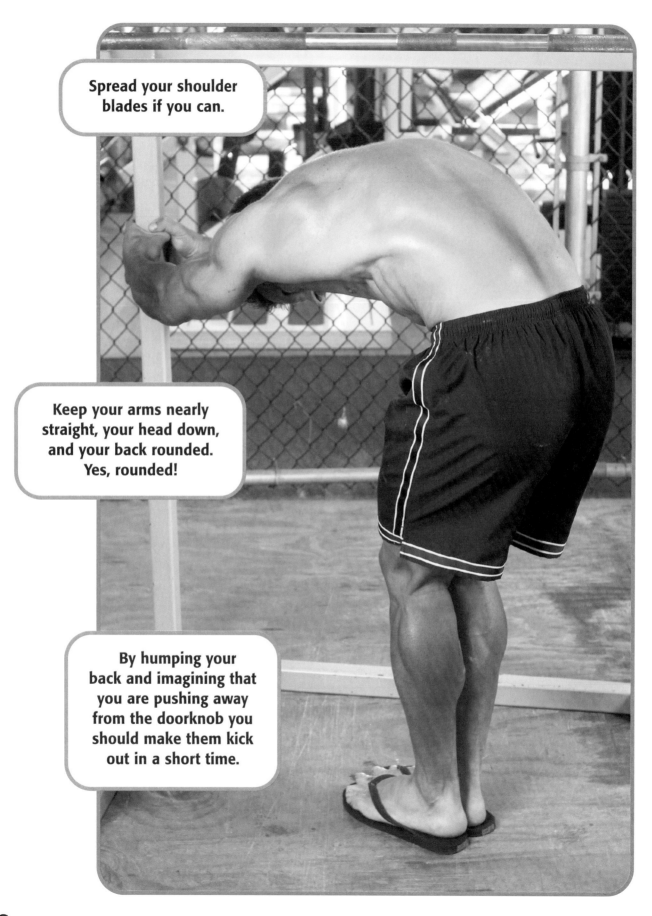

Question: Should I arch my back when working my lats?

Arching recruits the scapulae retractors or mid back muscles. You should do it most of the time to develop them and to ensure good posture.

But some round back lat work will do your wings good. Watch a professional arm-wrestler when he is backloading his opponent. His back looks exactly as yours does during the lat stretch I just described. If you look up an anatomy textbook you will learn that the lats assist in extending the spine. Round your back and you will pull on the latissimus' origins, thus stretching and loading them.

The safest exercise to incorporate round back lat training into is the one arm dumbbell or kettlebell row. Plant your other arm solidly on a bench to unload your spine.

Question: What should I do if I do not feel my lats working?

Quoting *The USMCRD Special Company Drill Instructor Guide to Pullups* , that I wrote at the Marines' request, "Controlled striking of the target muscles will teach a recruit or Marine to contract them more intensely. The strikes should not be painful, just noticeable. Do a pullup, assisted if necessary. After a brief rest do another one and concentrate on pulling with your stronger lats rather than the weaker biceps. Most likely you will have very limited success. After more rest, do another pullup and have your training partner chop your armpits from the moment you are about to start pulling until you are half way up. Note a greater involvement of the lats and greater ease of performing pullups."

Lats: the Secrets of the Russian Bodybuilding Underground

Bodybuilding was not encouraged by the Soviet government that considered it a vain and decadent 'bourgeois perversion'. Teenage street toughs who sought more muscle for their daily fights set up their own gyms or *kachalki* in apartment building basements. They were unheated and lacked the most basic equipment. Pullups from plumbing pipes and squats with a bunch of kettlebells hanging precariously on a rusty bar were normal. Mirrors were unheard of.

Lacking the means but not the drive, these comrades developed very impressive physiques and the strength to match. Frequently supervised by retired weightlifters who did not want to hang up their lifting belts for good, the kids followed the 'low tech/high concept' methods Russians are famous for.

No one heard of pulldown machines and other gimmicks in the golden decade of Russian bodybuilding, the 1980s, and that was for the better. Pullups were worked with a vengeance and the lats had no choice but grow. Muscles that were good for nothing but show did not impress street fighters. And every underground muscle head, including those who topped the scale at over 220 pounds could easily knock off at least twenty, dead hang, palms forward.

Lighter bodybuilders did – and still do – even better. In one of the former Soviet republics, Belskiy (2000) made a comparative study of the physical development and strength of experienced middleweight and light heavyweight athletes from different strength sports. Iron Curtain bodybuilders showed an average pullup performance of 23.8 repetitions. Just in case you start arguing that your muscular pecs are weighing you down, Russian powerlifters specializing in the bench press got an even higher score of 26.6 consecutive pullups! Even three event powerlifters, chafing thighs and all, were good for 22.5 pullups!

In other words, you have no excuse for barely being able to squirm a dozen jerky half reps with your strongest grip. Here is your guide to pullup excellence and elite lat development, three 'low tech/high concept' programs born in the basements of Russia in the last years of the evil empire.

Lyubertsi, a small town in greater Moscow, is Russia's "Muscle Beach" The boys in the basement gyms of Lyubertsi held a firm belief that a bodybuilder wannabe had to be able to do at least twelve to fifteen overhand pullups and forty to fifty pushups – or fifteen to twenty parallel bar dips – before he was ready to start training with weights. The following complex of exercises is similar to the programs employed in the *perestroyka* era basements to quickly bring a beginner up to that base level.

RUSSIAN BODYBUILDING UNDERGROUND BASE LEVEL PULLUP PROGRAM

Routine A

1. Parallel bar dips – 2-3xRM
2. Wide grip pullups – 2-3xRM
3. Wide grip pushups with the feet elevated – 2-3RM
4. Pushups with the feet elevated – 2-3xRM
5. Pushups – 2-3xRM
6. Hanging knee raises to the chin – 4xRM

Routine B

1. Wide grip pullups – 2-3xRM
2. Medium grip pullups – 2-3xRM
3. Narrow grip chinups – 2-3xRM
4. Parallel grip pullups – 2-3xRM
5. Parallel bar dips – 2-3xRM
6. Hanging knee raises to the chin – 4xRM

Perform two to three sets per exercise. Do as many perfect reps as you can. For the record, 'RM' or 'repetition maximum' means doing as many reps as possible in good form, not squirming till you fail!

David Whitley, Senior RKC, one strong man who casually plays with 106-pound "Beast" kettlebells and lifts his colleague, Master RKC Andrea Du Cane, overhead with one arm, clearly explained the difference between training to failure and training to the limit or RM on the dragondoor.com forum: you have got to push "until you complete the last rep, not conk out in the middle of it."

Have your training partner assist you if necessary. Recognize that 'assisted' reps and 'forced' reps are not the same thing. The partner should be acting as a pullup or dip assist machine and enable you to do your drills with confidence. No drawn out, shaky forced reps please! Shoot for five clean reps per set if you must resort to outside help.

Do not do any more reps than you can manage with crisp perfection. Commit to stop before your form deteriorates. And, very importantly, do not become a slave to numbers. The "I did ten reps last time therefore I will not settle for anything less than eleven today" mindset is a road to injury, no gains, and frustration. You cannot gain every workout; at least not once you achieve a decent strength level, the point of diminishing returns. And if you try you will be subconsciously cheating to make the reps. Before you know it your technique will be atrocious, with all the undesirable but logical consequences.

A conservative number of "Swiss watch precision" reps builds strength that carries over to all-out efforts with a very heavy weight. Bouncing and cheating for max reps does not. What you can get away with when you are handling a light poundage will not fly once the hard and cold reality of heavy iron sets in.

Take one of the greatest back exercises – correction, one of the greatest exercises, period – the deadlift. You could maximize the number of reps with a light barbell by jerking the bell from the floor – and then bouncing it off the platform between repetitions and not locking out the lift on the top. But if after a period of such 'training', you tried to apply yourself to a heavier, low rep pull you would either hurt your back when jerking the bar off the ground or simply fail the lift.

Powerlifters know that a heavy dead must be 'squeezed' off the platform and always do so even with light poundages. It sacrifices their rep count but they do not care; they know that they are getting stronger and that is all that matters. Come to think of it, a near zero potential for injury is nothing to sneeze at either.

Ditto with pullups Put on a flak jacket or hang even a small barbell plate on your waist and practice those cheater half reps. You will be stopped in your tracks, dangling on the bar like a helpless sausage.

Besides, you will not build any muscle by swinging and jerking on the bar like an ape. So record your reps, but do not try to top them at any cost. Form and substance over numbers.

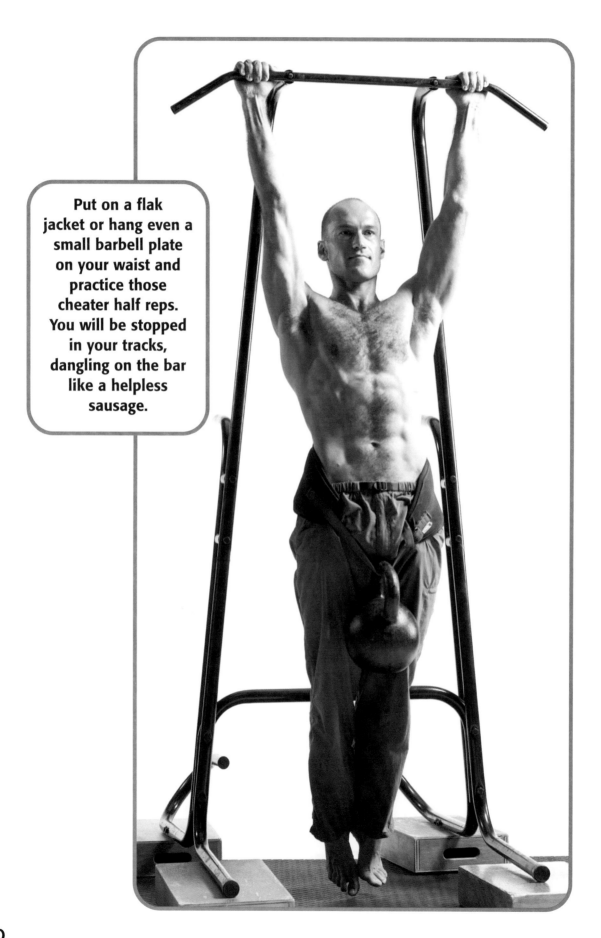

Put on a flak jacket or hang even a small barbell plate on your waist and practice those cheater half reps. You will be stopped in your tracks, dangling on the bar like a helpless sausage.

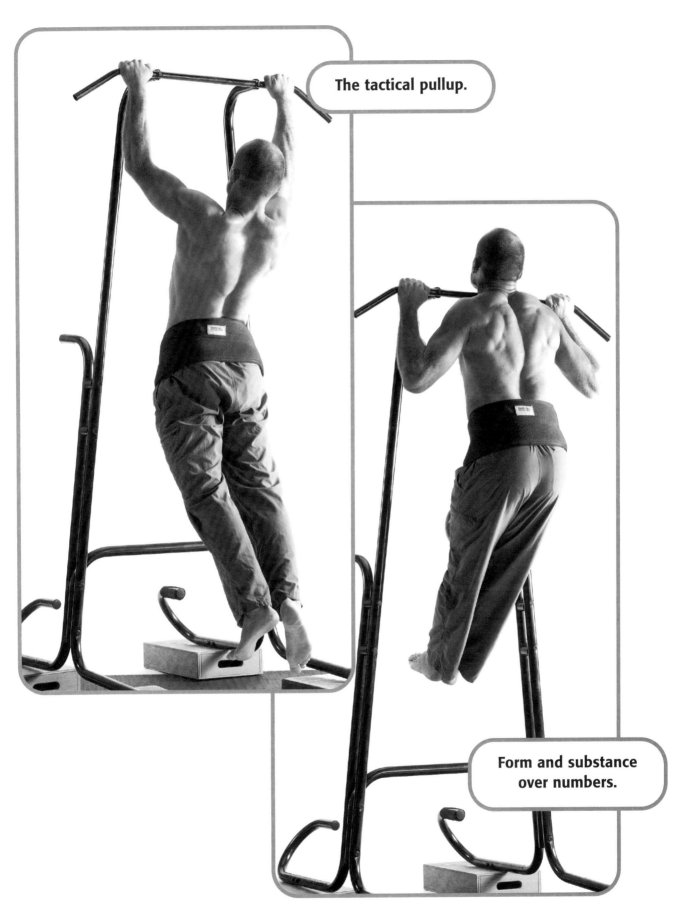

The tactical pullup.

Form and substance over numbers.

Wrap up with four sets of hanging knee raises to the chin. Get a full stretch of the abs and the hip flexors on the bottom and a full contraction on the top. The above routines were alternated daily until the trainee felt fatigued. Then he took a day off and carried on with the rotation. Sometimes he trained five days in a row and others only two.

Note that although you will be working the same muscles almost daily you will be alternating high volume and low volume days; this is a basic Russian approach to cycling or 'waviness' of loads. Needless to say, do no other upper body work for the duration of this routine, which is typically six weeks. Classic twenty rep squats three times a week will take care of your legs. Plug them in before the knee raises.

Proper pullup technique is of the essence. First you need to learn how to pull from your elbows rather than your hands, to really recruit the lats. Bend your elbows and raise them over your head as if you are about to perform a French press. Have your training partner press his or her hands against your elbows and provide resistance as your are bringing your elbows down in a semi-circle until they are tucked into your sides.

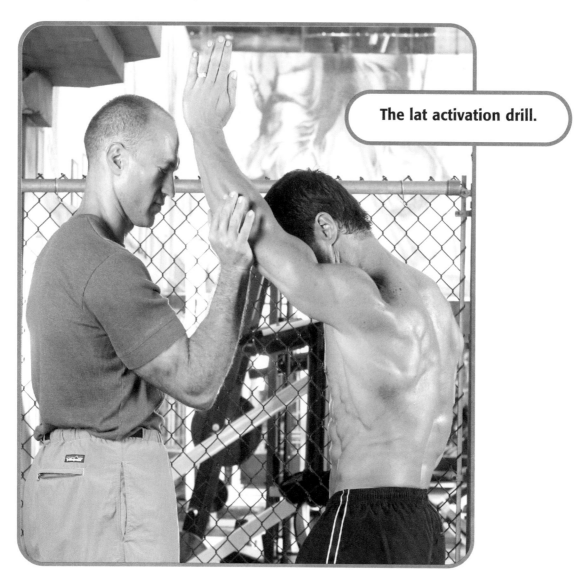

The lat activation drill.

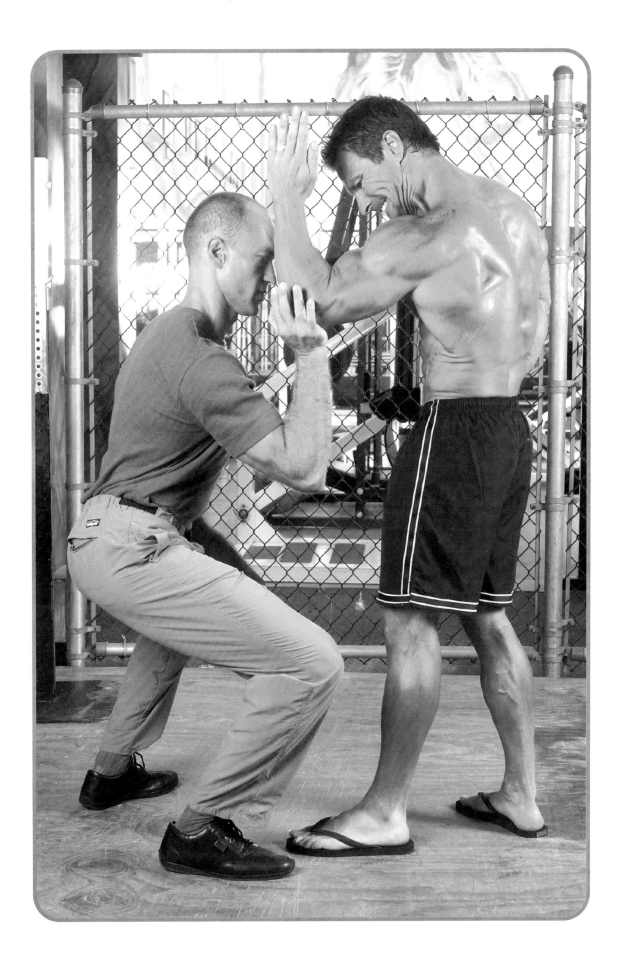

Now the same thing up on the bar. Get a shoulder width grip with your palms facing forward. Do not wrap your thumbs around, this will weaken the biceps and help you focus the effort on your latissimus. So will keeping most of your weight on your little and ring fingers rather than closer to your thumbs.

Onward and upward! You have not completed a pullup unless your chin has cleared the bar. Some units in the armed forces and law enforcement in the former Soviet republic Belarus even require that their personnel touch the bar with their necks. That way there is no doubt that you have completed a rep.

Going all the way down is also a must if you are going to claim a legit pullup. To protect your joints, squeeze the bar as you are about to hit the full stretch.

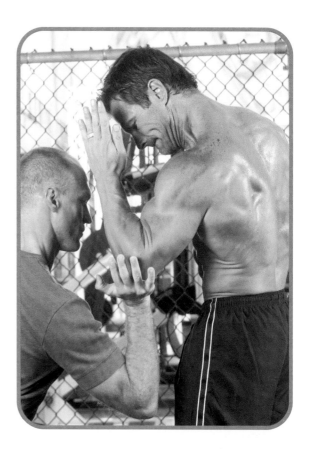

RUSSIAN BODYBUILDING UNDERGROUND ADVANCED LAT AND PULLUP SPECIALIZATION ROUTINE #2

Monday (heavy load/20 sets)

1. Wide grip pullups – 5xRM
2. Medium grip pullups – 5xRM
3. Bent over rows – 6x6
4. One arm kettlebell or dumbbell row – 4x12

Wednesday (light load/10 sets)

1. Wide grip pullups – 5xRM
2. Pullups on a V-handle – 5xRM

Friday (medium load/15 sets)

1. Medium grip pullups –1x15, with weight 5x10
2. Medium grip chinups – 5xRM
3. Narrow grip T-bar rows – 4x10

The second underground program from Lyubertsi is aimed at a more experienced bodybuilder. That means you should be good for at least twelve to fifteen clean wide grip pullups. Again, it's slightly modified, because the original included pullups to the back of the head – which can do a number on your shoulders and neck,

Soviet bodybuilders of the eighties were convinced that the lats were virtually impossible to overtrain and best responded to what they called 'the head on strike' – a brutal onslaught of pullups outlined above. The lat load was cycled according to the heavy-light-medium format. To avoid systemic overtraining other muscle groups were worked only once a week, which was quite unusual for the 1980s. Deadlifts were included.

When doing pullups use your bodyweight only unless otherwise specified. The V-handle can be found at a seated row machine. Take it off, hang it over a pullup bar, and do your V-handle pullups to the sternum. You will find that tilting your head back – and looking back as if you are trying to do a bridge – will help. Force your chest to the handles as if you are doing a bench press.

If you have no access to a V-handle, grab a standard pullup bar with a staggered grip and your hands close to each other. First pull up with your head on one side of the bar, then the other. Switch the hand position on your next set.

A word on the bent over row technique that prevailed in Russian underground gyms. Deadlift your barbell with an overhand shoulder width grip. Fold over until your torso is almost parallel to the ground, your lower back arched, your knees bent. Rest your forehead on a bench of an appropriate height to assure that you will not be cheating. Let your shoulders drop and move away from your body and the bell swing forward naturally before pulling. Taller bodybuilders with long arms may have to stand on an elevation or use small plates. Pull in a long arc and finish with the bell touching your lower stomach. Draw your shoulder blades together and flex your lats tight.

A tip for the T-bar row. Inhale and expand your rib cage as you are lifting; exhale through pursed lips on the way down. But never lose sight of the meat of these programs – pullups and lots of them.

Talk to anyone who has great lats. There is a pattern you cannot miss – all these comrades do a lot of pullups and would never contemplate using the lat pull-down machine for anything other than a place to park a towel or a water bottle. Now talk to the bodybuilders whose lats are non-existent. Without doubt you will hear excited speeches about how much burn they feel in their pits on the lat pulldown machine. Sherlock Holmes would call it a clue. Even Inspector Clouseau would. A lot of pullups is the only road to lats and everything else is just icing on the cake. Period.

QUESTIONS & ANSWERS:

IS THE DEADLIFT THE KING OF BACK EXERCISES?

Question: Is the deadlift really the cat's meow of back exercises, like you are saying?

Mike Mentzer used to think so. Charles Poliquin has named the deadlift the most underrated bodybuilding exercise. Mr. Olympia Ronnie Coleman pulls over 800 pounds. You can put the two and two together.

The sheer intensity of the dead smokes your whole back, from top to bottom. The lats keep the bar from getting away and – through a complex anatomical rig with the unpronounceable name of 'lumbodorsal fascia' – aid your electors in keeping your spine straight. The muscles between your shoulder blades keep your upper back in its proper alignment. The neck does not get to relax either. Few powerlifters do any direct neck work and even fewer can fit their bull necks into store bought shirts. The traps and the lower back… well, that is obvious.

To get the most out of the deadlift in the meat-building department start with 5x5 three times every two weeks. For instance, Monday, Friday, and Wednesday of the next week. Start light, for instance with a weight you could probably pull at least ten times, and add a couple of pounds every workout.

Pull conventional, that is with your feet about shoulder width apart or slightly narrower. Sumos are great for building glutes and hip power but are inferior to classic deads when it comes to back development.

DON'T FEEL YOUR LATS? – WE'LL FIX IT!

Question: I don't feel my lats when I do pullups, just my biceps. What should I do?

First, use the palm forward grip with your thumb not wrapped around the bar but tucked in next to the fingers.

Second, keep more weight and tension on your little and index fingers than on the middle and index fingers.

Third, start each pullup by 'tightening up your armpits'. Ask your training partner to give you a couple of light karate chops to your lats so you understand what 'tightening up' means.

Finally, instead of curling, visualize driving your elbows down. Near the top "pull your elbows to the ribs", as recommended by Charles Staley in his excellent book *The Science of Martial Arts Training*, rather than mindlessly muscle your way up.

The mind to lats connection is not an easy one to develop. Plan on spending months and even years finessing it. In the interim do not settle for a mullet lat routine of pull-downs and cable rows. When your armpits start chafing you will know it was worth it.

SPREAD YOUR WINGS AND MAX OUT ON THE PULLUP TEST WITH 'TACTICAL PULLUPS'

Question: I am a Marine and I want to max the PFT pullup test but I have a hard time clearing the bar with my chin towards the end of the set. Please help.

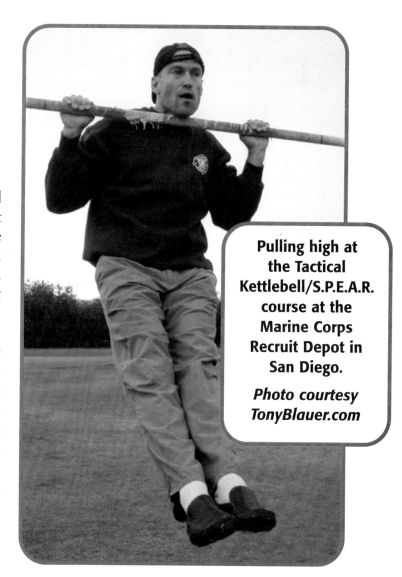

Pulling high at the Tactical Kettlebell/S.P.E.A.R. course at the Marine Corps Recruit Depot in San Diego.

Photo courtesy TonyBlauer.com

If you are familiar with the Tactical Strength Challenge, you know that it demands that the competitors touch the bar with their necks or chests to make a rep count. This technique comes from the spec ops units of the former Soviet Union.

Although the USMC test does not require you to do that, tactical pullups will dramatically improve your ability to do regulation pullups. Powerlifters help their competition pull by practicing deadlifts off a platform or by using twenty-five pound plates. The tactical pullup works the same way. When you are used to an exaggeratedly long movement, the 'regular' one feels short and easy.

You will have to cut your reps in the beginning; do not do any more pullups if you cannot touch the bar with your neck or upper chest. Increase your sets accordingly to keep the volume. For instance, if you used to do 5 sets of 10, do 10 sets of 5.

A couple of months later 'just' clearing the bar with your chin will feel like a piece of cake. Smoke your test, Marine!

ARE BENT OVER ROWS OVERRATED?

Question: I heard that you don't like bent over rows. How come?

In my opinion they over fatigue the lower back. BORs do not work it nearly heavy enough to get it strong but surely long enough to tire it out, and thus hamper the recovery of this slowest recovering part of your body. If you deadlift and/or squat heavy, this cannot be good news. Besides, I am yet to see good form on this exercise.

I suggest you focus your back training on pullups and deadlifts and throw in a few rows that do not get your lumbars' attention, as the icing on the cake. You have three basic options. One is the one-arm row with your free hand resting on your thigh or on a bench. The other is the chest-supported row off a bench that is popular with powerlifters. The third is Coach John Davies' 'renegade row'. Assume the pushup position on two kettlebells. Shift your weight to one bell and row the other. Any way you row, let the weight slip forward near the bottom of the movement, then bring it in back towards your waist in an arc.

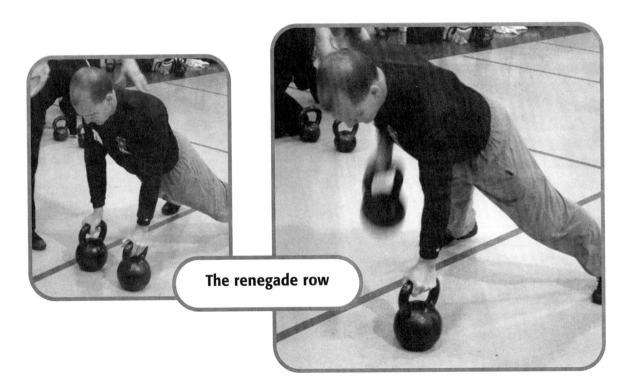

The renegade row

'INJURY PREVENTION BY IMPERFECTION TRAINING'

Question: Is it true that, for injury prevention, Russian coaches have their athletes do simultaneous bends and twists and other moves that I know are dangerous to the back. How is that supposed to work?

The late Dr. Mel Siff pointed out that the traditional injury prevention strategy of avoiding 'dangerous' exercises and excessive loads is inadequate. The scientist advocated 'injury prevention by imperfection training'. The following exercise for the lower back falls into that category. Deadlift a light kettlebell with both hands. Then slowly lower it to one of your heels. Straighten out and twist to the other side. Perform 2-3 sets of 15-20 reps. Never to failure, stresses Oleg Fetisov, a former Soviet ice hockey star – remember the movie *Miracle on Ice*? – and Russia's Minister of Sports, who endorses this exercise. And not on your first workout; build up slowly! The Russian authority promises that this drill "cannot be beat for building a powerful corset of ligaments and muscles. It will help a lot when you lift any weights, participate in contact sports, or perform complex gymnastic exercises." This drill is demonstrated in my DVD *Resilient*.

Taking carefully measured doses of 'poisonous' exercises to build up one's tolerance is not an exclusively Russian practice. Tommy Kono, former Mr. Universe and weightlifting Olympic and world champion, recommends 'the loosening deadlift' in his outstanding book, *Weightlifting, Olympic Style* (get your copy from CBass.com).

It is a fact that most trainees do not train their backs at all and those who do always lift with a tightly arched spine. Kono points out that such alignment, while necessary for safe and powerful lifts, leads to "overcontracting of the lumbars." "Imagine the muscles of your back as quality metal," says the iron legend. "If it is like cast iron then it is stiff and unbending and rather than bend under stress it would break. On the other hand, if the muscle is like a steel spring, well tempered, there is dynamic life and "lift" to it, and it has the quality to take punishment and still be flexible."

Start 'the loosening deadlift' with a very light bar in the deadlift lockout position. How light is light? – If you clean over 300 pounds, 110 will do, clarifies Kono. First lower your chin to your chest, and then roll your spine down one vertebra at a time. Keep your legs straight. Go slow and smooth. Breathe out as you lower the bell, something you would never do with the classic deadlift.

Reverse the movement once you have comfortably bottomed out. Straighten out your lower back, your mid back, and finally your upper back. Kono recommends 1-3 sets of 8-12 reps in the end of your workout. Before adding more weight it is better to increase the range of motion by standing on a block.

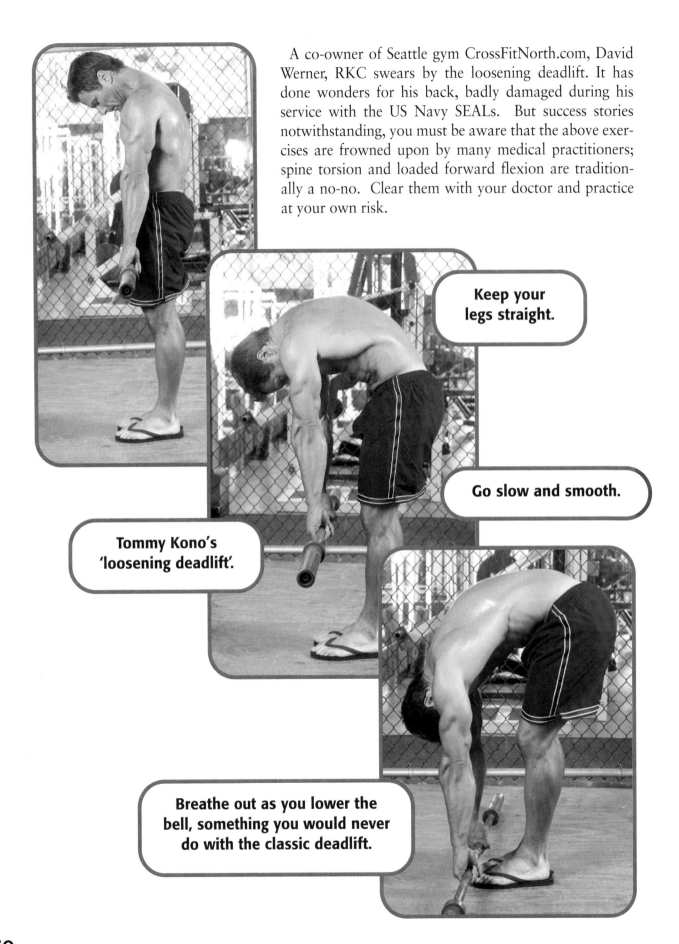

A co-owner of Seattle gym CrossFitNorth.com, David Werner, RKC swears by the loosening deadlift. It has done wonders for his back, badly damaged during his service with the US Navy SEALs. But success stories notwithstanding, you must be aware that the above exercises are frowned upon by many medical practitioners; spine torsion and loaded forward flexion are traditionally a no-no. Clear them with your doctor and practice at your own risk.

Keep your legs straight.

Go slow and smooth.

Tommy Kono's 'loosening deadlift'.

Breathe out as you lower the bell, something you would never do with the classic deadlift.

SOLUTIONS FOR A TIGHT BACK

Question: My back gets really tight after my bodybuilding workouts. Do you have any good stretches to loosen it up?

Provided it is not a medical condition, the following complex will do the job and then some. Three out of the five exercises are recommended by Valentin Dikul, a man as famous as Arnold Schwarzenegger in the countries of the former Soviet Union. A circus acrobat, Valentin took a bad fall and broke his back when he was seventeen. Dikul said no to the wheelchair and painstakingly rehabilitated himself. But he did not stop there. He proceeded to become a great circus strongman juggling 80kg balls and later – in his sixties! – a record shattering powerlifter. More importantly, Valentin has helped many people to reclaim their healthy backs.

1. Hang on to a pullup bar, palms over, and rotate your torso as far as possible clockwise and counterclockwise. 3 sets x 8 reps. I prefer doing this drill on parallel bars rather than a pullup bar.

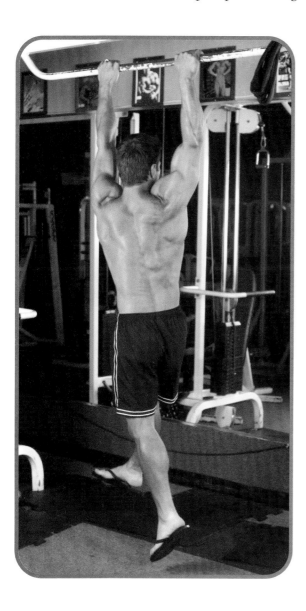
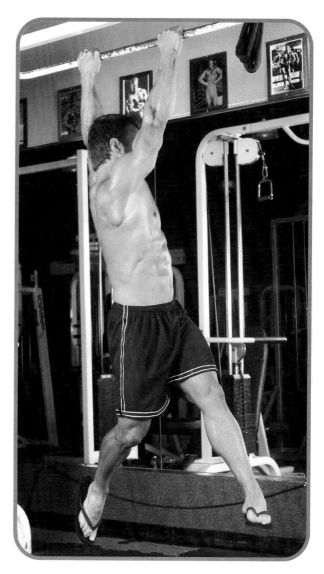

2. Hang on to a pullup bar, palms over, and raise your legs, the feet together, side-to-side. No swinging! – 3x8. Incidentally, Frank Zane used to do this exercise to cut up his midsection.

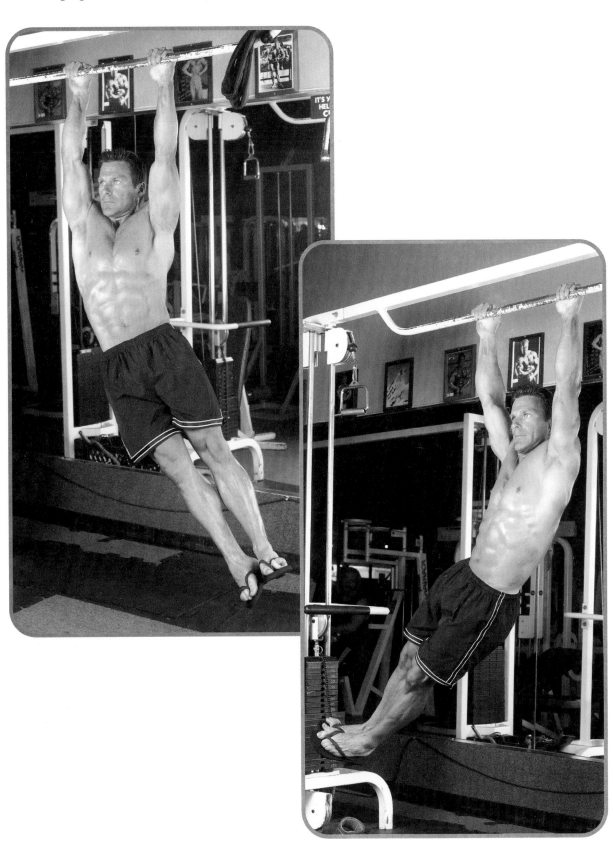

3. Hang on to a pullup bar, palms over, tilt your head back and maximally arch your back. – 3x8. Superset this exercise with the next one.

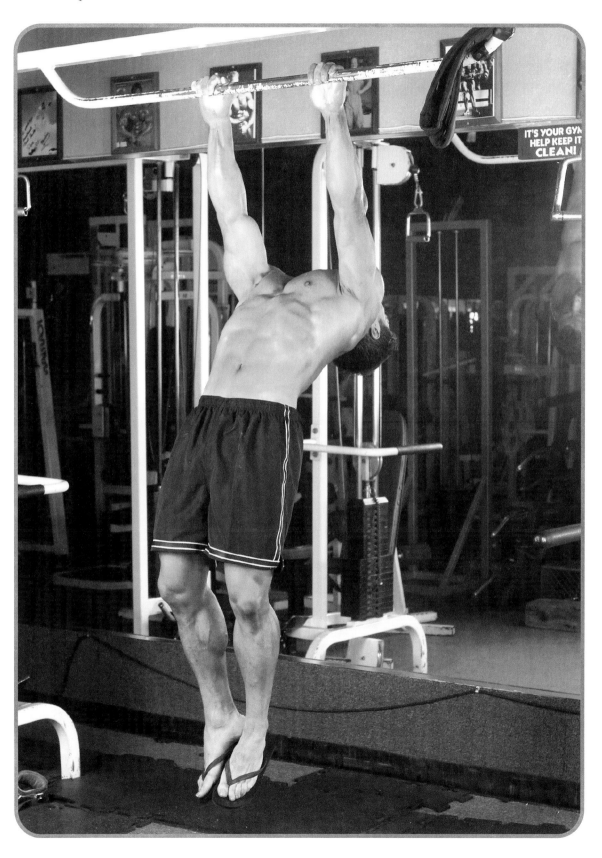

4. Hanging leg or knee raises. – 3x8. Russian powerlifting coaches believe that hanging leg raises following heavy lifting are not only beneficial to the spine but help normalizing the intra-abdominal pressure.

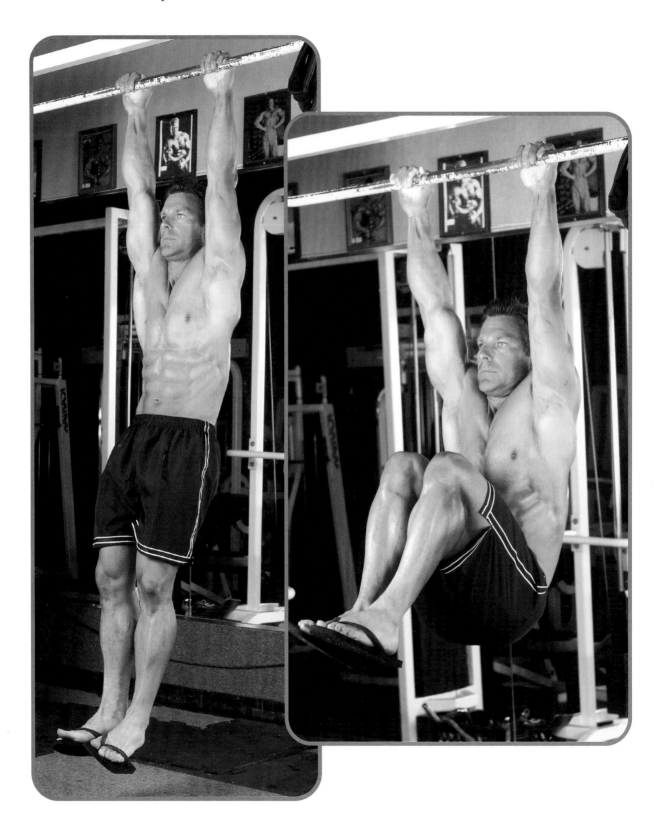

5. Hang on to a pullup bar, palms over, and move your straight legs like scissors back and forth. 3x8. This drill is recommended by Russian coach Mark Tartakovsky.

When you are done your back will feel alive. Guaranteed.

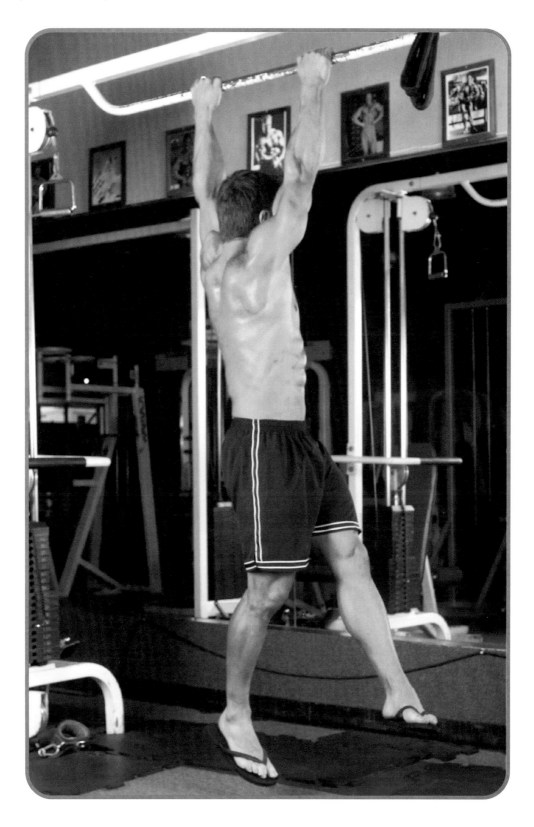

THE MCKENZIE METHOD FOR A HEALTHIER BACK

Question: What can I do to reduce the odds of a back injury when I am working out?

NOT lifting light. NOT avoiding squats and deadlifts. The first three things that come to mind are good technique, proper abdominal pressurization, and common sense, i.e. not lifting more than you can handle. To go the extra mile, follow the advice of the world-renowned physical therapist from New Zealand Robin McKenzie.

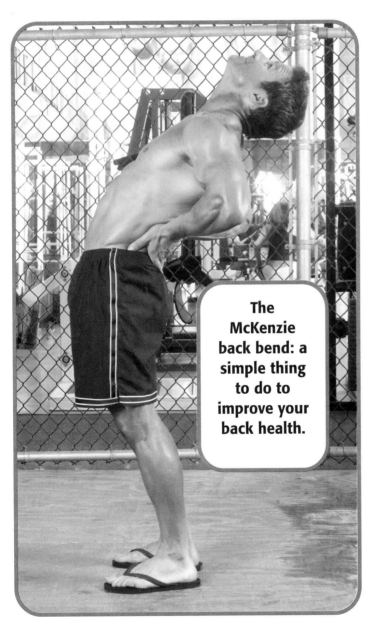

The McKenzie back bend: a simple thing to do to improve your back health.

McKenzie explains that most back pain is triggered by overstretching of the ligaments and the surrounding tissues. Which is in turn often caused by bad posture, especially the loss of lordosis, or the arch in your lower back. Stooping over, especially for long periods of time or with a weight, is bad news. McKenzie recommends performing five back bends immediately before and after lifting objects (think the deadlift, the bent row, the squat, etc.). "By standing upright and bending back before lifting, you ensure that, as you begin the lift, there is no distortion already present in the joints of the lower back."

Place your hands in the small of your back pointing your fingers downward and keep your legs straight. Bend back slowly using your hands as the fulcrum, pause for a second, and return to the upright position. Try to bend further with each successive rep.

Interestingly, back problems associated with bending over are most prevalent in the first four to five hours of the morning because, explains McKenzie, the discs soak up fluid during the night. So if you have a glass back you had better save your heavy lifting for later in the day.

McKenzie warns against slouching immediately after exercise of any sort, not just bodybuilding. Unexpectedly, this seemingly harmless act causes back problems in strong and healthy athletes. "After activity, the joints of the spine undergo a loosening process. If, after exercise, we place the back in an unsupported position for long periods, distortion within the joint readily occurs. This is true whether we sit in a slouched position or whether we stand, bending forward with our hands on our knees." The author of highly recommended *7 Steps to a Pain-free Life: How to Rapidly Relieve Back and Neck Pain* makes a point that just because your back started hurting immediately following a given activity, you should not automatically blame it. Things are not always as they appear to be; most likely it was your slouch. So avoid slouching after any vigorous activity and wrap up with the same five back bends.

How do the abs protect the back? or 'We build our own belt'

Question: I hear all the time how I am supposed to work my abs to protect my back but for the life of me I do not understand how this is supposed to work?

When scientists generated a computer model of the human spine they were shocked to find out the spine together with the back muscles and connective tissues could not possibly tolerate heavy loads without snapping in half. It turned out that it is the intra-abdominal pressure (IAP) that keeps you alive. Cresswell, Oddsson & Thorstensson (1994) suggested that "the increase in IAP is a mechanism designed to improve the stability of the trunk through a stiffening of the whole segment."

Imagine swallowing an empty balloon, then putting on a snug lifting belt and filling the balloon with air. Before you know it your waist becomes rigid, any attempt to flex the spine will be met with resistance from the compressed air.

So the belt is good, right? – Wrong. Powerlifting great Ed Coan reminisces, "There was a powerlifter by the name of Uri Spinoff from the Ukraine [former super heavyweight world champion]... I saw him squat 947 without a belt and he stood straight up. He didn't even bend forward. He did a squatting type of good morning with over 800 pounds. I asked him about wearing a belt and he just laughed, tapped his belly, and said, "We build our own belt."

The function of your abs is to do the belt's job of containing and maximizing the IAP. Of all the midsection muscles the transversus abdominis, a broad belt underneath the showy muscles, appears to be most responsible for changes in intra-abdominal pressure (Cresswell, Grundström & Thorstensson, 1992). The best way to build up your TA is Power Breathing.

But do not think that the undercover T.A. are the only ones fighting for your back. Your recti abdominis assist in upping the IAP when the load gets high. Work them with Janda situps. Cresswell, Blake & Thorstensson (1994) of famed Karolinska Institute in Stockholm, Sweden discovered that strengthening your trunk rotators also improves your ability to pressurize your belly "during functional situations." Drills such as Full Contact Twists cannot be beat for oblique development.

Power Breathing, Janda situps, and Full Contact Twists are all covered in my book *Bullet-Proof Abs*. If you want your midsection work to protect your back you will not bother with the 'burn' but train heavy, e.g. 5x5. Quit your job at the Home Depot and get some abs, man.

IS THE TRAP BAR BETTER THAN THE STRAIGHT BAR FOR DEADLIFTS AND SHRUGS?

Question: My gym got a trap bar. Should I replace the straight bar with it for my shrugs and deadlifts?

The trap or Gerard bar projects the weight right over your feet rather than in front of you. It is ergonomically better designed for shrugs than a straight bar. The movement is 'cleaner'. Besides, the fact that your hands face each other enables you to go heavier before resorting to straps.

The problem you are likely to face is getting the bar into position. You can load up a straight bar in a power rack; a Gerard bar needs to be deadlifted first. After a few months you are certain to shrug more than you can pull off the floor.

The trap bar deadlift is more of a squat than a dead. Therefore it will work your legs more and your back less, than a straight bar DL, so treat it as a leg exercise. Consider using twenty-five pound plates rather than forty-fives to further increase the leg stress.

If you are trying to build up your classic deadlift the trap bar will help to strengthen your start while doing nothing for the lockout. So do your Gerard pulls in addition to, rather than instead of, conventional deads.

Whether you deadlift or shrug, do not ever lean back! While dangerous with a straight barbell, it can be a disaster for your lower back with the diamond shaped bar. Flex your abs and glutes a la Janda situp when you are locking out, this will help.

The bottom line on the trap bar: a valuable piece of equipment but not a substitute for the classic barbell.

SECTION FOUR

LEGS

CONTENTS

Articles

- *Legs of Steel (the 'Strong as You Look' series)*
- *Hot Wheels by Summer!*

Questions and Answers

- *Can you build good legs with plyometrics?*
- *Training calves at home*
- *Russian farmer walk for stubborn calves*
- *Powerful legs without squats?*
- *How deep is your squat?*
- *High rep front squats?*
- *A shortcut to perfect squats*
- *"Squat, squat, squat"*
- *Shoulder friendly heavy squatting*

LEGS CONTENTS

Questions and Answers

- *No more bowing knees in the squat!*

- *Heavy lifting, easy on the knees*

- *Can you let your knees slip forward when squatting?*

LEGS OF STEEL
(THE 'STRONG AS YOU LOOK' SERIES)

1.   Parallel squat

2.   One-legged deadlift

3.   Pyramid deadlift

4.   One-legged dumbbell calf raise

Do you know what a 'mullet' means in powerlifting lingo? A sissy who trains his legs with leg extensions, leg curls, leg presses, and occasional high squats with Malibu Ken and Barbie poundages and a color coordinated belt. Whiny, pseudo-intellectual explanations of why and how deeper or heavier squats would hurt his knees and back are the sure ID of a mullet.

The following program is NOT for mullets. It will make you a better man or woman while forging the best legs of your lifetime. Enjoy the pain!

1. PARALLEL SQUAT

It should not surprise you that a leg specialization program builds on the foundation of squats. Not Smith machine squats, not nose bleed high squats, but powerlifting legal parallel squats. In case you 'no comprende' what 'parallel' is: the crease where your thighs meet your abdomen drops below the top of your knee. Anything else is wishful thinking. Ask a powerlifter to watch you and do not get mad if your best squat suddenly loses 100 pounds when you are forced to go the distance. You could also look online for a beeper that straps on to the top of your thigh and does not squawk until you have broken parallel.

> **This is parallel. Anything less is wishful thinking.**

The secret to breaking the parallel is pulling yourself down with your hip flexors. Here is how to learn this skill. Lie on your back with your legs straight. Place your hands on your hip flexors, right below your 'lower abs'. Have your training partner hold on to your ankles and provide some resistance. Arch your lower back – the opposite of a crunch – and press your tailbone into the deck. Slowly pull your knees all the way up to your chest against your buddy's resistance. Note the hip flexor contraction.

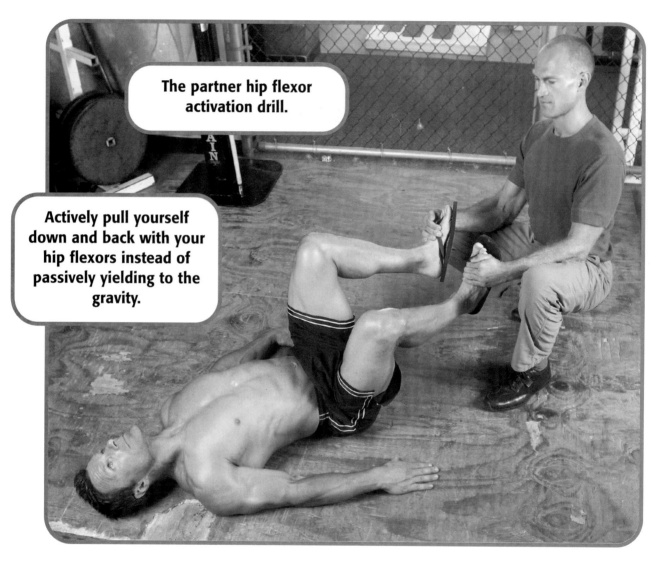

The partner hip flexor activation drill.

Actively pull yourself down and back with your hip flexors instead of passively yielding to the gravity.

When you squat recreate the above sensation: actively pull yourself down and back with your hip flexors instead of passively yielding to the gravity. You will instantly go deeper, improve your control of the weight, and tighten up the arch in your lower back. This results in a bigger, deeper, and safer squat.

But let us start from the beginning. Wedge yourself under the barbell. Keep the bar low on your back, there is no sense in scraping your vertebrae. Grip the bar close to your shoulders for better stability. Do not emulate heavyweight powerlifters; they hold their hands close to the plates because big and tight dudes cannot do it any other way.

Inhale, tighten up your whole body, and squeeze the bar off the pins. Face away from the mirror! Or else.

Back out while staying tight and breathing shallow. Did I mention, do not even think about wearing a belt? Consider it mentioned.

Set up your feet slightly wider than your shoulders, slightly turned out and tracking your knees.

Look straight ahead at a point that is level with your eyes when you are standing up. Keep your eyes on that spot for the duration of the set.

Take another breath, pressurize your abdomen, brace yourself even more, and pull yourself into the 'hole' – power speak for the parallel depth.

Keep your weight on your heels or on the entire surface of your feet, but never on your toes. Push your butt back to load the hamstrings and keep your shins as upright as possible. Never let your knees bow in.

Once you have hit the legal depth, grunt and push your feet down into the deck while driving your traps up into the bar. Make sure that your hips do not shoot up before your head. Enjoy the pain!

Recommended sets and reps: 3x6

Stay tight and keep your abdomen pressurized.

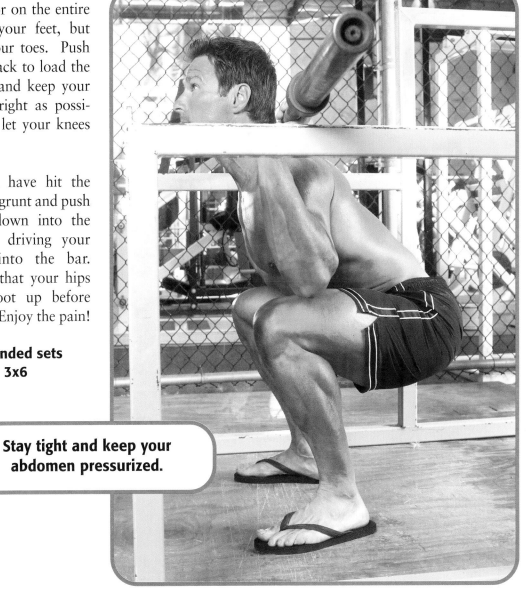

2. ONE-LEGGED DEADLIFT

The one-legged deadlift introduced by Harry L. Good in his 1940 course *The Keynote to Great Strength* is one of my favorite drills. It is an excellent assistance exercise for the deadlift and a hamstring blaster second to none. You will never give the leg curl machine another look once you have tried the one-legged dead.

You may pull almost any weight: a barbell, a pair of dumbbells or kettlebells, a sandbag. Face the weight with one foot centered and the other elevated behind you. Your shin should be an inch or so behind the bar. If you pull two bells stand between them.

Fold at your hip and semi-squat. Do not let your knee extend over your toes or buckle in. Grab the weight. Take a normal breath, pressurize, and lift.

Keep your weight evenly distributed on your foot. You do not need to be paranoid about the back arch; unlike its two-legged brother, this type of deadlift is very forgiving and lets you get away with pulling with a slightly rounded back. Two reasons: a much lighter poundage and an intense midsection contraction, 'a virtual belt', enforced by the one-legged pull's challenging balance.

You will find that you have to contract the glute on the working side very intensely to maintain your balance. Flex it to break the bell off the floor and cramp it even harder at the lockout. It will not take you long to realize that you have discovered one of the most effective glute exercises in existence.

If you start losing balance, catch yourself by landing your airborne foot. Carry on once you have got your equilibrium back. Unlike the regular deadlift, the one legged version enables you to lower the weight slowly safely so your neighbors will stop calling the police.

The one legged DL also does a fine job of strengthening your ankles, at least if you lift barefoot. Just grip the deck hard with your toes, keep the muscles around your ankle and on the bottom of your foot tight, and make sure that the inside of your foot does not buckle down towards the floor.

Another great advantage of the one-legged dead is it requires very little weight. That makes it an ideal leg exercise for a home or hotel gym.

Recommended sets and reps: 3x6 per leg

3. PYRAMID DEADLIFT

Russian powerlifters stand on two sturdy boxes, squat down in a wide stance with a weight in their hands and do a killer a squat-deadlift combo. It has a curious name of the 'pyramid dead-lift', probably because you are perched up on top of a tall structure. Boris Sheyko, the coach of the Russian National Men's Powerlifting Team, uses this forgiving drill to teach the perfect squat and deadlift form to beginners while developing the necessary flexibility. He has the lifter hold a kettlebell in straight arms between his legs.

A dumbbell would not work because it bumps into your body and does not allow you to stand up all the way. If you do not have a kettlebell you may use the low cable stack with almost any handle that does not hit your knees and two boxes or hard benches.

The exercise is much simpler than either the traditional SQ or DL because the weight is perfectly balanced below the musclehead's center of gravity; not above (SQ) or in front (DL). Which is why it is okay to practice for high reps; the form is not likely to deteriorate.

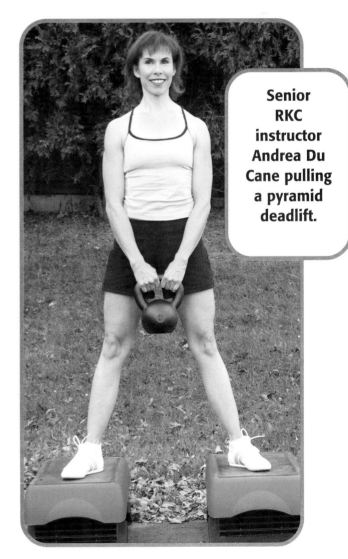

Senior RKC instructor Andrea Du Cane pulling a pyramid deadlift.

The keys to fine performance. Take a stance as wide as your flexibility allows and turn your feet out somewhat. But remember that your knees must always track your feet and never bow in! Look straight ahead rather than up or down. Do not let your hips shoot up before your head. Push your butt back and keep your shins close to vertical. Those are the basics. Now for the fine points.

'Pull your hips out of their sockets' on the way down as if you are pushing the walls apart with your knees.

Once you have gone down as deep as you can let out a sigh of relief and you will sink even deeper. Inhale on the way up. This peculiar breathing pattern would not apply to any power exercises with a lot of weight.

As your flexibility improves slowly widen your stance. Eventually an average sized trainee should be able to place his feet as far apart as the inside plates of a barbell.

Recommended sets and reps: 2x20-25

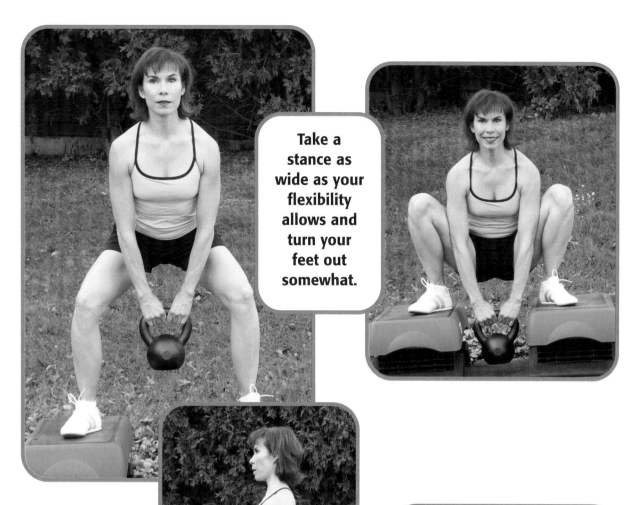

Take a stance as wide as your flexibility allows and turn your feet out somewhat.

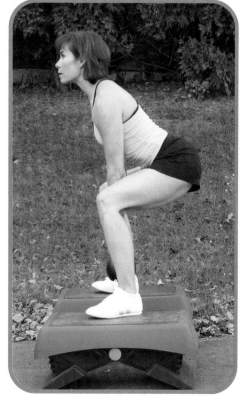

166

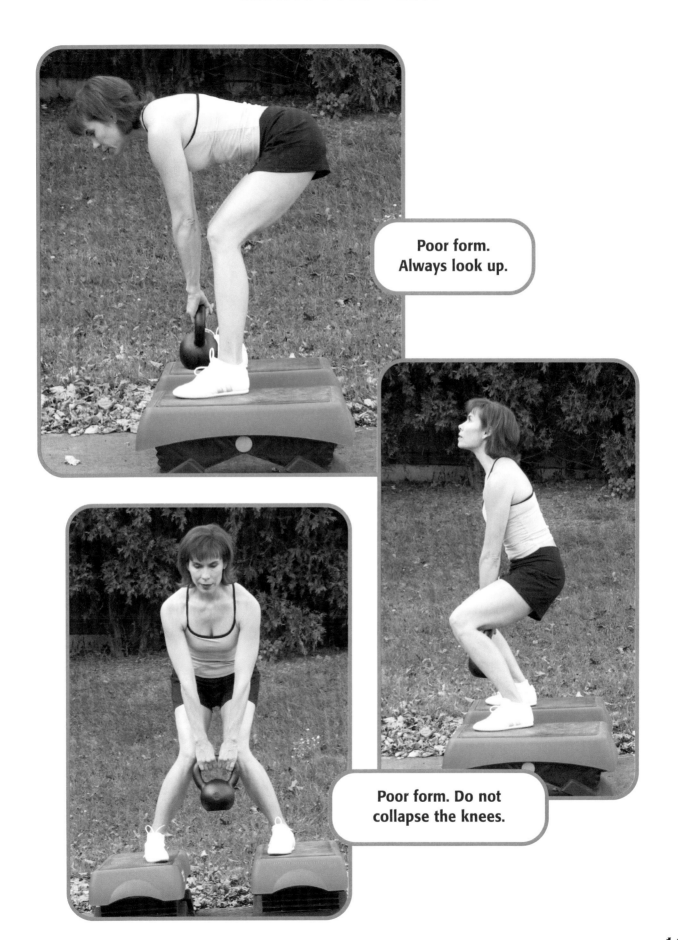

167

4. ONE-LEGGED DUMBBELL CALF RAISE

By now you should be pretty smoked. If you have been stuck in a rut in the calf development department you had better do the following calf workout some other time, for instance after your chest or arm session. If your calves are not too bad, finish the job now.

Nothing fancy, just the basic one-legged dumbbell calf raise. Stand on the ball of your foot on the edge of a step. Hold a dumbbell or a kettlebell in your hand on the working side hand. Hold on to something stationary for balance with your other hand.

Go down and get a good stretch. If you drew a line through your toes it would be parallel to the ground. In other words, keep your ankle at neutral and do not let your foot buckle in. Not complying could lead to health problems down the road. Ask your chiropractor for details.

Pause for a second – this will make the exercise harder and reduce the soreness – and push up all the way. Another pause. Another push.

For active recovery do an easy set or two of unloaded heel raises on both feet the day after.

Recommended sets and reps: 3x10 per leg

FREQUENTLY ASKED QUESTIONS ABOUT LEG TRAINING

Q: Should I squat with a towel? The bar hurts my back.

Somebody call the w-a-a-ambulance! A towel will make the bar dangerously unstable, at least with heavy weights. And since light weights are not worth squatting, just say no to the towel. Put some meat on your upper back and learn how to fit the bar snugly into the groove below your posterior delts. The Hise shrug outlined in the Back installment of the Strong as You Look series will help you with both.

Q: I love front squats but they hurt my wrists. What should I do?

First, never do more than three reps per set. Second, ask a weightlifter to show you how to rack the bar properly. If weightlifters are scarce in your parts get a copy of Arthur Dreschler's outstanding *Weightlifting Encyclopedia*. Kettlebell front squats rack very easily with average flexibility and can be safely done for high reps. I demonstrate the kettlebell front squat in the *More Russian Kettlebell Challenges* DVD.

Q: What is wrong with the leg press machine?

Where do I start? The leg press puts you in an unnatural position where your knees extend but your hips do not (your legs do line up with your body). In a study by Canadian researcher Digby Sale, strength gains on the leg press had no meaningful carryover to the squat, read a functional movement.

The hip sled can be dangerous, especially if you bring your knees too close towards your chest as is typical among muscleheads. Your tail comes off the pad and your rounded lower back has to bear the brunt of the unrealistic poundage. This type of flexion is the number one cause of disc herniations.

Last but not least, the sled and most other machines do not challenge your stabilizing muscles. With very few exceptions (e.g. Dr. Michael Yessis' gastro-ham-glute machine or Dick Hartzell's Jump Stretch deadlift platform) exercise machines belong on the junk pile of history next to Communism.

HOT WHEELS BY SUMMER!

You sport some decent pipes, pardner, and respectable pecs, but your scrawny and flabby legs look like they could have been adopted. Sure, you could get away with the tank top plus bulky sweats look in the winter. But you are not going to fool anyone when the Fahrenheits start peaking. Do not let the beach season catch you with your pants down! Get acquainted with the squat cage right now.

Fortunately, unlike some other body parts, legs can be transformed from soft mediocrity to awesome muscularity in a matter of weeks. But you will have to wave a tearful good-bye to leg presses, Smith machines, and other gimmicks and do some real work.

The following routine, although it contains only two exercises, the squat and a unique football drill, will do more for your paws in four weeks than all the chrome hardware at your gym in a decade.

Kick off your leg day with the 'renegade lunge', a cool drill from the arsenal of NFL strength and conditioning consultant John Davies. Stand sideways near a plank set at your waist level, for instance a power rack pin. Squat down until your head is lower than the plank and push off the leg furthest from the plank like a speed skater. Your body will lunge under the pin. Make sure that you are tracking your feet with your knees and that you are not doing anything exotic to twist and hurt your knees. Stay tight and in control; do not thrash around. And watch your head, Inspector Clouseau!

Stand up on the other side. Straighten out completely and push your hips forward. Squat down and go back under the pin. That was one rep. Do a total of three repetitions. Walk around and relax your legs for a couple of minutes. Pretend that you are shaking water off your legs like a dog, to release the lactic acid and tension. Russian athletes from all sports swear by such relaxation exercises (see my *Fast & Loose* DVD).

Lower the pin a notch and perform another set. Then lower it for one last time and do the last, third set. Every workout do three progressive sets, hopefully starting deeper every time until you have developed the flexibility and strength of a mutant.

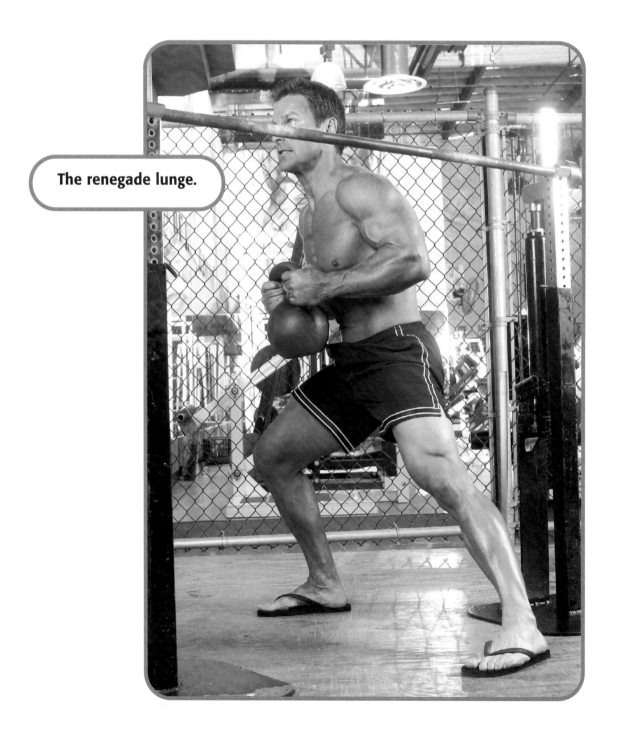

The renegade lunge.

Muscularity, symmetry, and cuts will come as a part of the package deal. So will the athletic ability. "From a sport specific standpoint," states Coach Davies, the author of *Renegade Training for Football* (Dragon Door Publications, May 2002), "I haven't found anything better to assist in lateral movements." If you are an athlete, a soldier, or simply living hard, you will benefit greatly from the renegade lunge. Jim Reading, the fitness advisor to the US Marine Corps base in San Diego, showed me 'the patch', an outdoor log structure where he puts his son and his baseball buddies through moves like the renegade lunge. We discussed rigging up a similar course for the Marines; limbo drills are a custom fit for infantrymen who spend a lot of time crouching down.

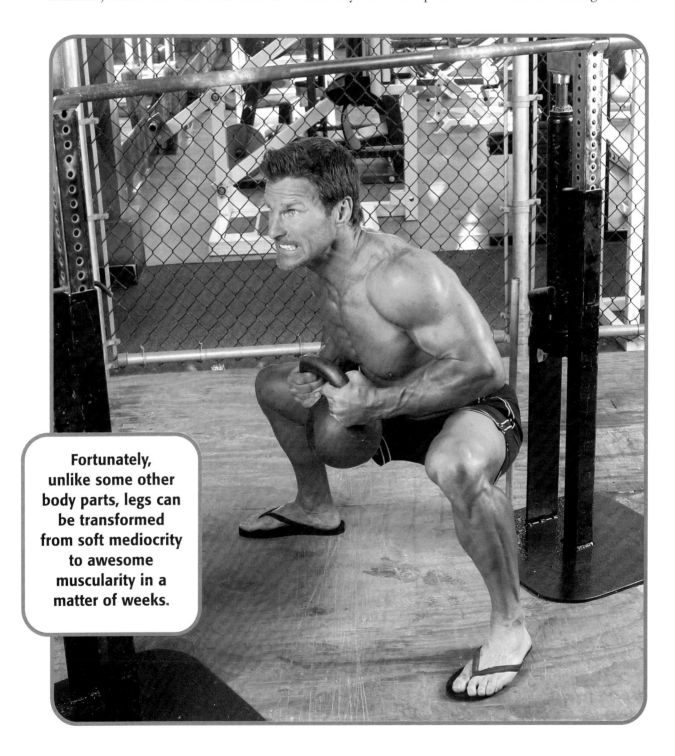

Fortunately, unlike some other body parts, legs can be transformed from soft mediocrity to awesome muscularity in a matter of weeks.

Although Coach Davies has his players hold a kettlebell in their hands for extra resistance I am sure he would make an exception in your case and let you get away with bodyweight only since you have fifty squats in your near future. That is right, tens sets of five! And to top it all off you will be doing it three times a week! Yes, you must go an extra mile for extraordinary and quick gains. No cowardice camouflaged with pseudo-intellectual discussion about overtraining is accepted. Just do it. Or else.

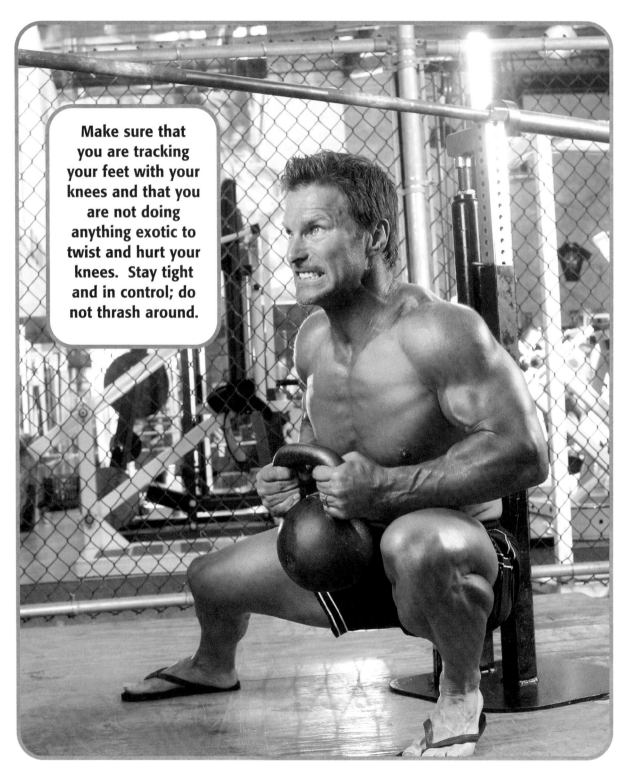

Make sure that you are tracking your feet with your knees and that you are not doing anything exotic to twist and hurt your knees. Stay tight and in control; do not thrash around.

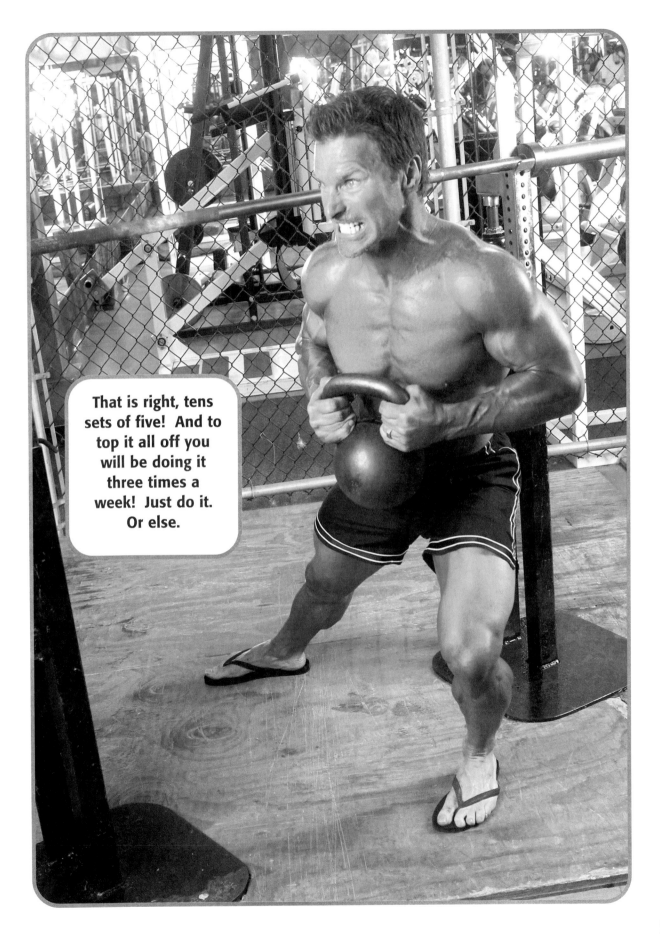

THE 'HOT WHEELS IN FOUR WEEKS' WORKOUT

Train three times a week, on Mondays, Wednesdays, and Fridays.
Start each workout with 3x3 of lateral limbo lunges. Follow up with squats.

Workout#	Squat sets x repetitions x poundage
1	10x5 @ 50%1RM
2	10x5 @ 50%1RM+5lbs.
3	10x5 @ 50%1RM+10lbs.
4	10x5 @ 50%1RM+15lbs.
5	10x5 @ 50%1RM+20lbs.
6	10x5 @ 50%1RM+25lbs.
7	10x5 @ 50%1RM+30lbs.
8	10x5 @ 50%1RM+35lbs.
9	10x5 @ 50%1RM+40lbs.
10	10x5 @ 50%1RM+45lbs.
11	10x5 @ 50%1RM+50lbs.
12	10x5 @ 50%1RM+55lbs.

If you have the energy finish each workout with your favorite calf exercise.

The bad news is, you will be doing more squats in one month than you have done in the last year. The good news, you will be starting out at only half of your max squat. If your squat PR is 250 pounds 10x5 @ 125 pounds is not exactly a killer.

Take brief breaks between sets, between thirty seconds and two minutes. The Monday workout will start easy but the pump will catch up in a hurry. Do not forget to load up on protein, calories, and sleep in the aftermath. If you do not get enough you will not grow.

You will be sore on Wednesday. Ignore it. Tell someone who cares. Add five pounds to your 50% and squat again. You will be adding a fiver every workout if your one rep max is between 150 and 250 pounds. If you squat less than 150 add five pounds every other session. If you put up between 250 and 500 pounds add ten pounds per workout. And if you squat more than five wheels your experience will tell you how much weight to add.

More soreness and another weight increase on Friday. Keep the pressure up and by the end of the second week you will not be getting nearly as sore. Forced to perform, your legs are adapting. And growing.

But before charging your squat cage, please review the following fine points on technique. The squat, although supposedly such a basic, is hardly ever done properly.

Start by finding a comfortable squatting stance. Do not emulate the stance of the biggest guy in your gym. His build, strength, and flexibility are different from yours and copying his groove will do you no good.

Here is how to find a squatting stance for your body only. Squat down on your haunches or as deep as you can. Shuffle your feet in and out and play with the angle your feet are facing out. Persist until you find a position where your feet are planted flat and solid and your knees are tracking your feet. You should be comfortable enough in this position to be able stay in it for a couple of minutes, without propping yourself with your arms against your knees. 'The catcher's crouch', is that what you call it?

Occasionally you may vary your squatting width for the sake of variety or addressing weak links but mostly stick to the stance you have just found, your safest and most powerful one. Keep in mind though that it might change as your flexibility improves and you add muscle mass to your legs. Retest yourself every couple of months.

Another comment on the squat technique. Do not confuse a 'straight' back with an 'upright' back. It is impossible to do a full, even a parallel, squat with an upright back if you keep your heels planted as you are supposed to and do not let your knees extend over your feet. It is plain physics and it is easy to test. Sit in a chair with your shins nearly vertical. Now try to get up without either bringing your feet underneath you or leaning forward. It will not happen, Comrade, you will land on your butt.

So quit challenging the natural law and do not be afraid to squat bent over, as long as your spine stays straight (not vertical). Start your squats by pushing your butt back as far as possible and sit back – not down! – at the point where your glutes cannot back up any more without toppling you.

Descend at least to parallel. That means until the crease on the top of your thigh drops below the top of your knee. Have someone check you, a big dude whom you cannot cower into sweet-talking you. You will be unpleasantly surprised that a big bite has been taken out of your squat PR once you hit the legit depth or the 'hole'. Many big-big bodybuilders who claim 700-pound squats cannot get up with 500 when forced to hit the legal depth. Join the recovering high squatters club.

It is very likely that in the beginning you will be unable to hit the hole in good form, even with a light weight. Either your knees will slip way forward and you will not be able to go any lower, your heels will come up, or your back will round and your butt will tuck in. Unless you are exceptionally tight you should be able to overcome this by contracting your hip flexors.

Here is how it is done. Stand on one foot with your knee up in the air. Push down on your knee with your hands and feel the muscles on top of your thigh tense up. Remember that feeling and try to reproduce it when you are descending into a squat. Literally pull yourself down with your hip flexors. You will instantly notice that you can hit a greater depth with better form and control.

Pay attention to the above tips and you will be rewarded with respectable squatting power, the legs to show for it, and superior training safety. Follow the outlined routine and be amazed at the improvement you will see in just a month.

There is no reason why you have to quit the 'hot wheels' program after four weeks. Stay on it as long as you can keep adding weight to your squats without increasing the rest periods beyond three minutes. Then you may choose to peak your squat strength with a basic powerlifting routine or switch to something altogether different. Leg power to you!

QUESTIONS & ANSWERS:

BUILDING LEGS WITH PLYOMETRICS?

Question: Can you build good legs with plyometrics?

No. True 'touch-and-go' plyos are meant to rewire your nervous system, specifically teach you to recruit your muscles more, with more power, and make a better use of stored elastic energy.

Less intense and more voluminous jump exercises will work though, provided you have healthy knees and your legs are already reasonably strong. Dr. Michael Colgan, the author of *The New Power Program* (applepublishing.com), points out that mountain runners develop huge lower legs by "whacking their calves with big eccentric downhill braking stresses". He recommends a radical regimen of downhill sprints to a bodybuilder lacking in the calf department.

For your quads try the jump squat variation popular with Russian kettlebell lifters. Clasp your hands behind your neck, keep your chest open, and quickly squat an inch or two below parallel. Immediately jump straight up; make sure to extend your body completely when airborne. Land on the balls of your feet, roll back on your heels as you are squatting down, and repeat. Maximum explosion is not necessary; the name of this game is sustained effort. This is NOT true plyometrics, after all. 2x10 is a good start. This exercise will spur new growth in your quads within days!

If you are interested in the complex science of plyometrics and want to know why the above exercises are not true plyos, read *Supertraining* by Mel Siff, Ph.D. available from elitefts.com.

TRAINING CALVES AT HOME

Question: I train at home and can't afford a Smith machine or a standing heel raise unit. All I have is a barbell and a squat rack. What can I do for my calves?

Here is an exercise from *Anatomy of Strength*, Dr. Arkady Vorobyev's classic text on bodybuilding. It may not be for everyone but if you have healthy shoulders and decent coordination you will make great gains with it.

Hoist a barbell on your shoulders as you would for squats. Staying inside your power rack with the pins set high for safety walk forward towards the wall – I presume that your cage is parked next to a wall – and make sure the barbell is comfortably sitting in the groove on your traps. Carefully let go of the bar with one hand while balancing it with the other. Work your arm over the bar and press your palm against the wall at your head level. Exercising caution, untangle your other arm and rest its hand on the wall as well. Step on a three to four inch solid block – and you are in the standing barbell calf raise business.

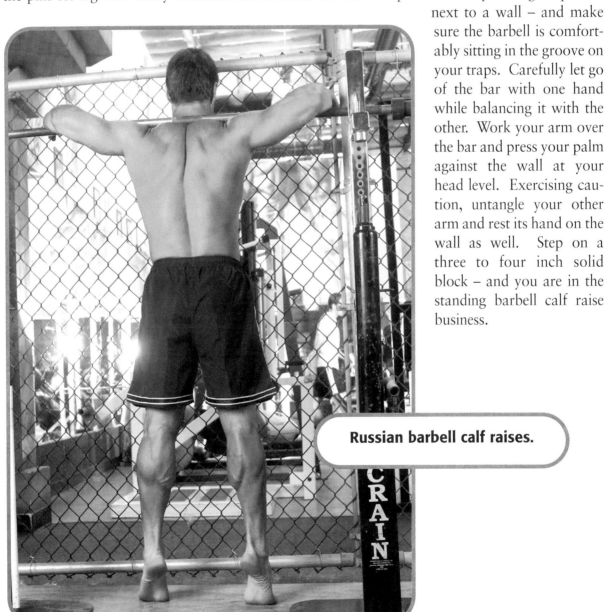

Russian barbell calf raises.

177

RUSSIAN FARMER WALK FOR STUBBORN CALVES

Question: My calves just don't grow no matter what I do. HELP!

Some Russian kettlebell lifting coaches recommend the farmer walk on the balls of your feet. Grab two bells, kettle or dumb, and go for it. Just walk around on your toes. For better results and greater ankle safety do the drill barefoot. It is even more special when practiced outside on uneven terrain.

Do not let your shoulders shrug up. Flex your tris and lats and push your shoulders away from your ears in the beginning. Then relax your upper body somewhat – but not your waist – while maintaining the described alignment. This will set your body in the most efficient position for the farmer walk.

Terminate each set before you drop the weights on your feet. It goes without saying that you will get a great grip workout in the process. Build up to five sets of two minutes each. Stretch your calves between the sets and afterwards. For obvious reasons this exercise belongs in the end of your session as a 'finisher'.

POWERFUL LEGS WITHOUT SQUATS?

Question: Can I build respectable legs without squats?

It depends on what you mean by 'respectable'. If you want to give Tom Platz a run for his money, the answer is a resounding 'no'. Nothing will maximize leg size as much as the basic squat. Nothing.

If you want your legs to be muscular and strong but you have no desire to go through a pair of dress pants in a couple of months, you can do it without squats. A stipulation: 'without squats' does NOT mean leg presses, leg extensions, leg curls, Smith machine squats, and other weenie moves! Following is a list of legit, hardcore, squat alternatives:

- The one legged squat or 'pistol' with a weight held in front or just the bodyweight;
- The front squat with a barbell or two kettlebells;
- The belt squat;
- The deadlift (a variety of stances are possible);
- The one legged deadlift with a barbell, two dumbbells or kettlebells;
- The saddle deadlift (also known as the Jefferson squat);
- The behind the back deadlift
- The Hack squat with a kettlebell.

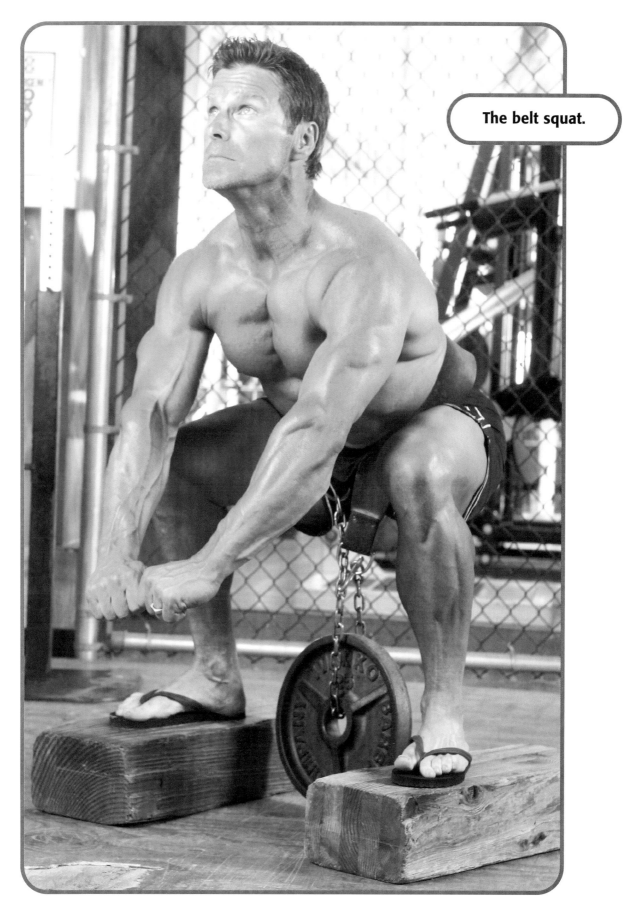

The belt squat.

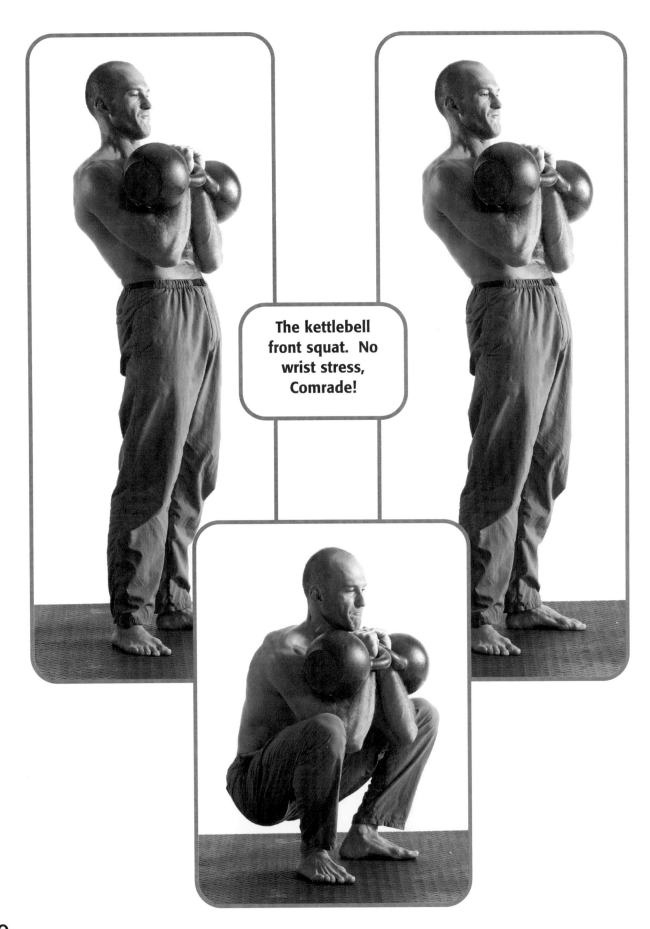

The kettlebell front squat. No wrist stress, Comrade!

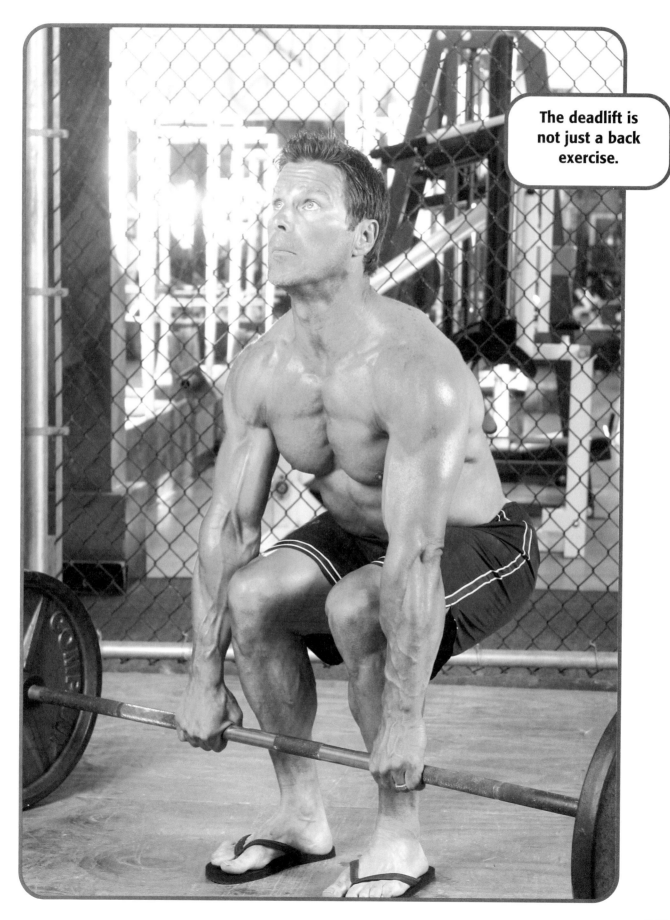

The deadlift is not just a back exercise.

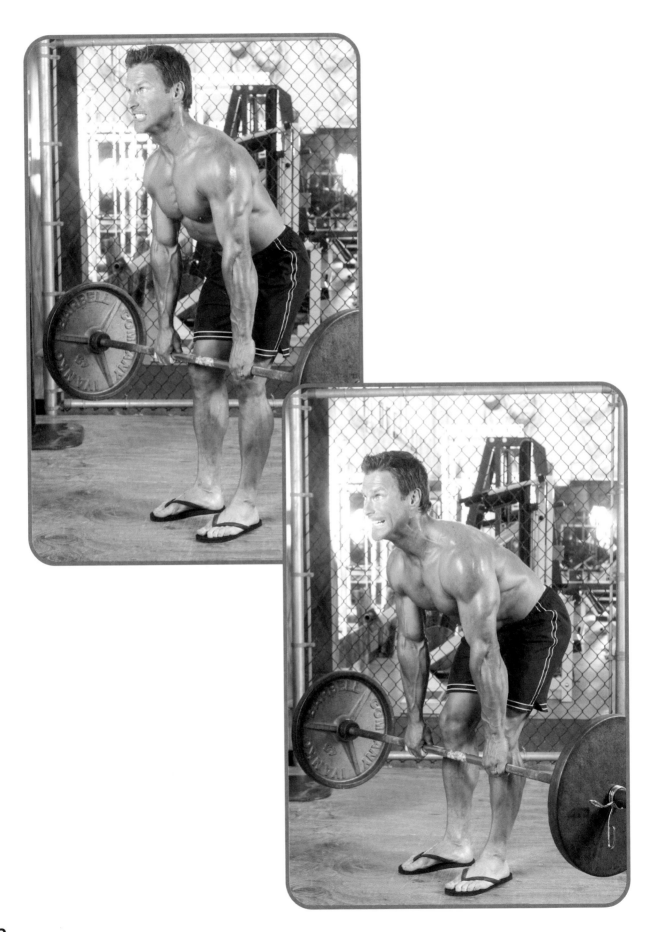

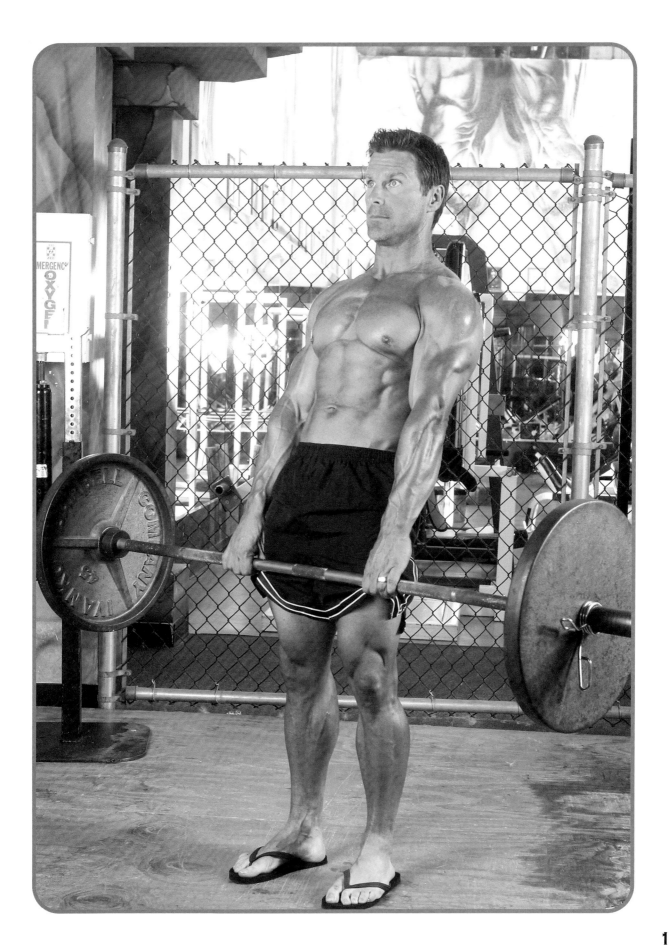

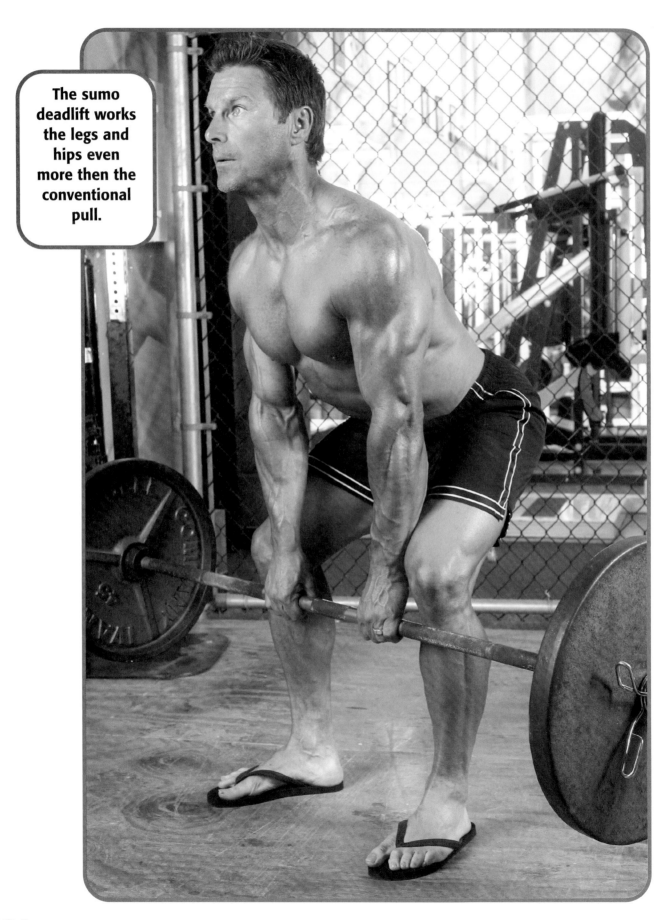

The sumo deadlift works the legs and hips even more then the conventional pull.

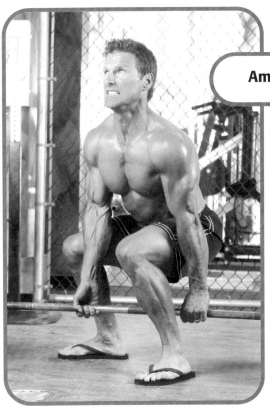

Americans call it 'the Jefferson squat'.

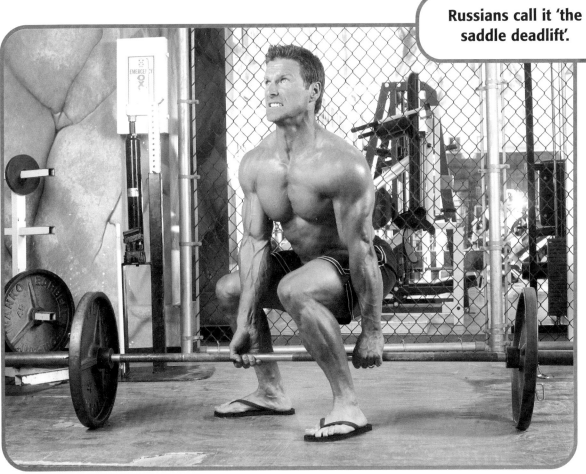

Russians call it 'the saddle deadlift'.

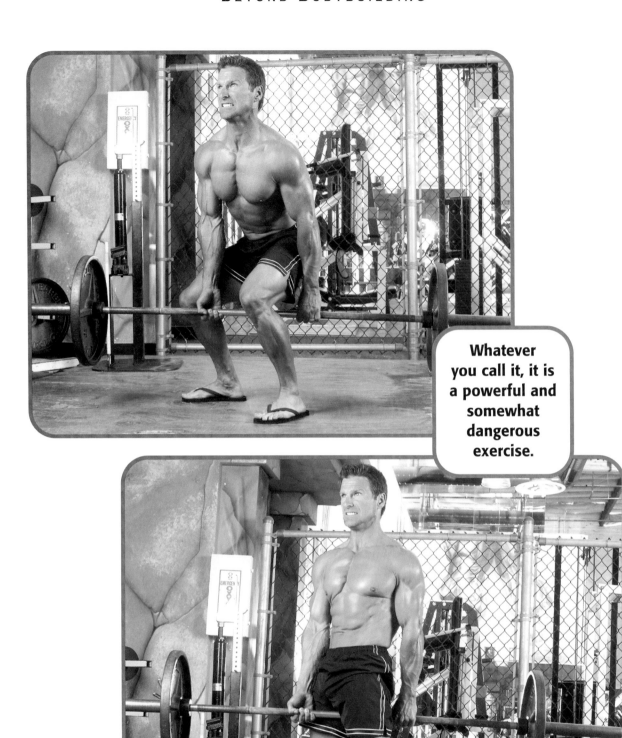

Whatever you call it, it is a powerful and somewhat dangerous exercise.

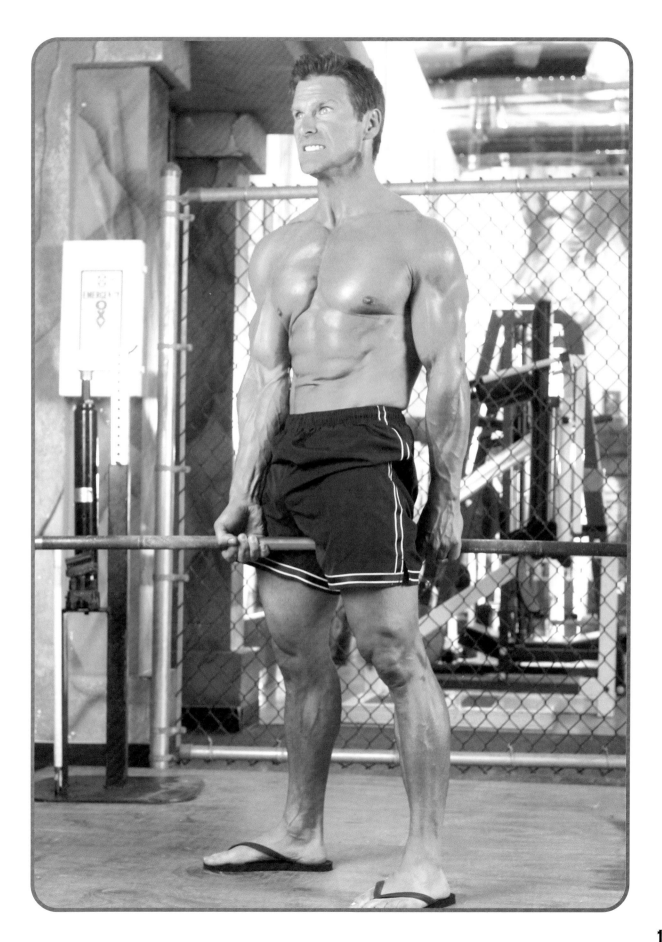

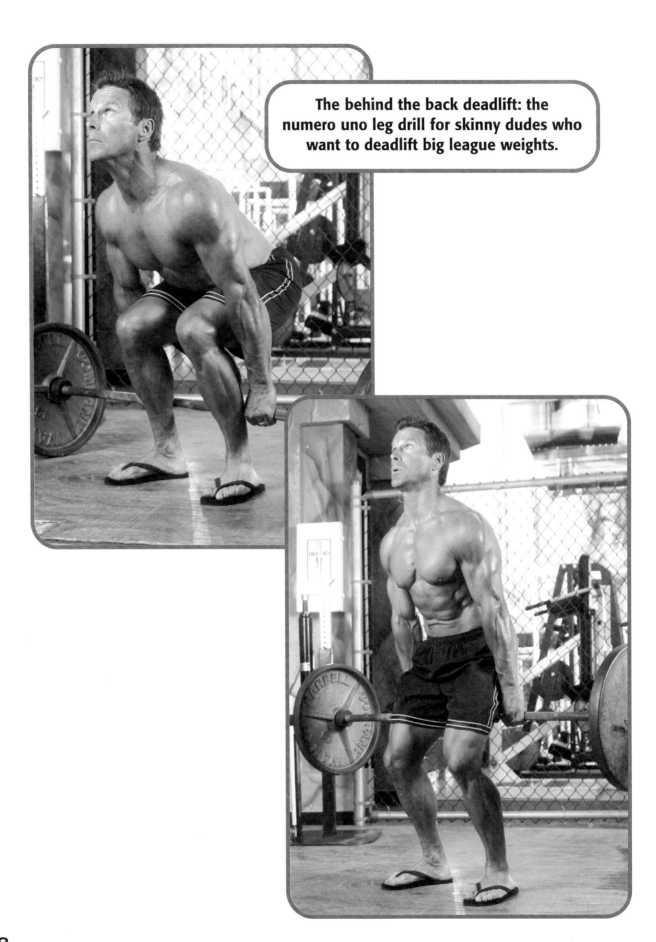

The behind the back deadlift: the numero uno leg drill for skinny dudes who want to deadlift big league weights.

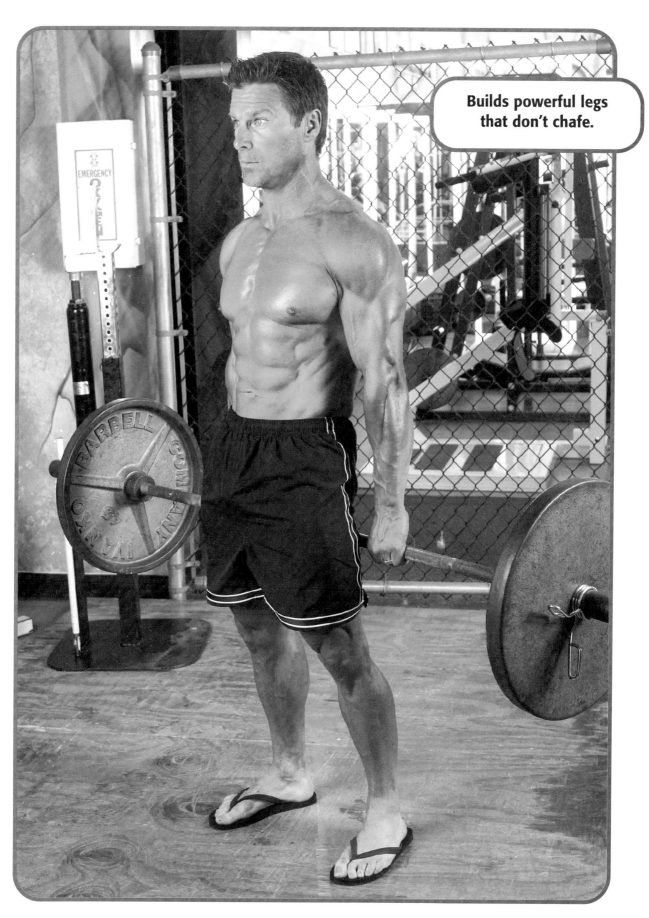

Builds powerful legs that don't chafe.

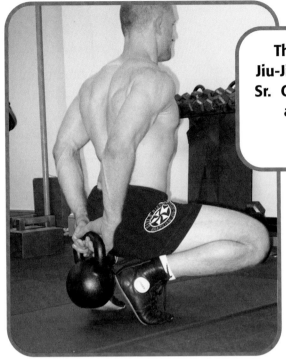

The Hack squat is a favorite of Brazilian Jiu-Jitsu world champion Steve Maxwell, RKC Sr. Go to Steve's Philadelphia gym Maxercise and become a better man or woman.

Photo courtesy Maxercise.com

There are some other good exercises that follow the same pattern: multi-joint and free weight. And if you are even contemplating a mullet routine (leg press + leg extension + leg curl) – slap yourself silly!

HOW DEEP IS YOUR SQUAT?

Question: Are full squats bad for the knees and back? And what is a 'full' squat anyway?

A 'full squat' means your hams are resting on your calves. Olympic weightlifters squat that way. A 'parallel squat' is deeper than you think. The powerlifting rules insist that unless the top of your knee is higher that the crease separating your thigh and your lower abs, it is not 'parallel'.

Regarding injuries to your knees and back, any depth squat could do when you do not know what you are doing. Full, parallel, and partial (anything above parallel) squats can be very safe and productive provided you have been taught the proper technique. The full squat is by far most technique demanding. Which is why it got the worst reputation, thanks to trainers' incompetence.

There are two issues. First is the back and hamstring flexibility required to keep a proper lumbar curve. Most bodybuilders are way too tight, their tails tuck in, and their backs get injured.

Second, once they get to the point a couple of inches above parallel, most bodybuilders do not know how to go down deeper safely. The answer is 'by pulling down with your hip flexors'. The muscle action is similar to the situp. If you are not sure what it means, watch my video *More Russian Kettlebell Challenges*.

The bottom line. For best development you should do all three types of squats. To squat safely you need to get flexible and technical.

HIGH REP FRONT SQUATS?

Question: I love the front squat. I feel that it hits my quads like nothing else. Unfortunately my wrists and shoulders give out after just a few reps and I just can't work my thighs hard enough. What is the answer?

The barbell front squat is a weightlifting exercise. It was never meant to be done for high reps. Three repetitions are about right. To make sure that you stimulate your fibers deep enough, just do more sets, for instance five to eight sets of three or ten to twelve sets of two. If you like higher reps use two kettlebells instead of a barbell. KBs can stay in the rack a lot longer than a barbell, with minimal or zero wrist and shoulder stress (not to be confused with discomfort).

When you front squat with a barbell always keep your elbows high. Mark Cannella, the head coach of the Columbus Weightlifting Club, recommends that you 'cork' or 'wedge' yourself under the bar as you are gripping it. The bar is a lot more likely to stay in place.

A note on the front squat depth: always go rock bottom. For reasons that are too complex to be discussed here, high front squats are too rough on the knees.

A SHORTCUT TO PERFECT SQUATS

Question: What is the quickest way to master the proper squat form?

Every coach has their own sequence and many of them work. I recommend starting with front squats plus good mornings. The front squats will teach you to pull yourself down into the hole with the hip flexors and to keep your stomach tight. The good mornings will teach you to push your butt back, to recruit your hamstrings, keep them tight all the way down, and not to be afraid to be bent over.

Another great thing about these two exercises, both of them have a great carryover to the back squat and the deadlift. Which means that your powerlifts will go up, way up, even if you do not practice them.

A good schedule is to train on Mondays, Wednesdays, and Fridays. Alternate FSQs and GMs every workout, for instance: Monday – GMs, Wednesday – FSQs, Friday – GMs, Mon – FSQs, etc. Practice both drills for five to eight sets of three reps. Start with very easy weights and add five pounds every workout. When you get to the point where you have to push the pedal to the metal in one or both exercises, switch to back squats. You will be pleasantly surprised with your form and power. Squat three times every two weeks for 5x5 and add five pounds per workout as before.

'SQUAT, SQUAT, SQUAT.'

Question: 'Squat, squat, squat.' This is a legs section, not a squat section!! Can't you talk about leg extensions and other exercises for a change?

I have mentioned deadlifts, haven't I? Chill and pay attention, dude. Instead of making up fancy routines of easy machine exercises why don't you get off your butt, get tough, and squat? Upper leg building is VERY simple: just squat. If you want to address a certain aspect of your legs just use a different type of squat. For more hamstring work do box squats or parallel squats with a three second pause in the hole (the bottom of a parallel squat in powerlifting lingo). Do Olympic or full squats for the quads. Wide stance power squats will take care of your hips and inner thighs. Just pick one and stick with it for six to eight weeks, then pick another. Add a calf exercise to balance out your legs and some posing for better cuts and you are all set. Keep it simple and make it hard.

SHOULDER FRIENDLY HEAVY SQUATTING

Question: My squat is going up but I am wary of adding more weight as my wrists hurt. Sometimes the shoulders and the elbows act up too. Am I doomed to squat light?

Change the way you carry the bar on your back. First, before you even get under, push your chest out as far as possible and pinch your shoulder blades together as if you are trying to hold a tennis ball between them. It will help if you visualize touching your elbows together behind your back. At the same time force your shoulders down, the opposite of a shrug. Fight the temptation to elevate your shoulders when you unrack the weight and during your set! Keeping your lats locked tight will help.

Get under the bar and let it lie in the groove naturally formed by your contracted upper back muscles below your posterior delts. Wiggle under the bar to get tight and comfortable before unracking the weight. Forget towels and padded bar sleeves, they just make the weight unstable on your back and cannot save your from discomfort on your heavy sets anyway. Besides, you might as well wear a T-shirt with a large 'I AM A MULLET!' sign on it. Develop a muscular upper back, keep it tight, and the discomfort from barbell pressure will be a thing of the past.

I AM A MULLET!

The grip width is an individual matter. Although generally the closer your hands, the more stable the load, most bodybuilders are too big and tight to grip the bar inside the power rings. Most heavyweight powerlifters have to grab it near the plates and it is not by choice.

You will be able to bring your hands closer – while minimizing or eliminating wrist and thumb discomfort – by taking a thumbless grip. Naturally, you will have to squeeze the bar tight throughout your set.

To end the shoulder joint discomfort, you will have to drive your elbows forward as far as possible, as you are unracking the weight – and keep them there. Do not lift your shoulders in the process! It is not easy but if the iron game was easy everyone would be playing it.

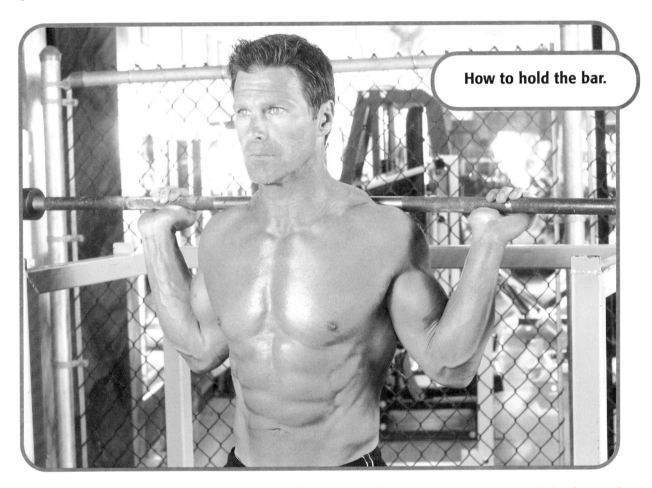

How to hold the bar.

The combination of the depressed and adducted scapulae, a tight false grip, and the forward elbow pressure will lock the bar tightly in place while unloading your beaten up joints. Some gym rats with good shoulders may also try drawing the elbows together, as in a chest fly, in addition to pushing them forward; this maneuver will immobilize your joints in one more plane.

Embarking on an intelligent shoulder flexibility program will help your squats big time. One effective exercise is the press behind the neck with an empty bar and a forward lean. Consider doing these before your squats. Start overhead with partial reps and gradually work them down.

NO MORE BOWING KNEES IN THE SQUAT!

Question: My knees tend to bow in when I squat heavy. How can I overcome this problem?

Some powerlifters recommend "spreading the floor" with your feet. A powerful technique, but don't you dare use it unless you are convinced there is enough friction between your shoes and the platform. If you feet slip or your ankle rolls, you are a goner...

A safer alternative is to 'screw' your feet into the platform, from inside out. Your feet should not move but you should feel a spiral of tension running from your groin to your feet. Your knees are a lot less likely to bow in. Plus, you cannot help noticing that some new muscles kick in. The result: an even greater strength and development.

A unique approach to strengthening the hip abductors in the squat specific way was invented at the Westside Barbell Club. Loop a sturdy rubber band around your knees –the WSB guys use Jump Stretch bands – and squat with your bodyweight.

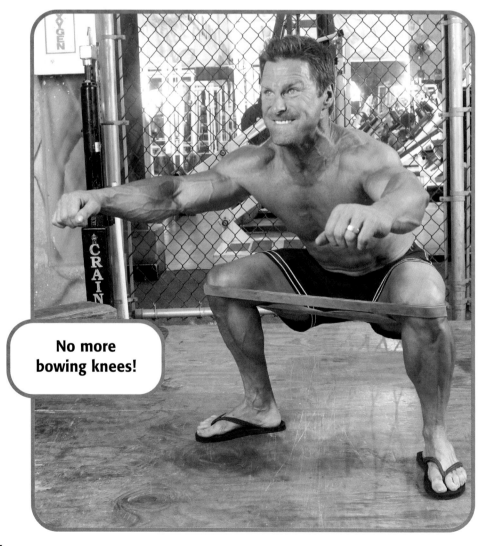

No more bowing knees!

HEAVY LIFTING, EASY ON THE KNEES

Question: My knees have been aching lately from my leg routine. My doctor says there is nothing wrong with me and the strength coach who watched me lift and checked my routine said I was all squared off. Do you have any ideas?

Drs. Apel and Latan, who once took care of the East German national weightlifting team, recommend that you do not do exercises back to back, that require deep knee flexion. Insert exercises that are easier on the knees – such as deadlifts and exercises for other body parts – between different types of deep squats. This is the standard operating procedure for the victorious Russian national powerlifting team.

Here is another tip for you. Slowly squat down rock bottom without a weight. Place the tips of your right index finger and thumb just above your right kneecap. Now slowly move your digits apart from each other: your finger will slide up to the top of the patella while your thumb will go down towards your quad. Slide them about four inches apart while pressing lightly on your skin, and then start over from the center. While you are doing this visualize that the part of your thigh below your finger and thumb is 'elongating' along with the movement of the digits to 'make more space for your knee'. Now try to recreate this 'open' sensation 'hands off' as you are slowly descending into the squat. Imagine that your kneecap is 'separating from your knee.' This voodoo sounding technique will noticeably unload your knees. It never fails in the RKC kettlebell instructor course.

CAN YOU LET YOUR KNEES SLIP FORWARD WHEN SQUATTING?

Question: I have been following your writings for a while and have seen you stress the importance of planting your heels flat and not letting your knees stick out forward in the squat many times. Now I see you recommend Hack squats in your interview with Outside magazine. What about those shearing forces? Have you switched parties?

Is it my conversion from a Commie to a running capitalist dog that gave you this idea? There is no inconsistency, Comrade. A properly performed Hack squat – the spine upright and the hands against the tailbone rather than under the thighs – imposes a brutal leverage. To give you an idea, you need to barbell squat at least 300 to stand a chance of hacking a 70-pound kettlebell. Senior RKC Steve Maxwell hacks an 88-pounder for reps. For kicks he challenged a couple of 600-pound squatters to try it. They could not stand up.

Pushing those knees forward with 70 and with 300 pounds are two very different ball games. Because the weight is light and the reps are low healthy knees should have no problem with Hack squats.

A couple of tips for powerful Hack squats. First, drive hard with your glutes, pinch an imaginary coin with your cheeks; it is the only way to remain upright. Contrary to the popular belief, Hacks do not isolate the quads. Second, flare your knees out, especially if you have long thighs. And third, you will master the movement quicker if you start from the top as in the regular squat rather than from the deck. Tense your glutes, open your chest and descend, insisting on keep your spine vertical. Looking way up will help. You should get the sense for the required balance and will have an easier time getting up. There is no dishonor in practicing without any weight first.

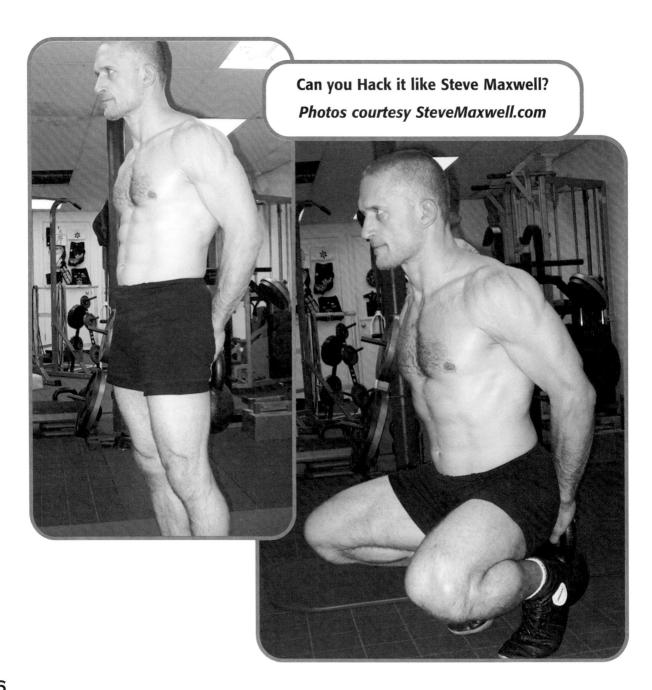

Can you Hack it like Steve Maxwell?
Photos courtesy SteveMaxwell.com

SECTION FIVE

NECK & SHOULDERS

CONTENTS

Questions and Answers

QUESTIONS & ANSWERS:

THE OLD-TIMER NECK BRIDGE

Question: Can you recommend any new exercises for a strong, muscular neck?

Not new in the real sense of the word, but sure new to the modern generation of bodybuilders. My friend and colleague Jeff Martone, RKC Sr. has brought it to my attention that old time physical culturalists had a unique way of performing the back bridge. I quote Sig Klein from his 1940s *Super Physique Body-Building Bar-Bell Course*:

"Lie flat on your back with barbell a few inches from your head. Grasp the bell with the hands shoulder width apart, being sure it is balanced properly. Then pull it over face to the chest and press bell up to arms length. Bring the knees up so that the feet are flat on the floor and close to the buttocks, raise your hips so that only the upper back, neck, and feet are on the floor. From this position push your body up until the upper back rises from the floor and all the weight is supported on the soles of the feet and the top of the head. From this position lower slowly until your back just about touches the floor, then rise again and repeat. Keep the barbell in upright position throughout the exercise. Inhale rising, exhale lowering." It goes without saying that you need a reasonably soft surface such as a wrestling mat.

Note that you are not getting as much range of motion as you would from the traditional wrestler's back bridge – which can be good or bad depending on your goals and neck health – but your neck extensors have to work very hard because of the poor leverage.

Unless you have been training your neck hard, you probably should perform the drill without any weight. Or hold a very light weight on your stomach or your chest. Also, don't 'jam' your neck in one spot; imagine that you are elongating it and 'wrapping it around' something.

Don't forget to work the front of your neck for a balanced development. Lower yourself into the bottom pushup position, rest your forehead on a padded surface, tense up your neck and stomach, and slowly take some weight off your hands. Breathe shallow, stay tight, and hold the position for a period of time.

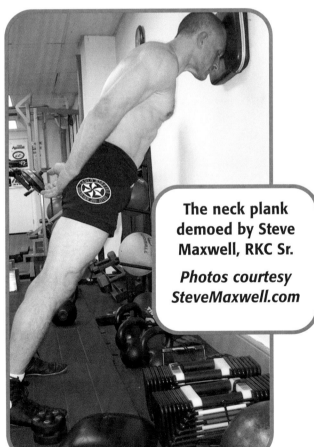

The neck plank demoed by Steve Maxwell, RKC Sr.

Photos courtesy SteveMaxwell.com

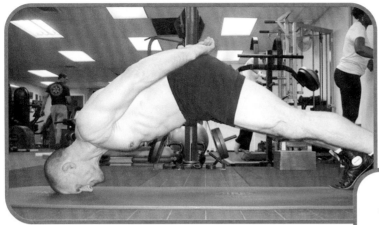

The neck plank and its variations demoed by Steve Maxwell, RKC Sr.

Photos courtesy SteveMaxwell.com

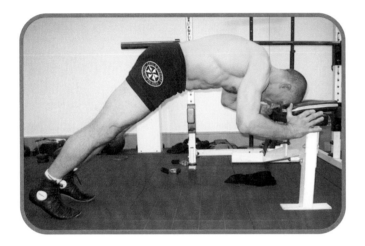

Keep unloading your hands as you get stronger, until your fingertips float above the ground just to spot you. Also bring your feet in until they are together. This will also challenge your abs. Lifting one leg up is even harder but you have to be extra careful.

Once you adapt, give more work to the muscles on the sides of your neck. In the above position, but with your hands solidly planted, slowly roll your head to one side and then the other. Flaring your neck, as if you are trying to maximize its size when being measured, will help you in this and many other neck drills.

As with most neck exercises, clear these with your doctor.

THE SECRET OF PAUL ANDERSON'S POWERFUL NECK

Question: I read that weightlifting and strongman legend Paul Anderson had the thickest neck in the history of the iron game. How did he build it?

The late strongman listed his favorite neck routine in his book *Power by Paul* (highly recommended reading, available from crainsmuscleworld.com). He would superset two exercises. The first one was the conventional neck extension with a head strap. Attach a conservative poundage to such a rig, place your hands on your thighs, and lean forward. Tilt your head back while looking up, then let it come down without overstretching the back of your neck. In his first set Anderson did 50 reps!

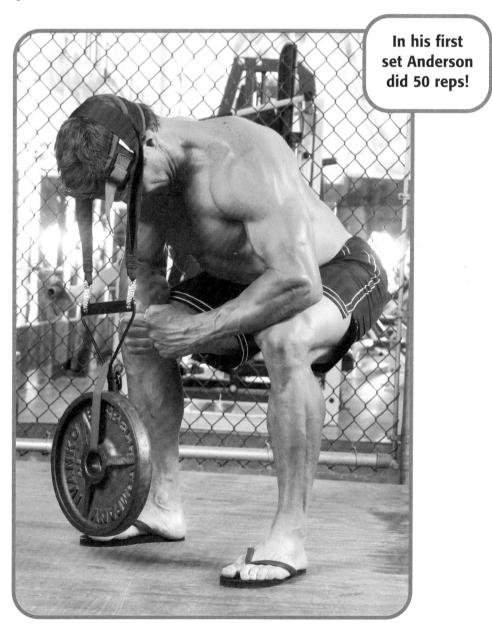

In his first set Anderson did 50 reps!

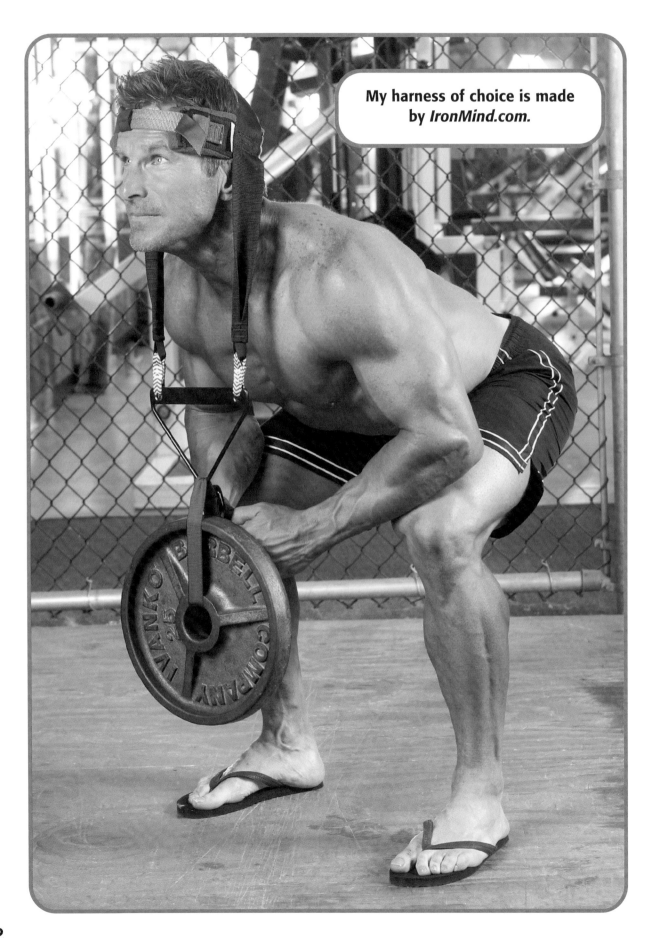

My harness of choice is made by *IronMind.com.*

The second drill was anything but conventional. Paul would pad a table, lean forward and rest his forehead and his hands on it. Then he would roll his neck side to side, from ear to ear, until he could not do it any longer. I do the same drill lying face down on the floor and like it even better.

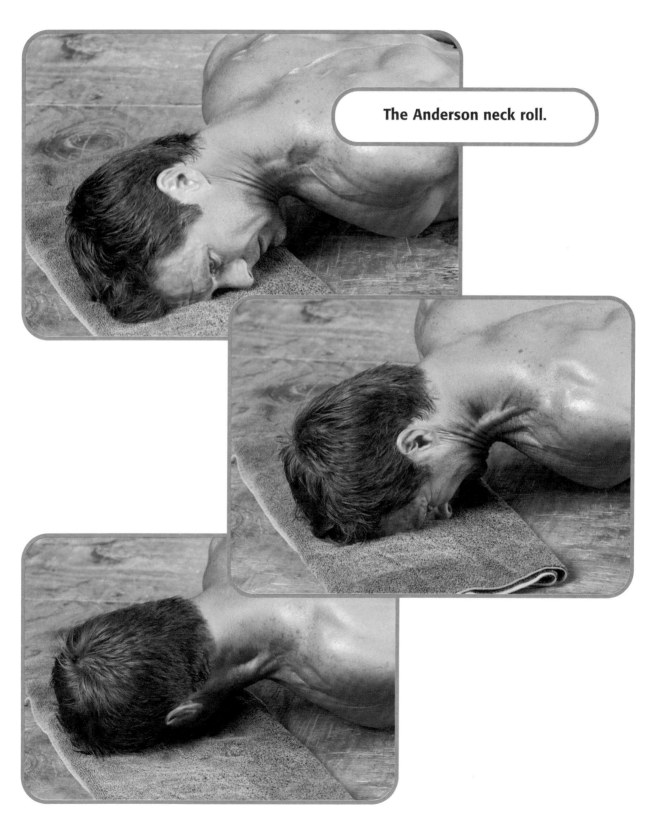

The Anderson neck roll.

203

After just a few seconds of rest 'the Wonder of Nature' repeated the superset. For the third set he increased the poundage on the harness so he was limited to 10 repetitions and wrapped up with another set of neck rolls for 'as long as he could endure'. Very powerful, efficient, and out of the box. Very Paul Anderson.

On a side note, if you are strong enough, you may want to try the floor neck roll in the low pushup position. Very challenging; make sure to spot yourself carefully with your hands and keep constant tension in your neck.

SHOULDER TRAINING ON THE TWENTY-REP SQUAT ROUTINE

Question: I have made great gains on the twenty-rep squat routine from Dr. Randall Strossen's book 'Super Squats'. Now how can I specialize on my shoulders without abandoning this squat routine?

I saw a question almost identical to yours in a 1947 issue of Peary Rader's *Ironman* and I could not answer it better than old-timer Charles A. Smith did. He suggested sticking to Monday-Wednesday-Friday squatting and clean-and-pressing EVERY DAY. "Most lifters use the THREE WORK OUTS a week system, some get in four workouts or five a week, but you will have no fear of staleness or of working too hard even if you press seven days a week seven times a day," stated Smith. "There is only ONE secret of success in pressing – and that is to press and press and press on each and every occasion you get near a bar. The record holders in the press actually use this method when they are in training to better their records."

Now before you holler 'Overtraining!' you must understand what type of press training was done in the good ole' days. The same author wrote an excellent article on power pressing two years later. "It has been said that only one man in 150,000 can press bodyweight," wrote Smith. "As we see it, there is no earthly reason why any man of a year's experience in weight training cannot perform this feat. The reason why the records in the press have reached such astonishing heights... is because of this intensive application of specialized training in the press. [Russian champion] Novak presses every day, likewise [American champion] Davis..." Isn't interesting that with all the 'modern advances' today you will have an easier time finding a bodybuilder who does not lie about his arm size than one who can clean and press his bodyweight?

George Walsh, a British physical culture authority from those days of better men, told the story of a young man who pushed his C&P up from 160 to 200 pounds in a year. 200 pounds may not sound like a lot if you have never pressed heavy overhead but let me put this in perspective for you. A 350-pound bencher friend of mine – and we are talking about a strict, paused, no assistance equipment BP – barely cleaned and pressed 155 pounds!

The young Englishman started by military pressing 115 pounds three times a day, each time in five sets of three. That is forty-five daily reps! Every day he added a tiny washer to the bar; the jumps were so small that they totaled barely a pound a week. Get mini-plates or just improvise them out of metal wire or something similar.

This classic method that flies in the face of all the modern day pseudoscience will do wonders for your delts, provided you do no other presses, shoulder, pec, and triceps work, keep your reps super low, and stay away from muscle failure. "…while high numbers of reps are successful with a few unusual men, the majority find that a more conservative number of repetitions are best." Walsh mentions another physical culturalist who totally failed on a similar system of training by doing too many reps per set, seven specifically (Isn't it funny that these days seven reps qualify as 'low'?). And "when he dropped to three reps per set, he was eminently successful." Some things never change.

THE SOTS PRESS: AN EXTREME SHOULDER WORKOUT WITHOUT AN EXTREME WEIGHT

Question: I am on the road a lot and I often end up working out in hotel gyms that only have light dumbbells and machines. Lateral raises hurt my shoulders; are there any compound shoulder exercises I can do under the circumstances?

Do the Sots press named after Victor Sots, an early 1980s world champion weightlifter from Russia. It is a hit at our kettlebell instructor certification courses. Senior RKC Jeff O'Connor can Sots press a pair of 106-pound kettlebells. What a killer blend of strength and flexibility!

Take a very light dumbbell or kettlebell – if you can military press an 88-pound kettlebell for reps you might or might not get a single with a 53-pounder in the Sots press! – clean it, and squat rock bottom. Make sure your heels stay planted. Press!

Why is it so hard? Because there is no way you can cheat. And because, in addition to the weight of the bell, you are dealing with the resistance of your tight antagonist muscles. You could say that you are driving with your parking brake on. Remove the brakes with strength-flexibility drills such as the Sots press and you will have an easier time pressing weights in conventional strength exercises. You will also put on new muscle. You cannot help noticing an intense and unusual contraction of the upper back and the triceps as you are suffering through the humbling and awkward Sots press. Variety is the spice of bodybuilding life; because the nature of the strength-flexibility overload is so different from that of your usual boring exercises you are guaranteed new growth.

A few tips. Work in multiple sets of one to two reps as your strength-flexibility quickly drops off. Do not get frustrated; the Sots press is what the doctor ordered for every tight bodybuilder, even if he has all the weight he needs for conventional military presses. Practice this drill for a few months – and your shoulders will be as square as those of the Red Army show-off troops on the October Revolution anniversary parade!

BUILD CANNONBALL DELTS YESTERDAY WITH AN OLD TIME STRENGTH FEAT

Question: I am sick of having puny shoulders! I will do anything to fill them out ASAP!

Repetition dumbbell or kettlebell cleans and presses will send you shopping for new clothes in a hurry. Since studly John Allstadt, RKC started hitting kettlebell C&Ps, he quickly gained twelve pounds of muscle even though he was not even trying to gain weight.

This exercise is so powerful that Ethan Reeve, RKC the head strength and conditioning coach at Wake Forest University, believes that repping out C&Ps with a pair of seventy pound kettlebells makes a much better strength test for football players than bench pressing 225 for reps.

Brooks Kubik, the author of *Dinosaur Training*, is also a fan of the repetition dumbbell clean and press. His website quotes famous pre-World War II strongman and bodybuilder Sig Klein who urged aiming high for cleaning and pressing a pair of seventy-five pound dumbbells a dozen times. According to Klein very few men could complete that feat. I am sure that in these days of bench and seated presses and glass backs that number has dropped even lower.

Clean the bells from a hang or a swing before each press. This is what makes this drill so productive. Cleaning before each press adds work to the delts, hits the shoulders and the upper back from a different angle, and also helps you to get tight before the next rep.

The business of 'getting tight' is very important. If you do more than a couple of repetitions from your shoulders your waist and the rest of your power base will lose its tightness. This results in mediocre presses and back injuries. When you reclean the bells before each press, you are forced to brace your body to accept the shock. It is like loading a spring before the press. Make sure to press without any delay or you will lose some tightness.

Henry Duval, an old-timer friend of mine, saw the famous weightlifter David Ashman practice his jerks with 500 pounds. He could not clean that weight by himself. Instead of simply taking the barbell from the stands set up at his chest level Ashman had two guys, one on each end of the bar, help him clean the weight in a precisely synchronized and dangerous effort. Ashman understood that he could never get tight enough under a dead weight sitting in the rack. If he was willing to go to all the trouble with a huge poundage, believe it that cleaning your bells before pressing them is worth it.

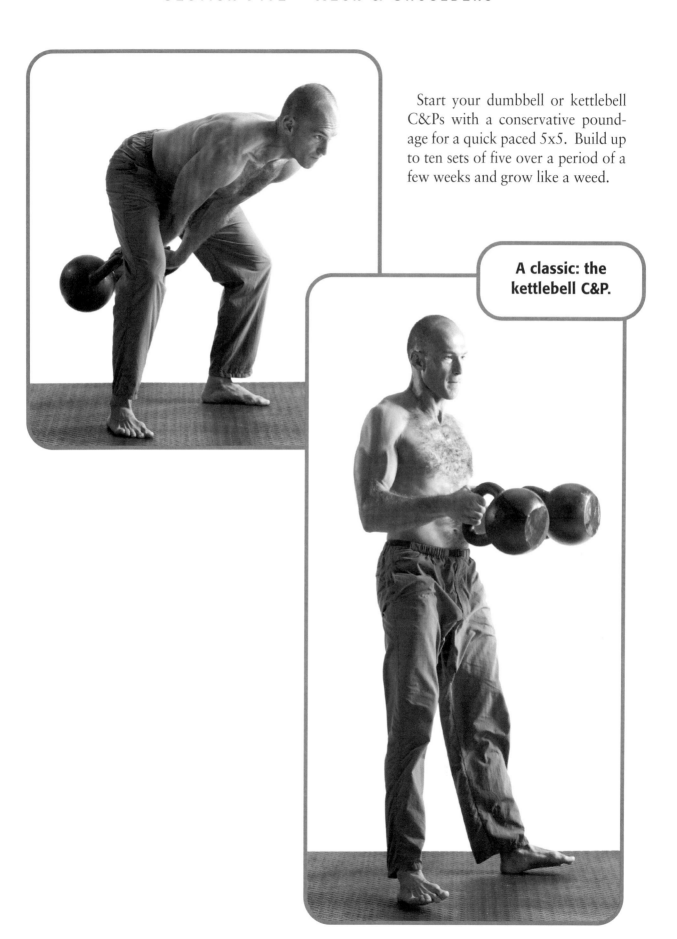

Start your dumbbell or kettlebell C&Ps with a conservative poundage for a quick paced 5x5. Build up to ten sets of five over a period of a few weeks and grow like a weed.

A classic: the kettlebell C&P.

The business of 'getting tight' is very important. If you do more than a couple of repetitions from your shoulders your waist and the rest of your power base will lose its tightness.

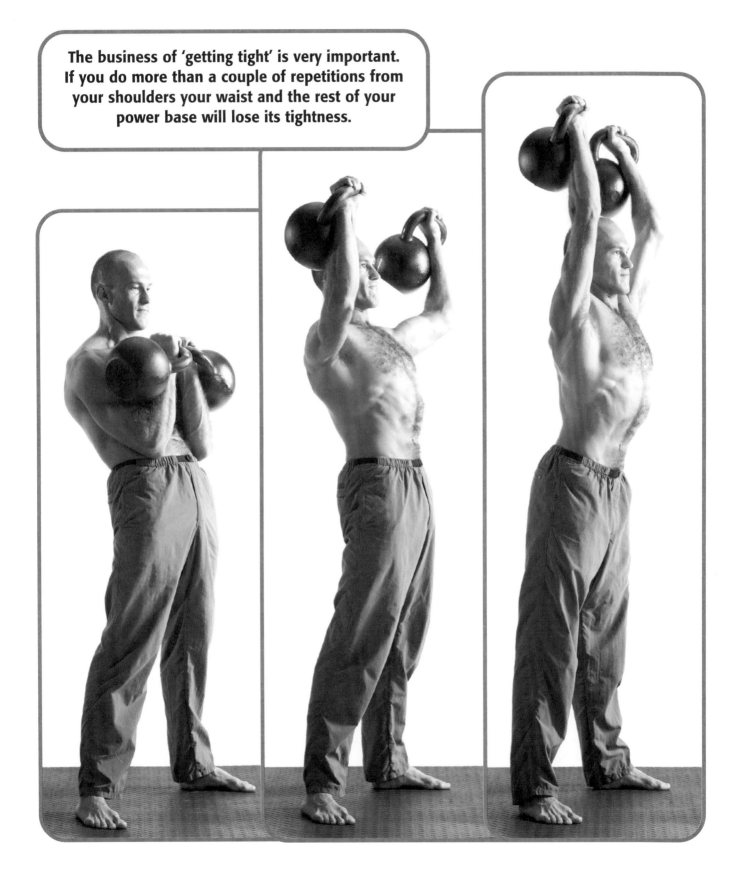

THE SHOULDER FRIENDLY SEE-SAW PRESS

Question: Because of an old shoulder injury my arm locks out slightly to the side rather than straight up when I press overhead. This severely limits my dumbbell press poundages. Any ideas?

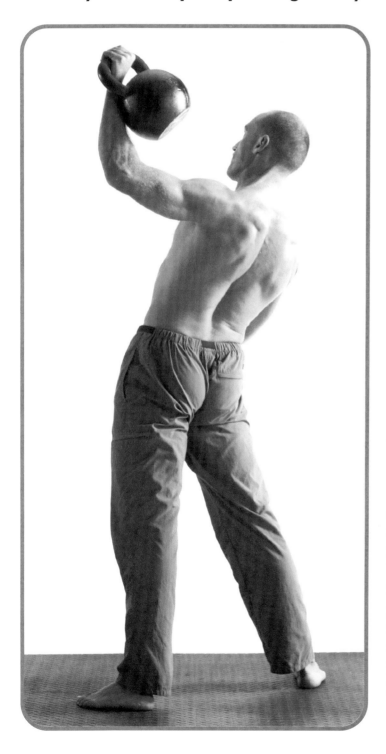

Try the alternate kettlebell or dumbbell press, but with a 'twist'. Imagine that there is an invisible connection between the bells, as if they are parked on the opposite ends of a teeter-totter. Say you have locked out the left bell overhead and your right is still at the shoulder. Now start actively 'pulling' the left dumbbell down. Visualize that it is pushing down on the teeter-totter and makes the opposite bell go up.

As the bell is coming up push your hips under it. Eventually your hips should move side to side in rhythm with your presses. You will discover that turning your feet out about forty-five degrees and spreading them wider than your shoulders will help. So will keeping your quads flexed and your knees locked.

I promise that you will love the see-saw press. It is very shoulder friendly and there is an awesome powerful feeling to it. Thanks to an obscure neurological phenomenon, you will be able to handle more weight for more reps than would be possible if you pressed the bells together or separately but out of sync. Another benefit is a solid oblique workout. Even your lats will get in on the action if you do it right. Enjoy!

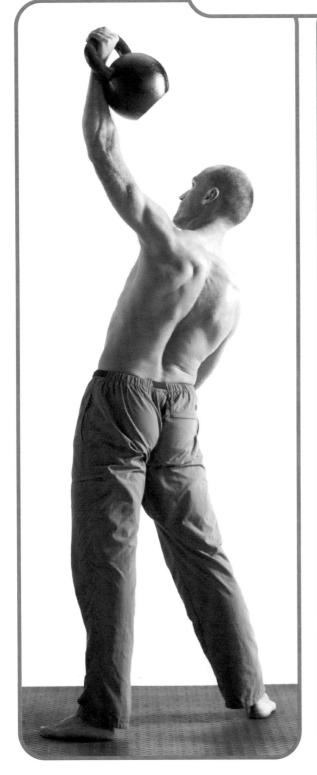
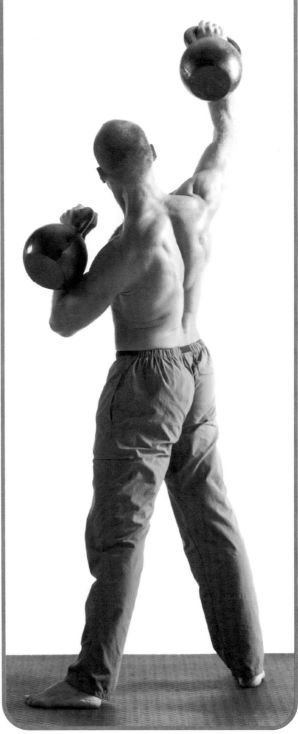

The kettlebell see-saw press: hard on the muscles, easy on the joints.

You will love the see-saw press. It is very shoulder friendly and there is an awesome powerful feeling to it.

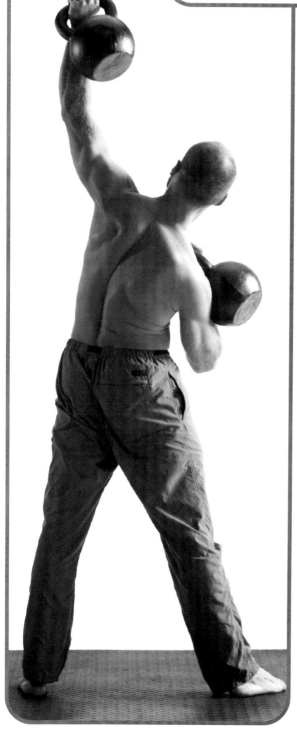
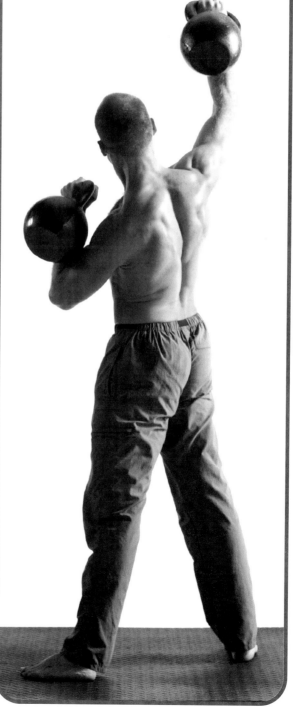

THE NECK AND TRAPS, THE HALLMARKS OF AN ELITE ATHLETE

Question: Do I need direct trap and neck work?

It depends. Powerlifters generally have very developed necks and traps just from deadlifts. Heavy explosive barbell shrugs as practiced by Olympic weightlifters quickly pack a lot of meat on both the neck and the traps. Just look at the photos of Russian weightlifting legend David Rigert.

If you wish to max out your neck size, add neck harness work to the above. Ironmind.com sells the best rig on the market. Certain sports demand highly specialized neck exercises that must be learned from professionals in your chosen sport. To give you an idea of sport specific neck training, here is an old school boxing drill I learned from boxing coach Steve Baccari, RKC.

"Lie on your stomach; place your hands under your jaw." Steve showed me how he makes a fist with one hand and sets it down on the ground, thumb up. Then he wraps the fist with his other hand. What you get is a comfortable cup to fit your jaw in. "Have a training partner place his hands on the top of your head and slowly apply pressure. Slowly open and close your mouth. This will strengthen your jaw muscles and help prevent your lower jaw from slamming into the base of your skull. Which is what happens when you get hit on the button, as they say in the sport."

Baccari demonstrates this drill on the *Power Behind the Punch* DVD available from dragon-door.com.

CANNONBALL DELTS WITHOUT DIRECT DELT WORK?

Question: Some bodybuilding coaches recommend foregoing deltoid exercises altogether. They argue that between benching and heavy back exercises your shoulders are covered. Is it true?

You have described a valid training approach. Indeed, heavy bench presses, pullups, cleans, etc. cannot help hitting your shoulders hard. They will grow. All you need to do is take a look at powerlifters.

If you decide to go this route, make sure that your back receives at least as much attention as your bench. And, if you forego the overhead lifts, you will have to spend plenty of time working on your shoulder girdle's flexibility. Iron rats who make the BP the cornerstone of their routine are notorious for not being able to scratch their backs without rubbing against the doorway – and having terrible postures. "Dude, are you sure you did not forget to take off your bench shirt?"

By the way, 'flexibility' does not mean lowering your dumbbells deeper during your dumbbell BPs; that just wrecks your shoulders. In this context 'flexibility' is the ability to raise your locked arms overhead slightly behind your ears and close to the head – and a few other angles that kettlebell lifters and Olympic weightlifters are good at and bodybuilders and powerlifters suck at.

SORE SHOULDERS NO MORE

Question: Between my chest work and my delt routine I tend to easily overtrain my shoulders. Should I do fewer sets?

Cutting the weekly volume might solve your problem but you need to see the big picture. Chances are, you are doing way too many sets and reps of junky, non-productive exercises: the pec deck, bench dips, etc. Cut those out and focus on the basics: various presses with free weights. Keep your reps low, four to six, and do not push to failure. If you insist, leave one isolation type exercise per body part in your routine, a strategy employed by many successful bodybuilders.

Always training on the nerve and never backing off, a typical bodybuilding sin, is another common destroyer of shoulders. I have said it many times: cycle! That simply means starting with a light weight and building it up over a period of weeks. Do not rep out with a light poundage in the beginning of the cycle; it is supposed to be easy.

Learn to 'keep your shoulders in their sockets'. Letting your shoulders shrug up or move forward during chest and delt exercises is very rough on the rotator cuffs. Visualizing that you are 'pushing yourself away from the weight' rather than pushing the weight up is an effective imagery for keeping your shoulders down.

LATERAL RAISES MINUS THE HEADACHE

Question: My neck gets tight after I do lateral raises and I get a headache. Should I use a lighter weight?

I am sick and tired of seeing every type of exercise discomfort being 'solved' by lightening the load. It is the path of least resistance – literally. Learn to perform your exercises properly!

When it comes to laterals, your problem is raising the bells too high and shrugging your shoulders. The dumbbells have no business going up higher than your shoulders in this drill. So keep your lats tight to keep your shoulder girdle down.

Also, use this effective imagery from martial arts. Instead of focusing on getting the weights up, visualize reaching out with your arms to the opposite walls. Basically, project your energy outward rather than upward. Not only will your neck give you a break, you are going to overload your delts more effectively and you are likely to be able to lift heavier bells.

A word on breathing. In this exercise you are better off inhaling steadily through your nose on the way up and exhaling on the way down.

FYI, the above tips apply just as much to bent over laterals. It goes without saying, keep your elbows locked.

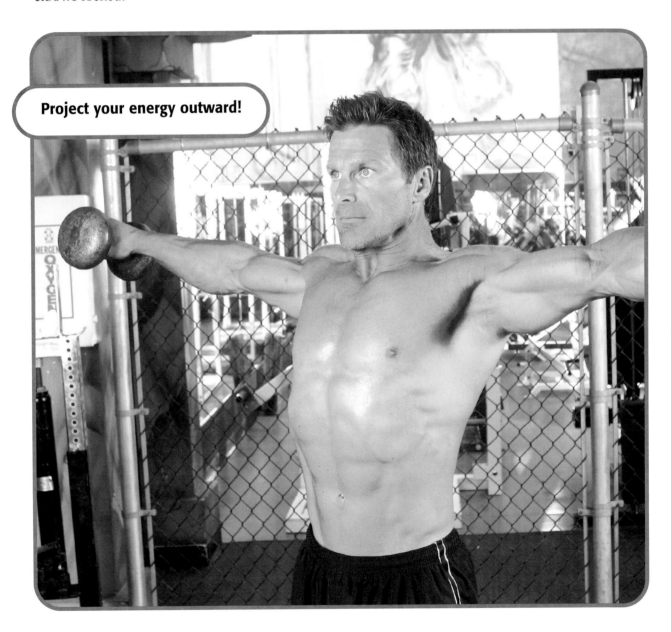

Project your energy outward!

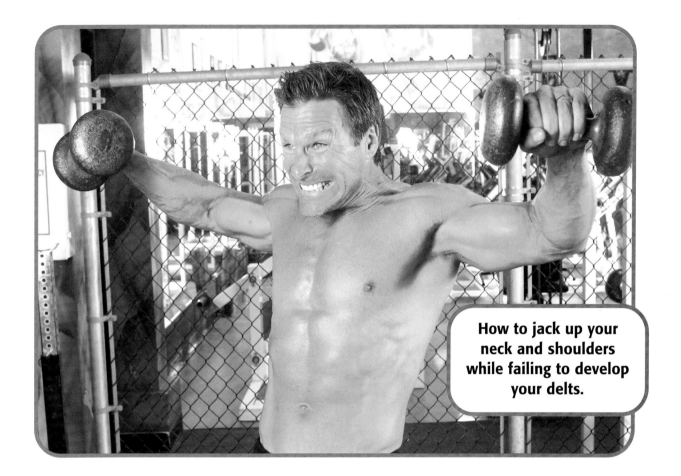

How to jack up your neck and shoulders while failing to develop your delts.

ALTERNATIVES TO THE PRESS BEHIND THE NECK

Question: I used to get great results from presses behind the neck but my neck and shoulders cannot take PBNs any more. Are there any safer alternatives to my favorite deltoid movement?

One option is to switch to military presses from the chest but make a point of leaning against the bar as it is passing your eyes and locking out in the PBN top position.

Another is to keep on pressing behind the neck but work one shoulder at a time. The one arm PBN does not require an Olympic weightlifter's flexibility.

Stick to the long Olympic bar; it is less likely, than a thick dumbbell, to wrench your shoulder back . Start the press with your elbow tucked into your side, as far back as comfortable. Keep the bar as much in line with your shoulders as your flexibility allows it. As the bar is passing your head, lean forward slightly to get a tight contraction of your posterior delts and the upper back muscles.

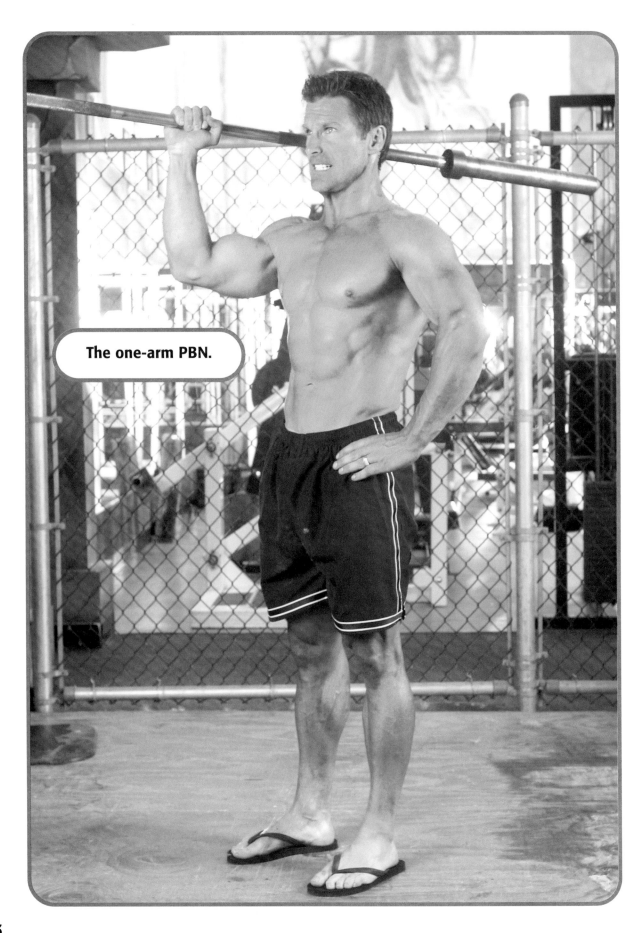

The one-arm PBN.

ROTATOR CUFF WORK –
IS IT WORTH THE TROUBLE?

Question: Is it a good idea to add rotator cuff work to my routine?

If you have an injury and your doctor tells you to – definitely. Otherwise, I do not see the point. Well-balanced training – not your usual mix of benches and curls – should take care of your cuffs. York Barbell Club legend Bill Starr recalls that in the days when iron rats did fewer benches and more heavy overhead work no one even heard of rotator cuff problems. In the Russian military, where pushups are not a part of the PT test and kettlebell snatches are, shoulder problems are almost non-existent.

Do a variety of overhead lifts, especially those demanding good flexibility and loading in planes unusual for a bodybuilder: side presses, military presses with a forward lean as the bar passes your head (the lockout looks identical to that of the press behind the neck), overhead squats, Turkish get-ups, etc. Also review your bench press technique. Stay healthy!

SEATED PRESSES FOR A TOUCHY BACK?

Question: My back hurts when I do standing barbell military presses. Should I switch to seated presses?

Forget it! Do not even think that switching to seated presses will solve your problem. Compare your spine and your legs to two springs in a series. If you remove one spring, the legs, the other, or the back, will get double the compression.

Russian scientist Robert Roman, recognized in the weightlifting community as the world's foremost expert on lifting technique, explained why some athletes have a problem with back bending during clean and presses. He said that when the waist muscles and the glutes are relaxed the athlete ends up literally pushing his torso away from the heavy weight, especially if he has a flexible spine. According to Roman, the solution is to keep the glutes and the midsection tight. Imagine that someone is about to punch you in the gut – that can be arranged! – and brace your stomach against the punch. At the same time clench your butt cheeks hard and tuck your butt under. The muscle action is identical to that in the Janda situp.

Another one of Roman's suggestions is to bring your feet closer together. This will further reduce the back bend. Consider going to the extreme and clicking your heels together as old timers used to do. Didn't you know that it was standing at 'At-ten-tion!' that gave the military press its name?

If you opt for the heels together style of military pressing squeeze your thighs together by flexing the adductors. Thanks to an obscure neurological phenomenon, this will amplify the tension in your abdominals. Your stability and power will go up even more.

SECTION SIX

ARMS

CONTENTS

Articles

- *Armed and Dangerous (the 'Strong as You Look' Series)*

- *The Top Ten Russian Arm Training Secrets*

Questions and Answers

- *Russian powerlifting triceps blaster*

- *Elbow friendly straight bar curls*

- *Forearm specialization for the pipe masters*

- *Clubbells™: for totally awesome forearms*

- *Build huge biceps with… the bench press!*

- *Are squats needed for big pipes?*

ARMED AND DANGEROUS
(THE 'STRONG AS YOU LOOK' SERIES)

1. Close grip bench press

2. Power rack barbell curl

3. Towel hammer curl/triceps extension superset

4. Barbell finger rolls

5. Straight arm wrist extension

1. CLOSE GRIP BENCH PRESS

A 1960s study by Travill revealed that unless you use maximal or near maximal weights two out of the three heads of your triceps are having a smoke break. In other words, the only way to get that horseshoe is by piling on some serious poundage. One of the best ways to do it is with close grip bench presses.

Although everyone is familiar with this move, a few words on the technique are in order. To learn how to align your hands in the safest and most powerful manner straighten out your arms, open your palms and bring your hands together. Your thumbs and index fingers will form a 'diamond'. Without changing the wrists' position slide your hands out until they are just outside the smooth part of the barbell. Grip the bar and unrack it.

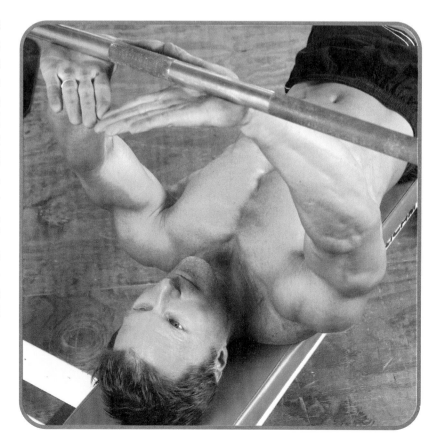

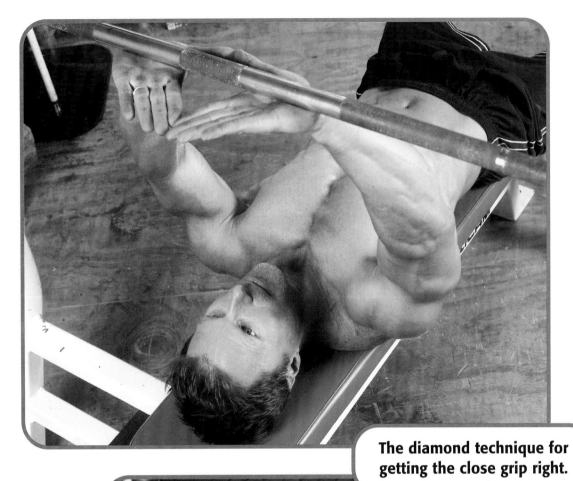

The diamond technique for getting the close grip right.

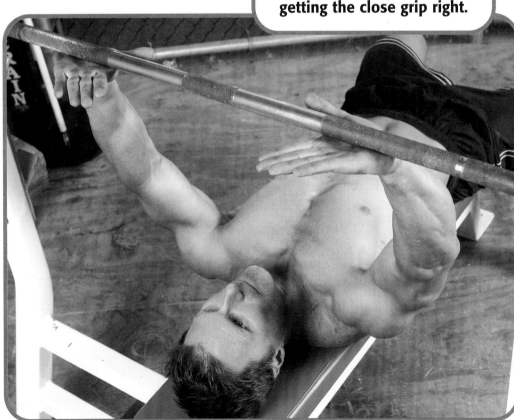

Keep your shoulder blades pinched together and your chest up. Squeeze the bar tight and imagine that you are trying to 'tear it apart'. If you have heavy-duty rubber bands, you owe it to yourself to try the following invention of the powerlifting Westside Barbell Club. Loop the band around your wrists. Push out with your straight arms to stretch the band, unrack your barbell and do your close grips. The inward pressure from the rubber cord will force you to squeeze the bar to pulp and 'tear it apart'.

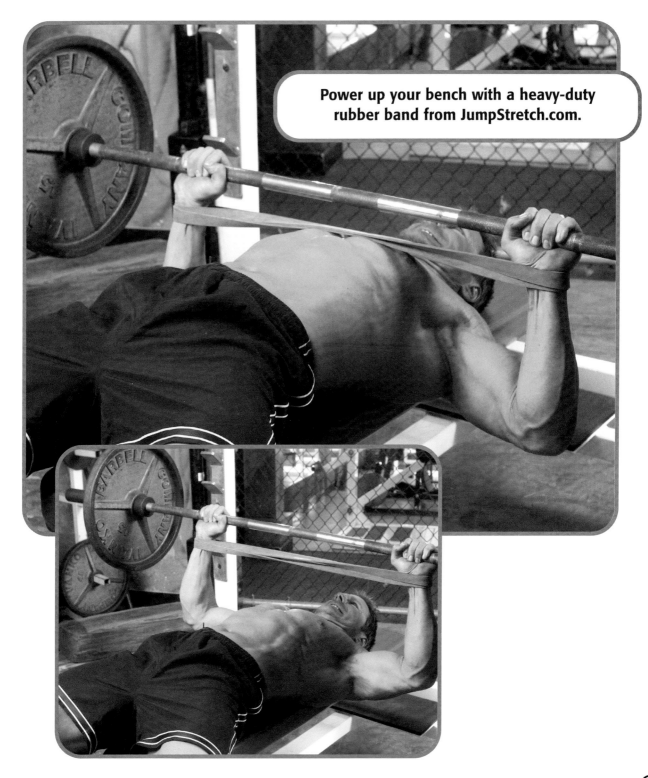

Power up your bench with a heavy-duty rubber band from JumpStretch.com.

Start with a weight you could probably press twelve times or so and do five reps. After a brief rest add ten pounds and do another five. Keep going up until you cannot get five clean reps, then work your way back down, still in fives.

Recommended sets & reps: pyramid up and down in sets of 5 reps

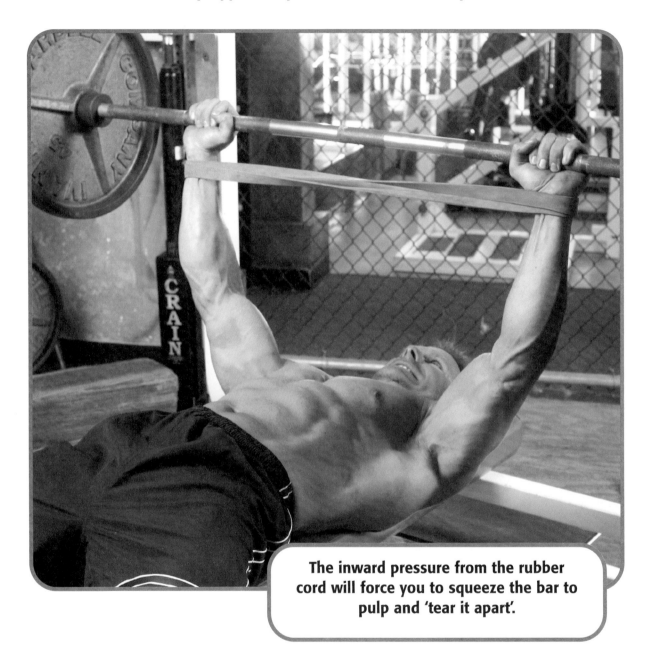

The inward pressure from the rubber cord will force you to squeeze the bar to pulp and 'tear it apart'.

2. POWER RACK BARBELL CURL

Few bodybuilders would argue that there is a better biceps builder than a heavy barbell curl. The problem is, most muscleheads curl with so much body English that only their chiropractors' accounts see any gains.

The answer is the power rack. It deprives you of the questionably luxury of starting your curls with a swing. Park an empty barbell on safety pins inside the cage. Set up the pins at a level where your arms are almost straight when you are grabbing the barbell. Keep your shoulders down when figuring out the depth and throughout the curl.

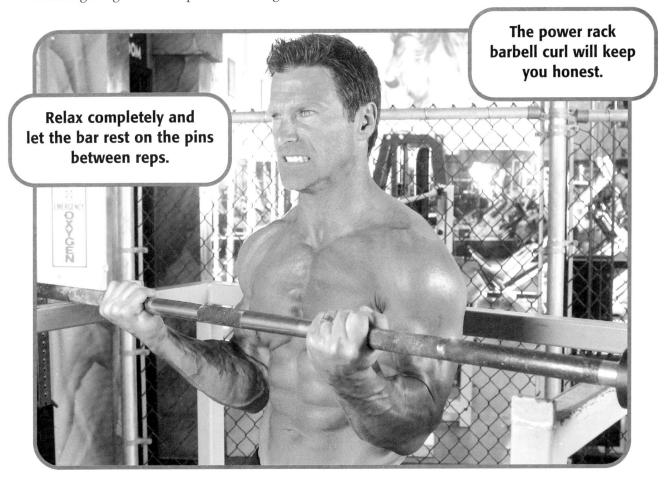

The power rack barbell curl will keep you honest.

Relax completely and let the bar rest on the pins between reps.

Load up the bar with a weight you can curl traditionally for fifteen reps or so. Stand inside the cage, take a breath, tense up, and curl. Relax completely and let the bar rest on the pins between reps. Do as many reps as you can in good form; stop before reaching failure.

Grab an upright of the power cage behind you and stretch your bis between sets. After a brief rest add five to ten pounds and do another set. And another one. Ideally, on your third set you will be able to do no more than three reps. But if you have reached the top of the pyramid in two or four sets it is okay.

Move the pins up one notch, unload the barbell and repeat the sequence. This should be plenty for your first workout. Each consecutive workout, add an extra level which translates into another three sets or so. If you find that this is too much, use good judgment and add a level every second or third workout – or even less frequently.

By the time you have worked your way up to two or three-inch partials you will have added some serious meat to your bis, not to mention some real rather than 'swinging' strength. And yes, finally you have a legit reason to curl inside a power cage! (You might find it amusing that S&C Coach John Davies, disgusted with bodybuilders who never use the squat rack for anything but curls, calls it 'the curl rack'.)

Recommended sets & reps: 2-4x3-10 per level

3. TOWEL HAMMER CURL/TRICEPS EXTENSION SUPERSET

You do not need any other curling exercise as long as you are following the above power rack curl routine. But if your arms still have some gas left – which I find highly unlikely – and you have built up tolerance to high volume training finish them off with the towel hammer curl/elbow extension superset. You may use a towel fed through the handle of a kettlebell or a rope on a low cable stack.

Start by doing strict hammer curls with a good contraction on the top and a complete extension on the bottom. Immediately turn around and do triceps extensions. Do not let your elbows flare.

Rest for no more than thirty seconds and repeat the superset. And one more time for good measure.

Recommended sets & reps: 2-3x5-10

4. BARBELL FINGER ROLLS

When elite rock climber Todd Skinner met Soviet climbers for the first time on the World Cup circuit, reports Eric Hörst in Flash Training, he was amazed at their finger strength – 'contact strength' as they call it – and the size of their forearms. The Russians reluctantly revealed their secret: heavy barbell finger rolls.

Pick up a barbell as you would for curls; make sure the bar has rotating sleeves. Open your palms and let the bar roll down until it almost falls out of your fingers. It is a good idea to do this drill in a power rack. Bring the bar back up using your finger strength; do not flex your wrists!

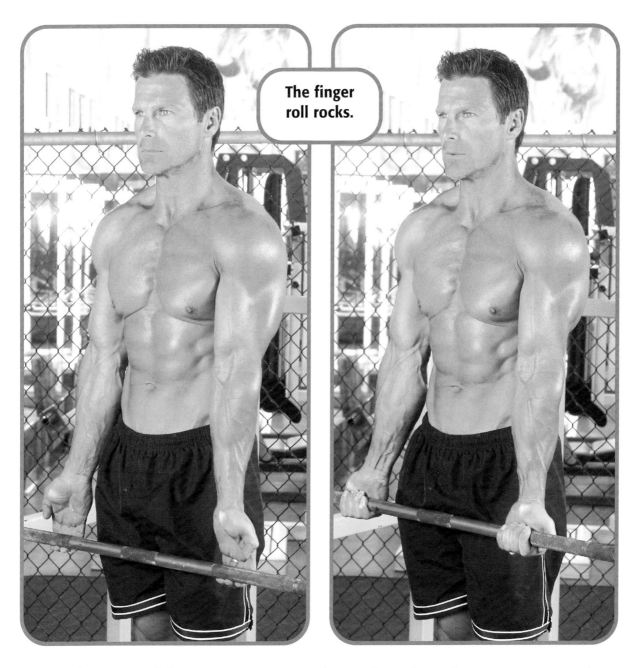

The finger roll rocks.

Do six heavy sets of three to six reps resting three to five minutes between your sets twice a week. Climbers new to this exercise typically start with a poundage equal to their bodyweight, but you must keep in mind that their Popeye forearms are already supremely conditioned, so be more conservative. An eventual goal: reps with 150% of your bodyweight. Who said that forearms should be trained with high reps and sissy weights?!

The barbell finger roll is a power drill. If you find that you are too smoked from all the curls to do it heavy, move the finger rolls from your arm day to a non-pulling workout, e.g. following your legs or benches.

Recommended sets & reps: 6x3-6

5. STRAIGHT ARM WRIST EXTENSION

Well-developed wrist extensors on top of your forearm will go a long way towards reducing the odds of elbow tendonitis. Here is an unusual way to train them.

Grab a light dumbbell in one hand or a barbell in both and lay your arms across a preacher curl bench or a similar elevation. The bar should be at your shoulder level or even higher. Now do your reverse wrist curls while keeping your elbows straight. You cannot help noticing a greater stretch on top of your forearm.

Instead of mindlessly muscling the bell up, imagine that you are performing a palm strike. Your triceps will tense up; let them.

You may do this drill between sets of finger rolls or in the end of your arm workout. Do 5x5 starting very light and build up to 5RM in a few weeks.

Recommended sets & reps: 5x5

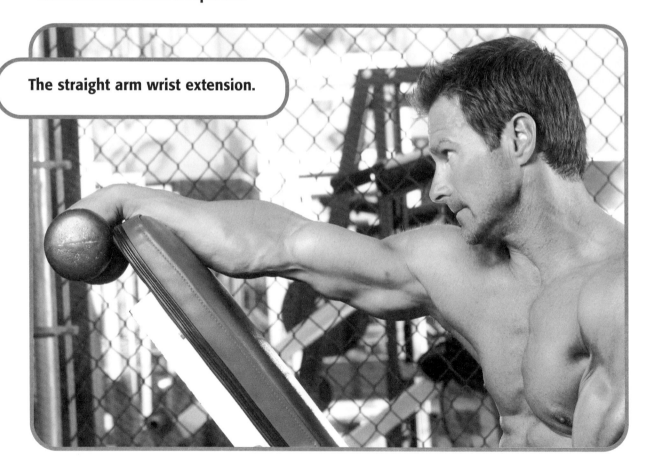

The straight arm wrist extension.

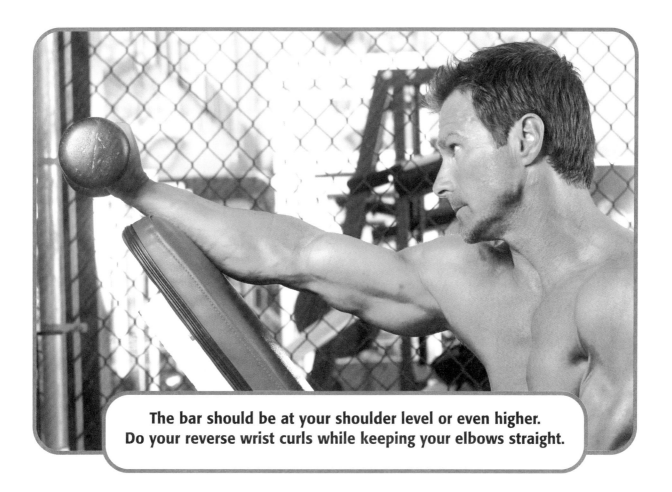

The bar should be at your shoulder level or even higher. Do your reverse wrist curls while keeping your elbows straight.

FREQUENTLY ASKED QUESTIONS ABOUT ARM TRAINING

Question: My shoulders tend to come up when I curl heavy. It hurts them and I don't feel much in my bis. Should I reduce the poundage or what?

What you need to do is push your shoulders away from your ears and lock your lats in place before curling. Then, instead of aiming to bring the bar up, visualize that you are trying to push your body into the ground by pressing away from the bar. This imagery is so critical to safe and powerful curling that I will say it again: push your rigid body straight through the ground by pressing away from the bar.

You should feel pressure in your feet and tension in your abs if you do it right. Chances are, not only will your shoulders will stop getting aggravated, your curl poundage will suddenly go up.

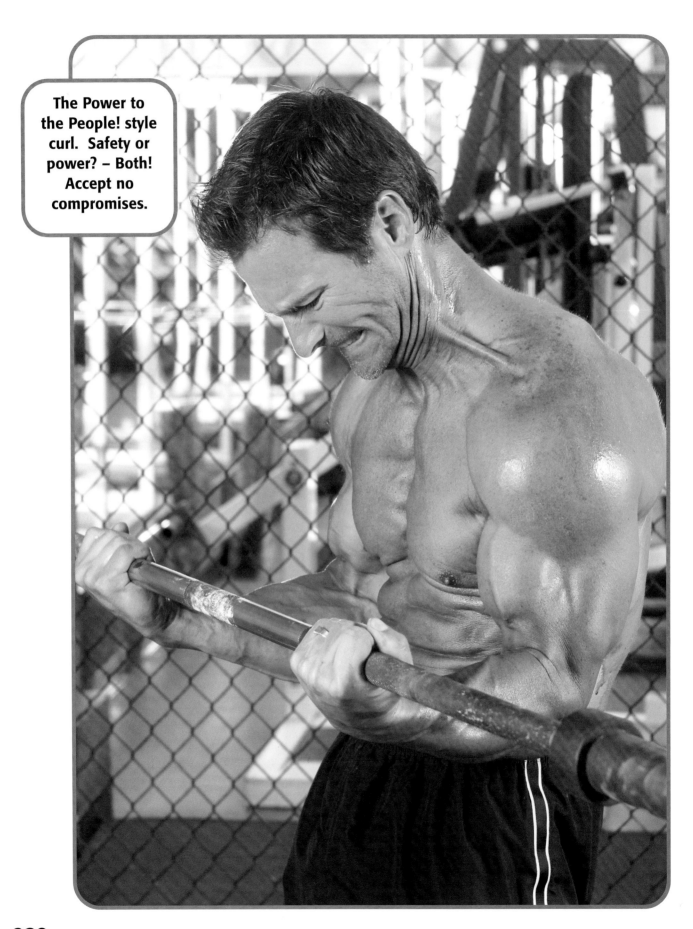

The Power to the People! style curl. Safety or power? – Both! Accept no compromises.

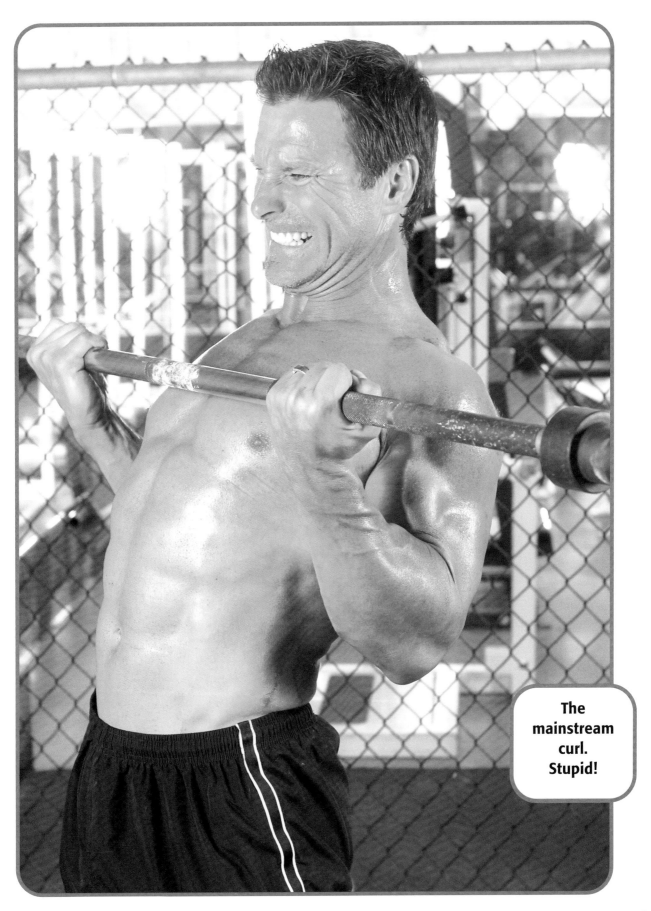

The mainstream curl. Stupid!

Question: Do I have to fully straighten out my elbows when doing curls?

Unless the exercise clearly specifies a partial range of motion (e.g. the power rack curl in this feature), the answer is yes. Failing to get a full extension leads to 'contracture' or loss of flexibility usually associated with aging, a lame curl 1RM, and an elbow prone to injuries during curls, pitching a ball, etc.

Straighten out your arm actively, by contracting your triceps, and stay tight on the bottom. Especially pay attention to these tips during preacher curls. These have been unjustly blamed for many tendon injuries. The blame belongs to the routine failure to extend the elbows on the bottom. The bodybuilder loses flexibility and develops an unbalanced strength curve: he is extremely weak at the very bottom because he never goes there. Then one day the muscle head hits heavy preacher curls, hits muscle failure, and the barbell boldly goes where it has never gone before – to complete elbow extension. Pop! goes the tendon and the biceps rolls up like a curtain.

Get a full extension in your curls, lower the weight with your triceps, stay tight, and do not train to failure. Long live your pipes!

Question: My elbow hurts when I do skull crushers, French presses, and similar triceps exercises. What should I do?

Provided it is not your doctor's problem, you could try a couple of things. First, squeeze the bell hard, especially with your little and ring fingers: keep the 'energy' on the 'triceps side' of the arm. This will take some load off your elbows and make you stronger at the same time. Second, bulge your biceps when you are getting close to the bottom of the movement; this cushion should help. Third, and I hate to state the obvious, do not bounce.

And if this does not help, you have another 100 triceps exercises to choose from, so don't sweat it if you are forced to say goodbye to one.

Question: I want to be able to do dips but I am not strong enough yet. Should I do bench dips?

Bench dips, where you park your feet on a bench and press up from another bench behind you, is one of the worst things you could do to your shoulders, short of being roughed up by a Brazilian Jiu Jitsu expert. You could tear your pecs too.

If you want to work up to dips do assisted real dips. Get a sturdy and long bungee cord (I recommend one from Jump Stretch), loop it around the parallel bars, stretch it and stand on it. Dip! The band will help you up through the hard lower half of the dip. Be careful; if the cord slips you could be heading for trouble. Keeping your abs tight will help you stay balanced.

Power to you!

THE TOP TEN RUSSIAN ARM TRAINING SECRETS

Comrade, did you know that Russian wrestler and strongman Ivan Poddubny sported a pair of twenty-one inch guns nearly a century before steroids? Wouldn't you want to learn the Russian arm training secrets?

The following Top Ten, old timers' intuitive discoveries plus cutting edge modern research, are guaranteed to put up to two inches on your arms in just a couple of months provided you back them up with big eating and a solid nine and a half hours of sleep a night.

BICEPS

1. Squeeze your 'bells to pulp when doing biceps work.

Make a fist. A white-knuckle fist! Do your feel how tension spreads from your forearm into your biceps?

According to the neurological *Law of Irradiation*, a contracting muscle spills its excitation over into its neighbors. Just the opposite of the silly and impossible notion of isolation, irradiation is a 'muscle software' that fortifies any effort. Due to an abnormally high number of nerves in your paws, anything that happens with your gripping muscles deeply affects your whole body – especially the nearby bis and tris. You can take an advantage of this powerful neural program by putting a hard squeeze on your barbells or dumbbells. The tension in the biceps will be off the charts. The result: unbelievable gains.

2. Always contract your abs and glutes when working your bis.

This bizarre maneuver also takes advantage of irradiation. In case you think that getting more juice into your arms by clenching your cheeks is preposterous try this party trick. Give your friend the hardest handshake you can muster. Shake off the tension, rest for a minute, then repeat the test. This time, in addition to trying to demolish your fellow muscle head's claw, flex your glutes as if you are trying to pinch a coin, and brace your abs for an imaginary punch. Expect an 'Ouch!'

In addition to powering up your curls, the ab and glute contraction will insure that you do not lean back during your curls. Power and safety, accept no compromises!

3. Lower the weights actively with your triceps.

Cramp your biceps on the top of the curl and actively lower the weight with the power of your triceps. You should feel that you are stretching a rubber band inside your bis.

Stay tight, do not relax even when you have reached the bottom – and by the bottom I mean the full elbow extension!   Reverse the movement of the tightly wound muscle spring by squeezing your barbell or dumbbell.

This unusual technique dramatically improves your control of the iron, especially on the bottom of the curl ROM. Finally you shall be able to blast your muscles instead of the tendons.

4. Perform Loaded Passive Stretches for the biceps between sets.

In a nutshell – or "in a nutcase" as I used to say in my early years in America – stretching the target muscles with weights between your sets of bodybuilding exercise will make you grow.

Right after each set of a biceps drill sit on an incline bench with a pair of moderately heavy dumbbells and let them stretch out your pumped guns. Do not relax your muscles as you are instructed for conventional stretches. Do not contract them in the isometric stretch fashion; just let them be. This is the so-called 'loaded stretching' technique from Russia, a remarkable tool for adding muscle and power.

Stretch for ten seconds right after each set. If you take long rest periods between your sets, stretch once more a minute before the next set.

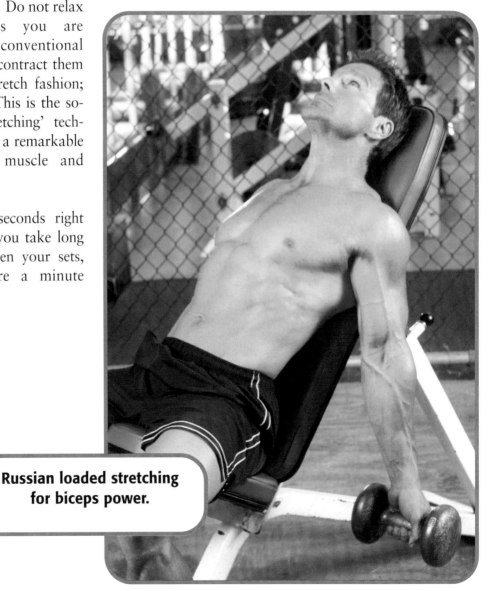

Russian loaded stretching for biceps power.

5. Periodically work both your biceps and your triceps with high sets of low reps, e.g. 10x5, not to failure.

If you boil the *energetic theory of muscle hypertrophy* down to gym speak, you will learn a powerfully simple growth formula. "If you get a pump while training with heavy weights you will get big."

Both fatigue and tension need to be present to turn on the cells' growth machinery. Fatigue is caused by high volume, or a lot of reps performed in a workout. Tension is a function of the weight. They appear to be mutually exclusive. If you say nuts to the tonnage and crank out a zillion reps with Malibu Ken and Barbie weights, you will not generate sufficient tension. If you push towards the other extreme and follow a powerlifting peaking workout of singles and doubles, near-maximal weights, and plenty of rest in between, the muscular fatigue will be minimal and the pump non-existent. And if you go to failure on all your sets, the amount of weight you can use, and therefore the tension values, will be severely compromised after the very first set.

The exact arm workout practiced by 'show' units of the Soviet paratroops, the ten sets of five minus muscle failure formula is your way out of this Catch-22. Relatively low repetitions enable you to handle heavier than usual poundages. And because all sets are terminated a rep or two before you bite the dust you will be able to do plenty of sets and get a great pump. Rest for one to two minutes between the sets to maximize the effect. When you have added at least an inch to your guns make sure to drop me a line on the dragondoor.com training forum.

TRICEPS

1. Rest the weight on the base of your palm and lose the gloves.

Place the load on your hand – from a barbell, a dumbbell, a triceps pushdown bar, or even the floor if you do pushups – on the spot at the very base of your palm, below the little finger. It is the spot karate masters use for crushing their opponents or stacks of bricks.

When pressure stimulates the *mechanoreceptors* at that site, they send a command to the triceps to contract more intensely, as so-called *positive support reaction*.

The poundages on all your triceps exercises will jump upward in the very first session. You do not need to be a Ph.D. to realize that a heavier weight, lifted for the same number of repetitions, will stimulate greater strength and size gains.

It is obvious that you should not wear workout gloves in order to take advantage of this phenomenon. Senior RKC Jeff Martone quipped that a person lifting weight has as much business wearing gloves as a blind man reading Braille.

2. Do close grip bench press lockouts for the medial head

A powerlifting favorite, a four-inch close grip bench press lockout in a power rack, builds thick and ripped horseshoes without delayed gratification.

If your gym does not have a free-standing bench that you could park inside a power cage, you may lie down on the floor. Keep the tension on the tris: squeeze the bar off the pins, do not throw it or jerk it. Push your chest out and press your shoulders into the bench or floor if they are dear to you. It helps to visualize that you are pushing yourself away from the bar into the bench rather than pressing the bar up, a winning imagery from powerlifting.

3. Build the long and medial heads at once with triceps extensions/pullovers

This unusual combo enables you to handle heavy weights safely and sparks awesome growth.

Lie on the edge of a bench with a barbell – preferably an EZ bar – in your hands. A close grip is in order. Press the weight off your chest and lock out the elbows to get in the starting position.

Inhale and bend your elbows to a ninety-degree angle, as if you are about to do skull crushers. Maintaining the square elbow angle carry on the drill as a pullover. Lower the bar behind your head as deep as you can go safely. The key to preventing injuries is to keep your upper arms and forearms parallel throughout the drill. Whenever your elbows flare out your shoulders might get hurt!

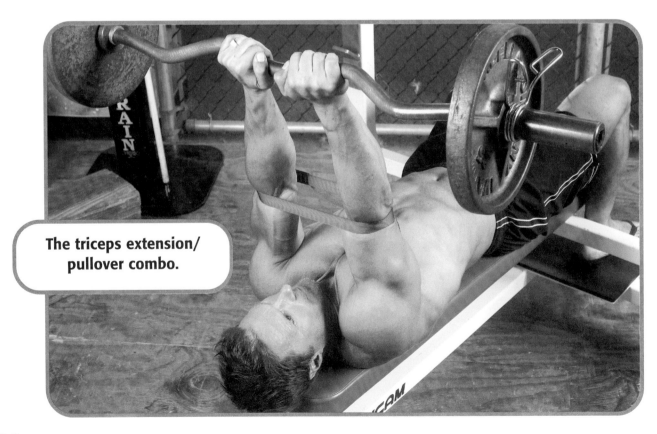

The triceps extension/ pullover combo.

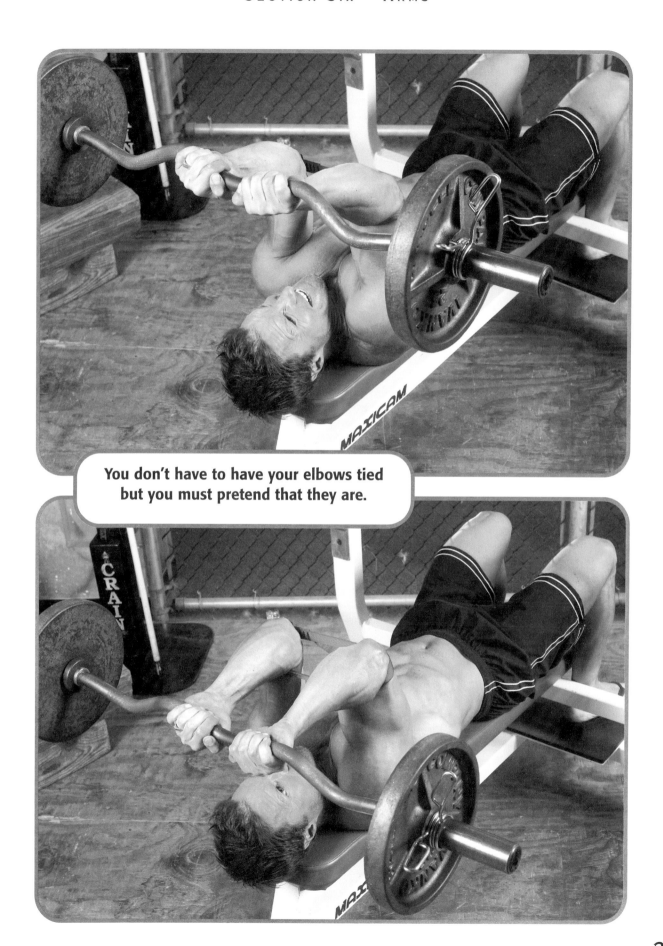

You don't have to have your elbows tied but you must pretend that they are.

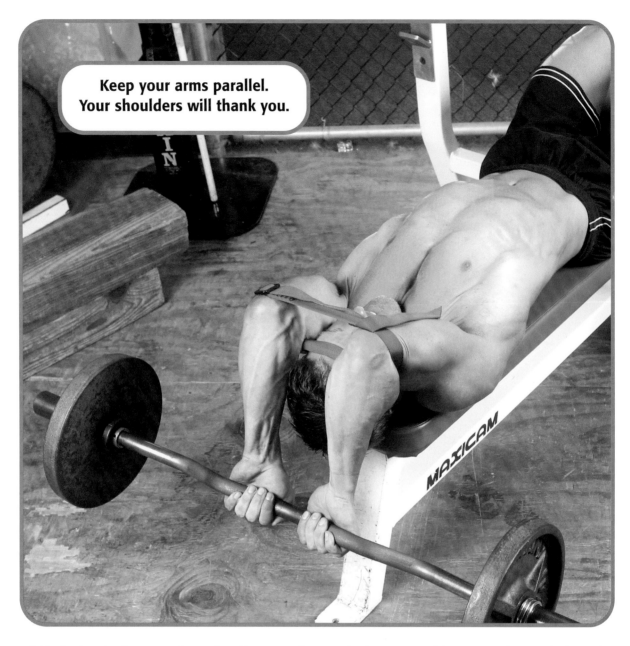

Keep your arms parallel.
Your shoulders will thank you.

Lift the bar in the opposite order. Do not relax on the bottom and keep your lats and abs tight.

4. Rip the lateral head to shreds with the curl grip bench press

This unusual press is the numero uno exercise for the lateral head of your triceps, or the outside of your arm. It also happens to be very easy on the shoulder joint because the arms are tightly 'screwed' into their sockets. If you have a shoulder injury, for example torn rotator cuffs, you will appreciate this drill as an alternative to regular benches.

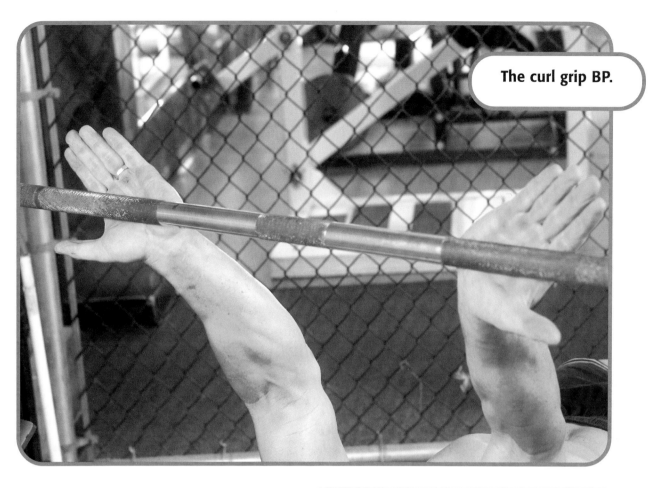

The curl grip BP.

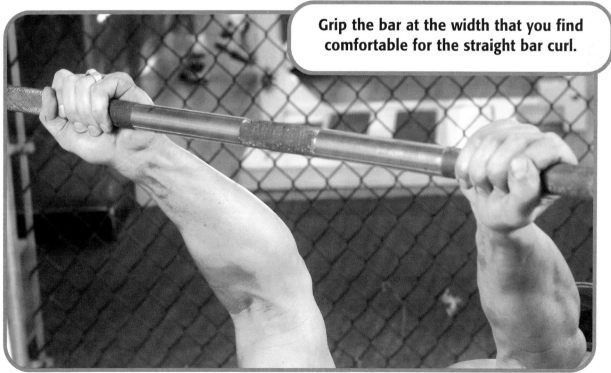

Grip the bar at the width that you find comfortable for the straight bar curl.

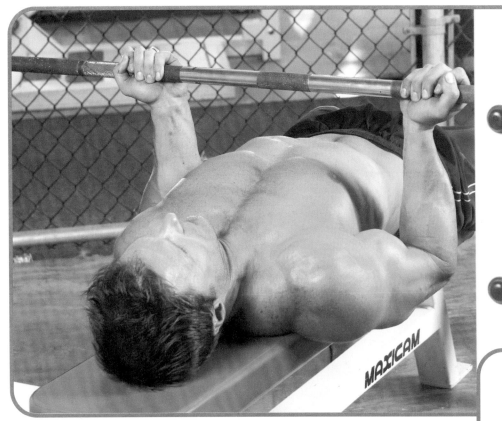

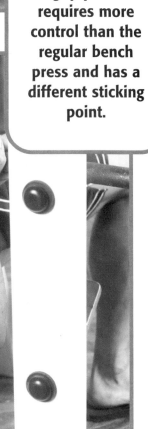

The reverse grip press requires more control than the regular bench press and has a different sticking point.

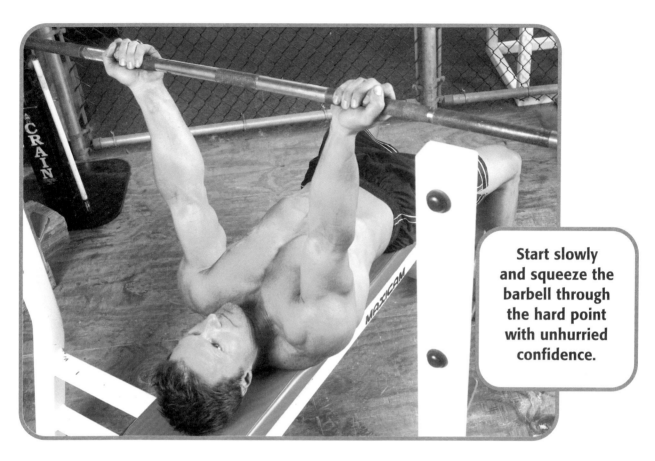

Start slowly and squeeze the barbell through the hard point with unhurried confidence.

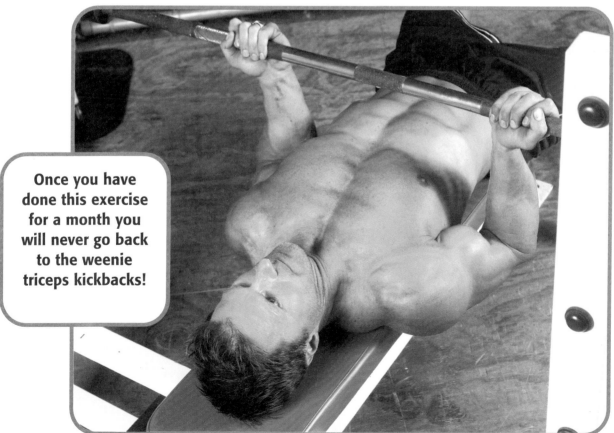

Once you have done this exercise for a month you will never go back to the weenie triceps kickbacks!

Grip the bar at the width that you find comfortable for the straight bar curl. Do not hang any plates on the bar until you find the right position. You will notice that your arms naturally go out to the sides instead of coming straight down. Turn your fingers out slightly and let the bar lie in the grooves of your hands to hit the power spot on the fleshy base of the palm and to avoid stressing out the wrists.

The reverse grip press requires more control than the regular bench press and has a different sticking point. Beware that the bar jumps off your pecs, as spry as if you were wearing a bench press shirt, and dies halfway up. The solution is not to gun the weight off your chest, in the attempt to outrun the sticking spot with momentum, but to start slowly and squeeze the barbell through the hard point with unhurried confidence.

Be certain to have a spotter who will unrack and rack the barbell for you and save you in case you lose it. Or you could do the drill alone, by pressing off the pins set in a power rack right off your chest.

Once you have done this exercise for a month you will never go back to the weenie triceps kickbacks!

5. Train your triceps heavy.

Eugene Sandow, George Hackenschmidt, and other old time Russian greats rarely if ever did high rep triceps work yet they sported symmetrical and well cut up 'horseshoes'. These early bodybuilders instinctively knew that the triceps needed very heavy stimulation. In the second half of the twentieth century science caught up with their intuitive discovery. A study by Travill found that the brunt of the triceps work, regardless of the exercise and the loading angle, is performed by the medial head. Only when the resistance gets very heavy do the lazy lateral and long heads do kick in. Which explains why many bodybuilders, especially ladies, find it so hard to define their tris: they favor light weights and high reps in their training 'for the burn'. The only road to a symmetrically developed triceps is through heavy weights, period. Do multiple sets of five on all your triceps drills and the DEA might knock on your door looking for juice, Comrade!

A time yellowed Russian poster shows a wide-eyed boy feeling the flexed biceps of an athlete with the letters 'C.C.C.P.' – the U.S.S.R. – proudly stenciled on his tightly stretched tank top. The blond giant Slav with Mr. Olympia pipes could have been a twin of the Russian boxer in Rocky IV – had he not been born half a century before Dolph Lundgren. *"Do you want to be just like him?"* demands the poster with Stalin's directness, *"–Then train!"* Train, do not aimlessly 'work out'. Go for the bull's eye with vengeance and knowledge. I provide the knowledge, you the vengeance.

QUESTIONS & ANSWERS:

RUSSIAN POWERLIFTING TRICEPS BLASTER

Question: What triceps exercises should I do for a big bench?

Igor Zavyalov, a Distinguished Coach of the Russian Federation in powerlifting, recommends the following unusual drill. Lie on your back on the floor with a barbell behind your head and do triceps extensions. Rip the weight off the floor! According to Zavyalov, this exercise is meant to build the triceps explosive strength that is a must following the bench press pause on the chest. But you would be smart to start out slow and tight and gradually, over a few weeks, add the acceleration into the equation.

You will have a better control of the bar if you focus on blasting the weight straight up, as if you are benching, rather than towards your feet. When you have locked out – throw the weight back! Yes, throw it rather than control the negative. And do not change your mind at the last moment; you do not want to start resisting a weight that has picked up some serious momentum.

Keep your elbows stationary; the Russian coach insists that you lighten up the load if your exercise evolves into a combo of the triceps extension and the pullover. Do three sets of 6-8 reps focusing on the good form rather than the poundage.

An important point: this drill is for experienced iron rats with pain free elbows. In the golden age of Russian bodybuilding, the 1980s, there was a strong belief that a muscle head had no business doing direct triceps work until he could bench 150% of his bodyweight. At that point triceps assistance helps to blow past the point of diminishing returns; before that it just overtrains the triceps.

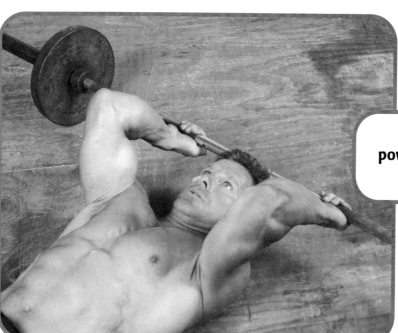

The Russian powerlifting triceps blaster.

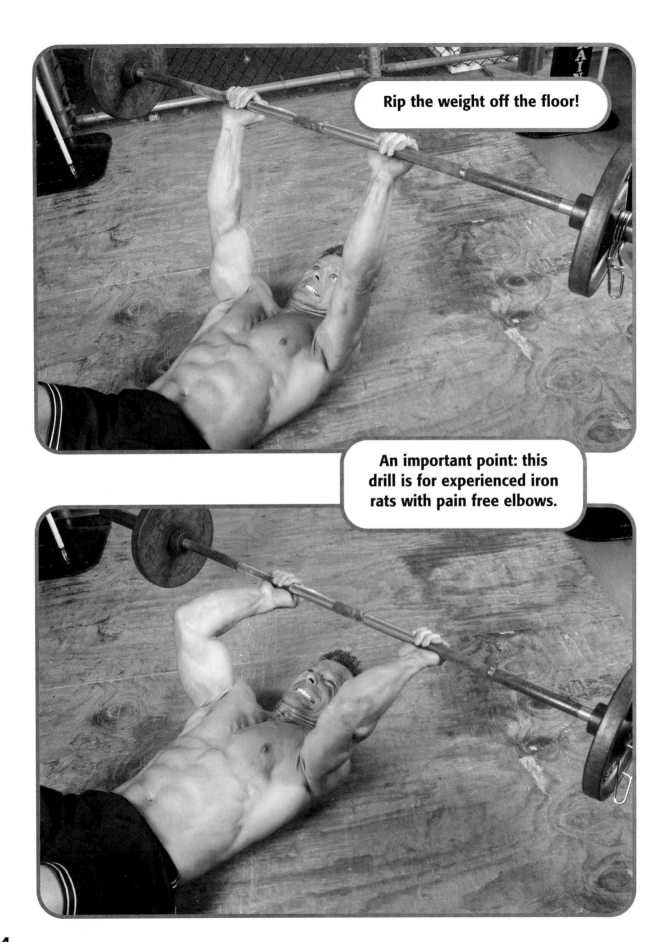

ELBOW FRIENDLY STRAIGHT BAR CURLS

Question: Straight bar curls bother my wrists. Should I switch to an EZ curl bar?

You could. Or just change your grip on the straight bar. Let your arms hang straight by your sides and then supinate your wrists, that is make your palms face forward as they do on the bottom of the curl. You will notice that your hands naturally move a few inches away from your body and your fingers point slightly out. Do not touch that dial; go over to the bar and pick it up with that exact grip. Curl. Chances are your wrists and elbows will give you no more trouble.

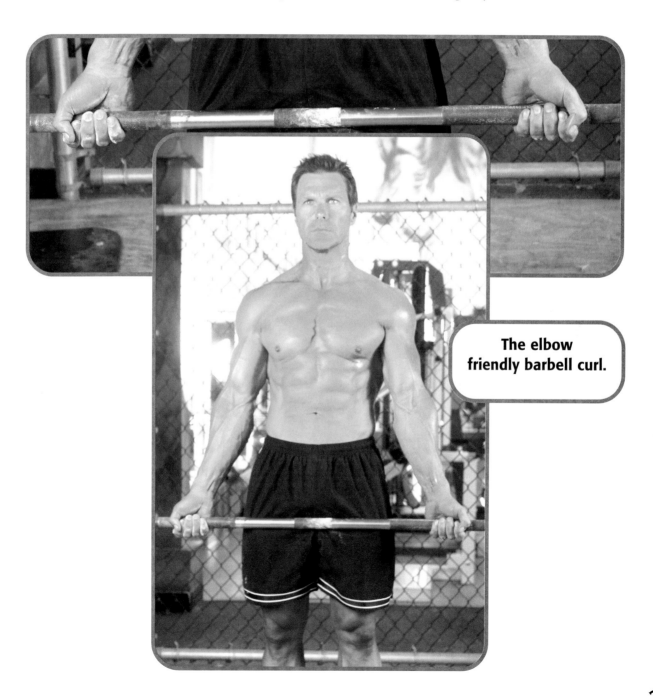

The elbow friendly barbell curl.

FOREARM SPECIALIZATION FOR THE PIPE MASTERS

Question: No matter what I do, I cannot get my biceps to grow any more. I have tried biceps specialization, squat specialization, all sorts of shock treatments; all in vain. Any desperate measures for a desperate bodybuilder?

Ease off on your curls and go on an intense grip and forearm specialization routine. "Surprisingly, I also gained almost an inch on my biceps, which now measured nearly 18 inches for the first time in my life," reported British Dr. Alan Radley in *MILO: A Journal for Serious Strength Athletes* after an intense stretch of specialization on grip feats. "…Please note as well that this progress is in a guy with nearly twenty years of heavy weightlifting experience…"

Heavy forearm specialization is a powerful old time secret of building loaded guns. Understand that forearm specialization does not mean doing a lot of high rep wrist curls and reverse wrist curls. You need to work the many muscles of the forearm from a variety of angles. Wrist pronation, supination, adduction, abduction, finger flexion and extension… The many degrees of freedom a human hand provides will never let you get bored with your forearm training.

To give yourself a taste of an effective forearm training drill grab a barbell plate in one hand, your fingers below on the smooth part and your thumb on the top. If you cannot find a plate to fit your strength you may sandwich a few small plates, fives or tens, together. Press up with your fingertips and curl! Do not let your wrist bend back, keep it rigidly in line with your forearm.

Go heavy and never do your Popeye work as an afterthought of your biceps work. Train your forearms at least three times a week in a separate workout or together with an unrelated body part, e.g. quads, calves, or abs. The best source of hardcore grip and forearm drills is John Brookfield's book *Mastery of Hand Strength* available from ironmind.com. John shows you many unique moves with such common items as sledgehammers and bricks. Iron Mind also offers a variety of top quality grip and forearm training tools.

CLUBBELLS™: FOR TOTALLY AWESOME FOREARMS

Question: I heard that old-fashioned Indian clubs are making a comeback and making a splash in the martial arts world. Do they offer any benefits to a bodybuilder?

I have passed your question on to Scott Sonnon, Master of Sports, USA National Sambo Coach who is responsible for the recent renaissance of the Indian club. Here is what I learned.

The clubs originated in ancient Greece and made their way to Persia. There they became favorites of wrestlers and strongmen. India was the next stop; this is where 'the Indian clubs' got their name. They were imported into the US from Britain in 1862. John Heenan, a famous Civil War era boxer stated that "as an assistant for training purposes, and imparting strength to the muscles of the arms, wrists, and hands, together in fact with the whole muscular system, I do not know of their equal. They will become one of the institutions in America." They did. Club swinging went on to become an Olympic sport and endured until the 1932 Olympics in Los Angeles where Americans cleaned everyone's clock. Recently a champion martial artist brought the Indian club back as a sleek Clubbell™ available from www.clubbell.tv.

What can Indian clubs do for a bodybuilder? – "Muscle building athletes use clubbells to get a high-octane pump on the forearms and shoulders because no other equipment targets all four aspects of grip strength: crushing, stabilizing, pinching, and driving strength," explains Sonnon. "Substitute clubbell exercises for barbell and dumbbell wrist curls at the end of your training. Here's a super-fast and simple club program to blast your forearms at the end of a heavy day:

Head Casts: 2 sets of 15 – 25 reps

Inward Pendulums: 2 sets of 15 – 25 reps

Wrist Casts: 1 set to failure."

THE HEAD CAST

Pick up the club with a tight grip and hold it like a torch for a few seconds. Tilt the bell towards you and let it rest on your shoulder, then raise your elbow. Keep raising it until it points straight up. Don't lean back. You will end up in the position similar to the bottom of a dumbbell French press. Before the club touches your back, explode upwards. Hold the bell above you, like a sword ready to fall, for a couple of seconds. Lower the club slowly until it is in front of you and start over.

THE INWARD PENDULUM

Swing the club from side to side and diagonally. Grip the ground with your toes and death grip the bell.

THE WRIST CAST

Lift your elbow as if you are holding a shield. Your upper arm should be parallel to the ground. Slowly yield with your wrist without moving your arm or shoulder. The club will slowly move towards you until it rests on your biceps or deltoid. Regrip, pressurize your breath, and slowly leverage the club back to the shield position.

Scott Sonnon recommends the above routine three times a week and a name change to 'Popeye'.

BUILD HUGE BICEPS WITH... THE BENCH PRESS!

Question: What is the best exercise for building a huge biceps?

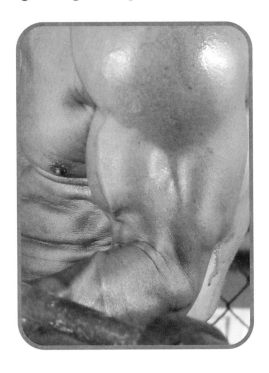

It is a matter of opinion. Mine says the wide grip bench press. Before you decide that I am nuts, check out the pipes on the top powerlifters and humor me for a few weeks.

A 'wide' grip means the max legal powerlifting grip, your index fingers touching the outside of the power rings. Going wider invites wrist problems or worse. Keep your shoulder blades pinched together. Keep your shoulders down and force your rib cage out. Squeeze the bar but imagine that you are 'pushing from your armpits' rather than your hands.

Do these benches for 5x6 three times a week. Limit or eliminate the rest of the chest and biceps work. Measure your pipes six weeks later and drop me a note on the forum.

ARE SQUATS NEEDED FOR BIG PIPES?

Question: I hear everyone saying that you cannot build big arms without heavy squats and deadlifts. Is it true?

I would love to tell you 'yes' because I like making people miserable, but it would not be true. Although heavy powerlifts will definitely help your big pipe quest, eighteen-inch guns have been built without a squat rack or a deadlift platform in sight. Just look at guys such as national arm-wrestling champion Jason Remer who sports a great bodybuilding physique. Although these days this rare gentleman athlete is serious about training his whole body, a couple years ago Remer won his first national title with no lower body work at all.

But before you let your squat rack get overgrown with spider webs you need to know one thing about Jason's training. Unlike a typical curl artist who bounces, pumps, and burns with sissy weights and high reps, the arm wrestling champ treats his curls as serious strength training. He lifts heavy, slow, and tight. A perfect and conservative triple with 150 pounds is a routine set of barbell curls for Jason Remer.

One of the top professional arm benders in the Midwest, Marty O'Neal has seventeen-inch pipes at 176 pounds of bodyweight and the height of 5'11". When I met the up and coming Marty about a few years ago he was wiry but certainly not bursting out of his sleeves. In other words, it is not just the genetics. It is the training: heavy curls plus arm-wrestling which is the ultimate in 'time under tension'.

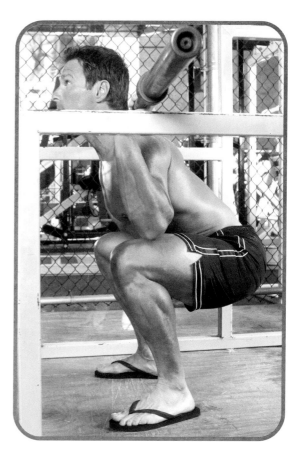

The bottom line. Big and strong arms can be built on a narrow specialization program. But there is no way around heavy weights and good form.

SECTION SEVEN

CHEST

CONTENTS

Articles

- *A Chest to Stand a Glass on (The 'Strong as You Look' Series)*

Questions and Answers

- *Old style pecs*

- *"I don't want my pecs to look like breasts!"*

- *How to train for 'old-timer pecs'*

- *Pecs without a bench*

- *Having a hard time recruiting your pecs? – We'll fix it!*

- *Powerlifting secret of pec power*

A CHEST TO STAND A GLASS ON (THE 'STRONG AS YOU LOOK' SERIES)

1. Bench press

2. Hand clap pushup

3. Incline dumbbell press

4. Floor fly

1. BENCH PRESS

There is no need to get cute and reinvent the wheel, the bench press remains the number one builder of pecs to stand a glass on. But in order to get the most out it I insist that you study the following fine points in technique.

Lie down on the bench and force your chest out to the max while drawing your shoulder blades together and pushing your shoulders down towards your feet. Performing a 'pullover' with the bench uprights will help you get into that position. The above is essential for max power, greatest pec overload, and shoulder safety.

Plant your feet like you mean it. Take a deep breath and brace your whole body as if you are about to get punched – that can be arranged! – and unrack the barbell. Flex your pecs hard on the top and literally pull the bar into your sternum with your lats. At the same time, keep pushing your chest out as if you are trying to meet the bar halfway. Your pectorals should feel a tight stretch as they are being loaded like rubber bands.

Trying to inhale with a heavy barbell compressing your ribcage is an exercise in futility, so hold your breath on the way down. Pause for a second when the bar touches your chest. Do not relax, stay tight and ready for a blast-off.

Squeeze the weight off your chest and push it towards your feet as if you are doing a decline press. Thanks to Louie Simmons, this technique has saved many pecs and shoulders in the powerlifting community. You will get best results if you imagine that you are *pushing yourself away* from the bar, sort of wedging your body between the weight and the bench. You will feel tightness and pressure in your upper back if you do it right. When you approach failure you will be pleasantly surprised that the bar keeps inching up, persistent and stable, as if in a Smith machine.

When the reps get hard and you hit your sticking point grip the bar hard. Simultaneously flex your glutes, abs, and grunt – imagining that you are sending energy from your stomach into your fists. The effect of this martial arts technique is nothing short of amazing. At a course I just taught at the Albuquerque Police Academy, an instructor benched twelve clean reps with his seven-rep max. His results are typical.

Before heading down for another rep make sure that your scapulae have not slipped out. If they have, pinch them together. If the weight in your hands is too heavy to allow it, rack the bell and continue your set in the rest-pause fashion. Enjoy!

Recommended sets & reps: 5x5

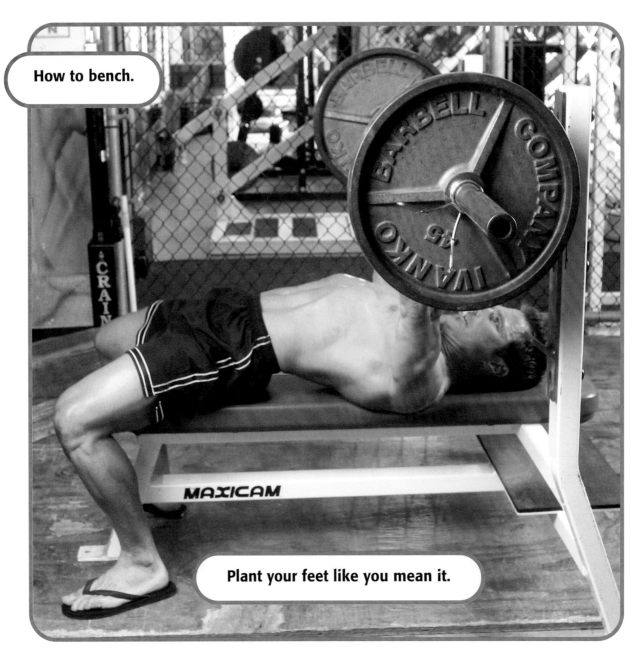

How to bench.

Plant your feet like you mean it.

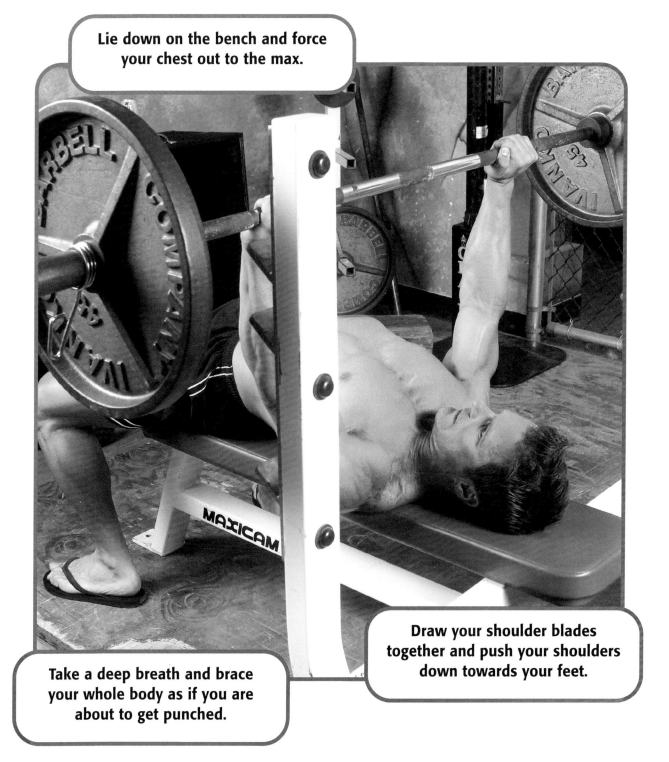

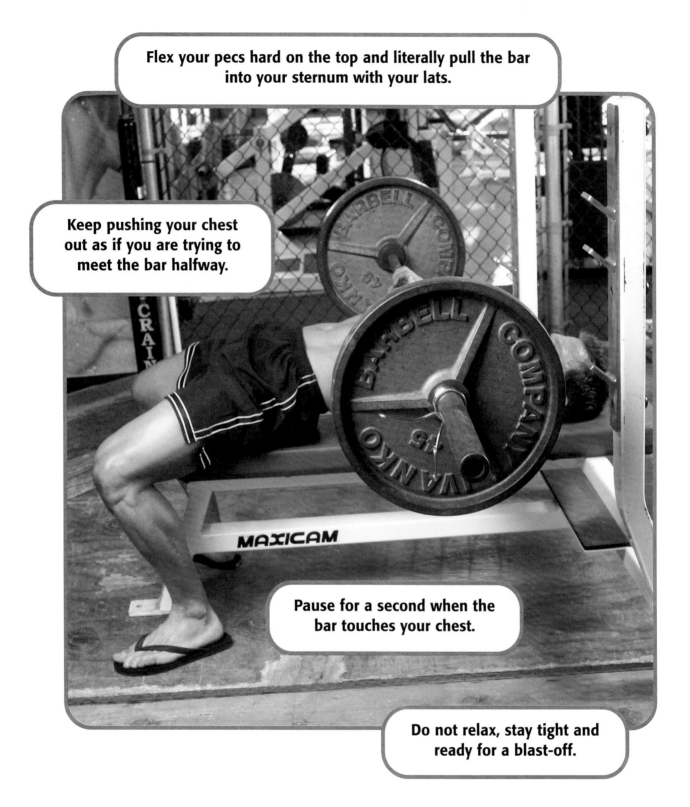

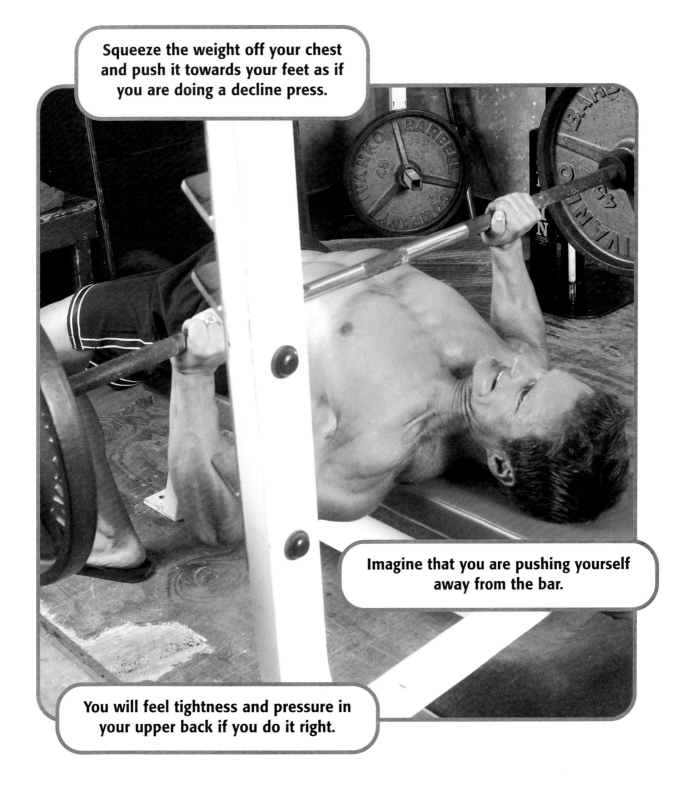

Squeeze the weight off your chest and push it towards your feet as if you are doing a decline press.

Imagine that you are pushing yourself away from the bar.

You will feel tightness and pressure in your upper back if you do it right.

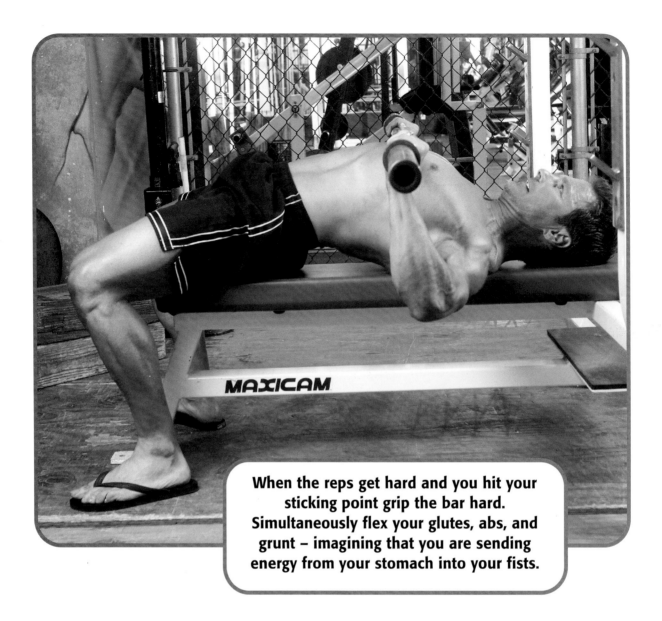

When the reps get hard and you hit your sticking point grip the bar hard. Simultaneously flex your glutes, abs, and grunt – imagining that you are sending energy from your stomach into your fists.

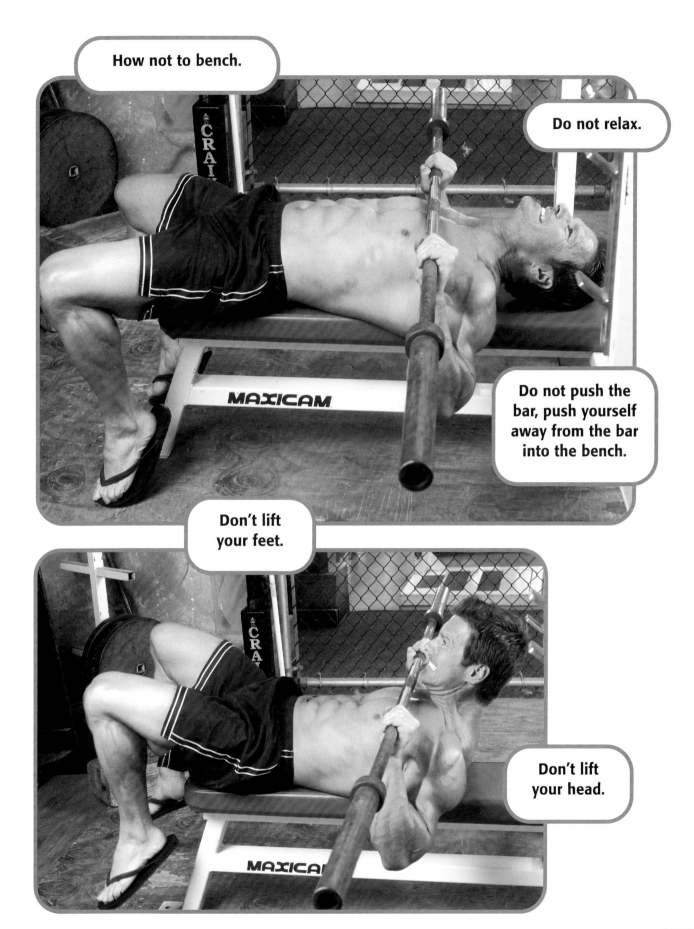

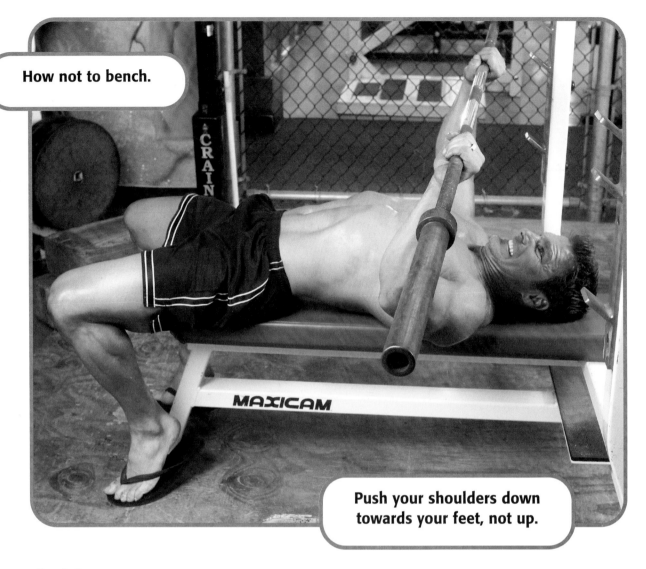

How not to bench.

Push your shoulders down towards your feet, not up.

2. HAND CLAP PUSHUP

A favorite of many power athletes, this exercise will quickly pack slabs of beef on your chest, thanks to the extreme and unusual overload it generates. If you are not strong enough for the mainstream version of the drill, you may do it off your knees or even against a wall.

Assume the pushup position with your hands and feet slightly wider than your shoulders – and your elbows out. Keeping your weight on the bases of your palms, drop until your chest almost hits the ground. With as much hesitation as you would have displayed had you touched a hot stove, explosively push up and clap your hands. Land back on your hands and carry on. Have enough sense to stop before your kisser is in danger of a plastic reconstruction.

A cool karate technique will help you recruit your pecs to the max. In the Russian Special Forces we were instructed to pretend that we were punching with our elbows rather than our fists to tap into the powerful torso muscles and keep our arms fast and loose. Do the same, push down straight from your elbows.

Even when you get really good at these, do not attempt to jump higher by straightening out your elbows; your chest muscles will respond best to short powerful bursts in the stretched position. Unlike some power athletes, a bodybuilder has little to gain from pursuing studlier variations of the drill such as clapping multiple times or clapping over his head. Just keep adding reps.

Start out with one set of ten, give or take a few, and build up slowly. Fifty is a worthy goal to shoot for.

Recommended sets & reps: 3x10

3. INCLINE DUMBBELL PRESS

In the olden days – when weightlifters trained with incline presses to simulate the Olympic press – the incline bench was just a long board you could lean against while standing on your feet. It was a great setup, very easy on the spine. Unfortunately, most modern incline benches make a bodybuilder sit down with an extreme arch in his back. Which is one good reason to do your inclines with dumbbells that force you to use a lot less poundage than a barbell.

You may vary the incline angle, for instance start steep and work your way down to the flat dumbbell bench press using the same poundage and brief rest periods. The improved leverage will be making up for the fatigue. But this is just one of many options.

As before, start on the top with your pecs flexed, your rib cage elevated, and your shoulders pulled down and back. Unlike the heavy barbell bench, the dumbbell press will enable you to get in a big breath on the negative. Push your chest up with all your might.

Dr. Fred 'Squat' Hatfield of ISSA.com offers a cool tip to advance the development of your pecs by light years: let the bells drift out slightly as if you cannot make up your mind whether you are doing presses or flies. Your pectorals will have to immediately get to work to prevent the dumbbells from crashing to the floor.

Get a good stretch on the bottom but do not overdo it, your shoulders are vulnerable in this position to overstretching.

Keep your scapulae pinched together – very important! – and push the weights to the top with your pecs. Flex your pecs hard at the top and come back for more.

Recommended sets & reps: 3x6

4. FLOOR FLY

It is impossible to isolate a muscle and keep everything else relaxed. Definitely not with any meaningful poundage. An attempt to do so is futile and dangerous. On the other hand, intelligent use of 'non-involved' muscles in a single joint exercise such as the pec fly will deliver greater power, safety, and mass. I explain this phenomenon of *irradiation* in my book *Power to the People!* Following, is the power bodybuilding technique for a single joint exercise, in our case the fly.

Lie down on the floor face up, spread your arms wide and grab a couple of dumbbells with your palms facing up. Why on the floor and not on the bench? Mostly for variety's sake, but also to enable you to handle greater poundages without the fear of ripping your shoulders out.

Straighten out your legs and keep your feet together. Maintain a slight bend in your elbows for the duration of the set.

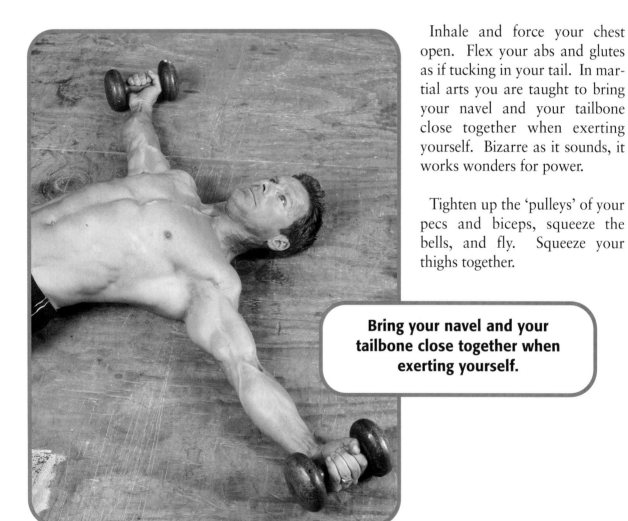

Inhale and force your chest open. Flex your abs and glutes as if tucking in your tail. In martial arts you are taught to bring your navel and your tailbone close together when exerting yourself. Bizarre as it sounds, it works wonders for power.

Tighten up the 'pulleys' of your pecs and biceps, squeeze the bells, and fly. Squeeze your thighs together.

> **Bring your navel and your tailbone close together when exerting yourself.**

You may land in the same spots or vary the stress by lowering the dumbbells straight out, slightly above your shoulders, above your head, by your hips, or anywhere in between.

Totally relax for a second when you have parked the weights on the floor. Inhale, tighten up, and carry on.

You will love this power fly. It's a single joint exercise that expresses a totally unique combination of strength, flexibility, and control – of the kind you'll find in gymnastics.

Recommended sets & reps: 3x10

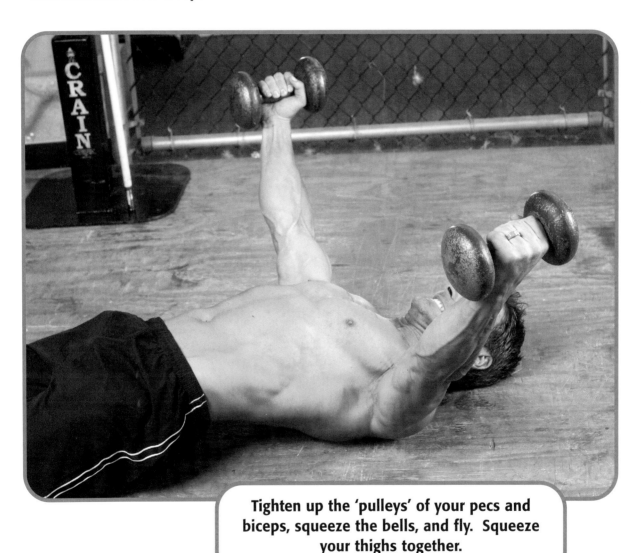

Tighten up the 'pulleys' of your pecs and biceps, squeeze the bells, and fly. Squeeze your thighs together.

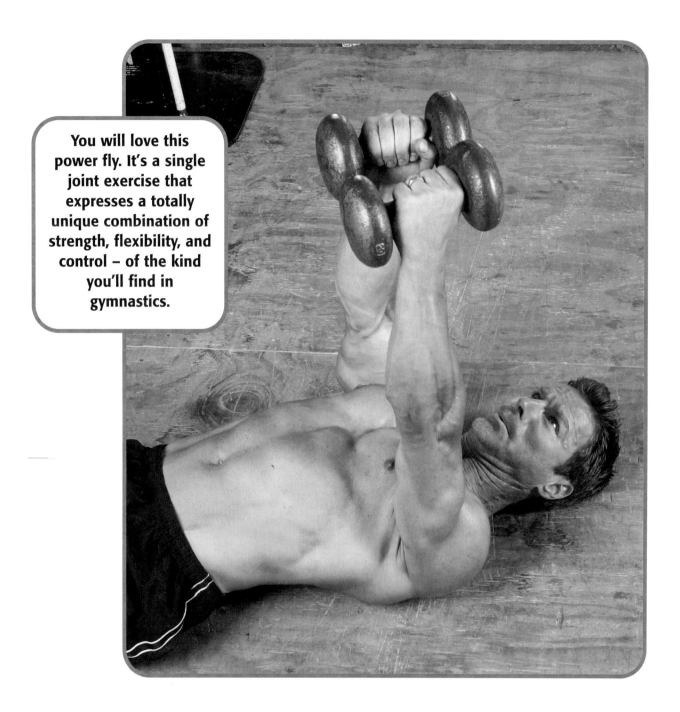

You will love this power fly. It's a single joint exercise that expresses a totally unique combination of strength, flexibility, and control – of the kind you'll find in gymnastics.

QUESTIONS & ANSWERS:

FREQUENTLY ASKED QUESTIONS ABOUT CHEST TRAINING

Question: Should I keep my feet on the bench to isolate my pecs?

Folding your legs on your belly like a dead cockroach will have an effect opposite to the one you desire. When your feet come up your back flattens, sinks your ribcage, and shifts the load from your pecs to your shoulders. So stand on your feet with confidence.

Question: Is arching my back during benches going to hurt it?

It depends. A reasonable arch is essential for pre-stretching the pecs. You will get such an arch by taking a deep breath and expanding your chest. Most bodybuilders' backs should have no problem with it. On the other hand, wedging your feet under the bench halfway to your head and bridging could be bad news. You could easily roll a basketball under tiny Russian ex-gymnast, turned world bench press record holder, Irina Krylova. Don't try to emulate her. Generally, if you plant your feet flat, rather than rise up on your toes, your arch will be just right.

Question: Should I do decline presses?

Your lower pecs will get all the work they need if you simulate the decline press on your flat benches, by lowering the bar to your sternum, almost your stomach, and pushing it towards your feet rather than your face. You will be safer too, as your shoulders will not be tempted to shrug towards your ears, as they have a tendency to do during decline presses.

Question: What can I do to prevent pec tears?

The primary causes for pec tears are steroid use and overtraining. It may shock you but there are a lot fewer pec tears among powerlifters than among bodybuilders! Any doctor working with iron athletes will offer you convincing statistics.

Although powerlifters push much heavier poundages, unlike bodybuilders they never train to failure, they keep their reps low, and they avoid overstretching the pecs and shoulders. Lifters also say no to zillions of junk sets of cable crossovers and cycle their loads. Follow the time-proven strategies above from your iron brothers and your chances of a pec tear will drop to next to nothing.

OLD STYLE PECS

Question: You have convinced me not to pursue huge pecs and to go with the old time bodybuilder's broad shouldered look. But I want SOME pecs – and overhead presses, dips, and pullups don't appear to stimulate them enough. Did the old guys do anything else?

There was another secret to the old-timers' pec strength and striations: bending horseshoes, nails, and similar manly feats. Few people practice this manly art in our soft age but the few who do sport awesome chests. Did you know that Marine vet Clark Bartram, whose photos you see in this anthology, is one of them? If you are ready to take on this challenge, get *Mastery of Hand Strength*, a book by John Brookfield available from IronMind.com.

Brett Jones, RKC Sr. is the eleventh man in the world to bend Iron Mind's famous Red Nail™.

Photos courtesy BreakingStrength.com and IronCoreLaJolla.com

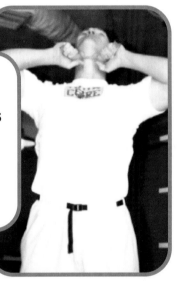
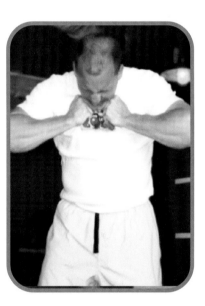
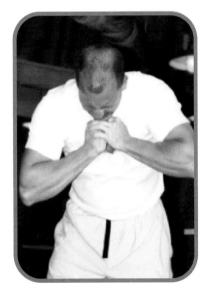
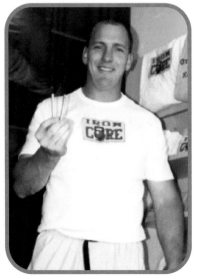

If you doubt that you are going to get around to it, there are free weight exercises that will have a similar effect on your chest. In the Soviet Special Forces we used to hold a kettlebell between our palms in such a way that it was supported by the inside pressure alone, rather than cupped by the fingers underneath. Then we would hammer curl and military press it. This drill has many cool applications. "This is exactly how I lock in my firearm!" commented a member of the Secret Service Counter Assault Team at a recent kettlebell instructor course. Arm-wrestlers also swear by it.

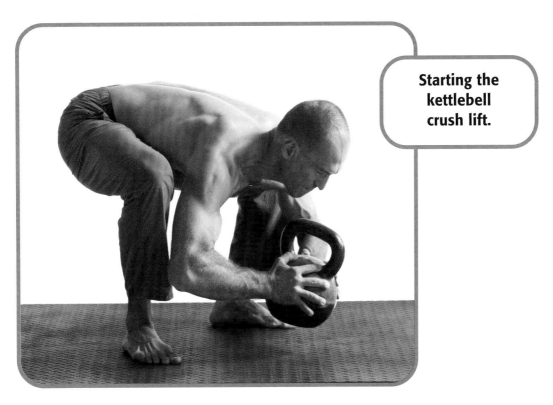

Starting the kettlebell crush lift.

Grip master John Brookfield invented a variety of similar exercises with a stack of bricks; see his other book, *The Grip Master's Manual*, for descriptions. Ex-gymnast Brad Johnson performs amazing feats of rafter pullups aided by the same drill with a pair of barbell plates sandwiched together. "Grab two smooth barbell plates and perform hammer curls with the plates sandwiched between the palms of your hands," wrote Johnson in his article on dragondoor.com. "Attempt to generate as much chest, bicep, lat, and shoulder tension as possible by pressing inwards. I performed two sets of 3-5 reps with two 25-pound plates. As I learned to generate more inward force against the plates, I extended the rep by pressing upwards (military press) after finishing the curl. I was very careful to lift the weights slightly in front of my body just in case the weights slipped." Inside pressure work tends to shorten the pecs, so make sure to stretch them thoroughly afterwards.

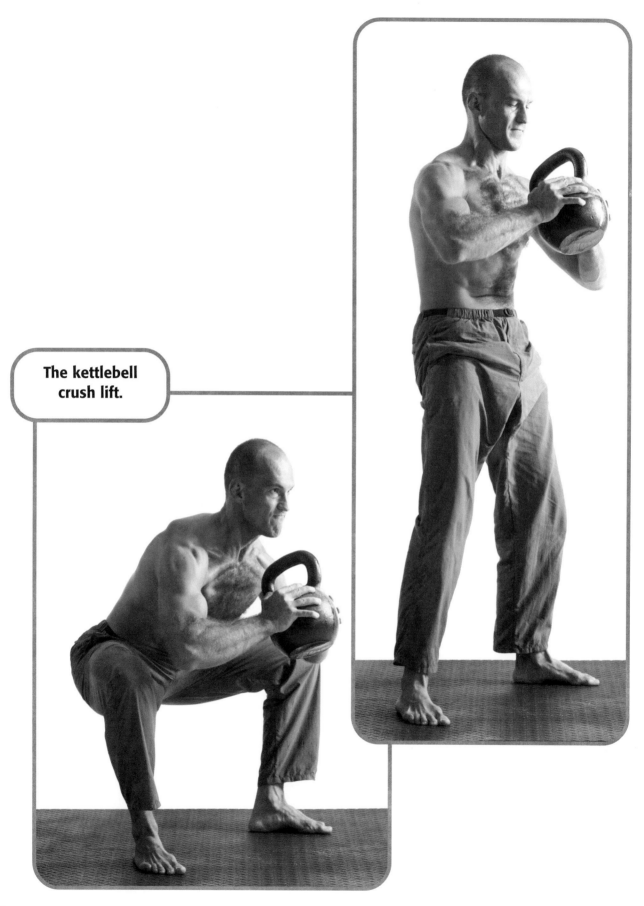

The kettlebell crush lift.

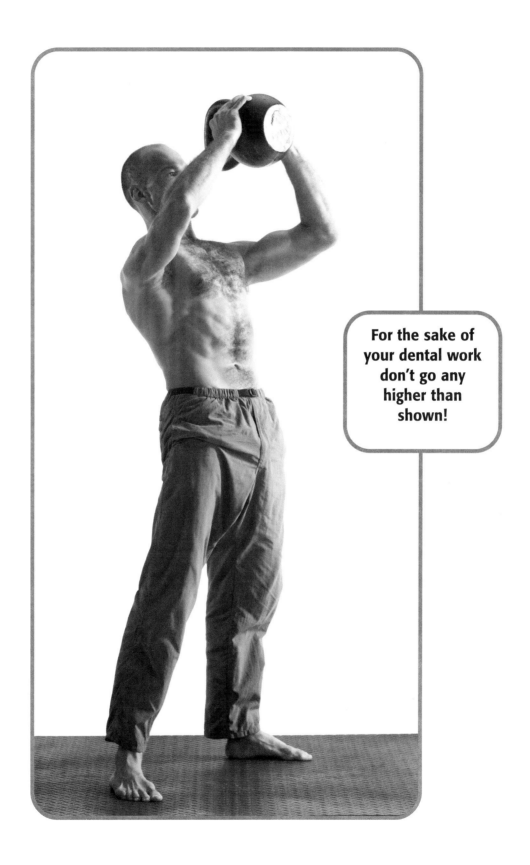

"I DON'T WANT MY PECS TO LOOK LIKE BREASTS!"

Question: Is it true that decline bench presses could give me drooping, breast-like pecs?

Yes. Especially as you grow older. There is no convincing reason for a bodybuilder to do decline presses at all. And even the ever so popular flat bench could do the same to some bodybuilders.

Strength coach extraordinaire Bill Starr gives a sensible old school piece of advice. Don't bench except on an incline. No declines, no flats, just inclines. Your pecs will acquire a square, gladiator body armor look to them. And because the flats and the inclines are similar enough exercises, should you decide to test yourself on the flat bench, you will do quite well.

If you are hooked on flat benches, a good compromise is to practice them only for very low reps and low sets, e.g. 54321 or 5x3. That approach builds a lot of strength and little mass. Then pump it up on an incline. This gives you the best of both worlds: a big bench and pecs you would not be embarrassed by, even in your old age.

Needless to say, the recommendations to avoid decline presses altogether and to do just a moderate volume of flat benches are just opinions. But hanging pecs are a fact.

HOW TO TRAIN FOR 'OLD-TIMER PECS'

Question: I have a quaint notion that bulging breasts are a female sexual attribute and have no place on a man. Ditto for chafing thighs. I dig the physique of an old time bodybuilder like Eugene Sandow. How should I train?

Old timers did not squat or bench. These two exercises are largely responsible for the modern look that you describe. Men like Eugene Sandow and Siegmund Klein concentrated on a great variety of overhead presses, including the awesome yet long forgotten side press and bent press and pulls: deadlifts, snatches, and cleans, one and two arm. The result was a physique built along the lines of Laurent Delvaux's statue *Hercules*: broad shoulders with just a hint of pecs, back muscles standing out in bold relief, wiry arms, rugged forearms, a cut-up midsection, and strong legs without a hint of squat-induced chafing. Different strokes for different folks.

PECS WITHOUT A BENCH

Question: I train at home with dumbbells. Is there any way to work my pecs without a bench?

I can think of at least three.

If you have a flexible and healthy spine you could sit on the floor with your knees bent and rest your upper back and head on a sturdy box, one to two feet tall, parked against a wall to avoid sliding. The exercise you will end up doing is a cross between a flat and an incline press. The great John Grimek used to do it before exercise benches were invented.

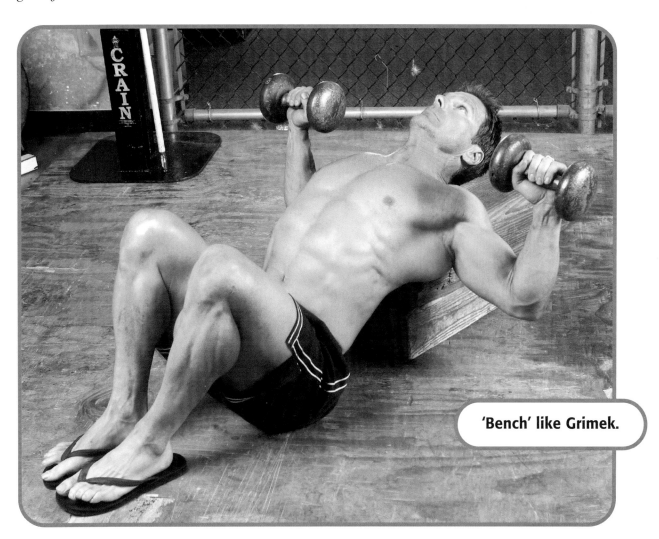

'Bench' like Grimek.

Another fine exercise is the floor press. Sit on the floor with a pair of light dumbbells at your shoulders and carefully lie on your back. Straighten out your legs and open your chest. Muscle out the bells with your triceps power until your elbows are locked. You are ready for the floor press.

Carefully lower the weights until your elbows or, if you have more meat on you, your triceps, rest on the floor. Take care not to slam the elbows into the floor, control the movement all the way down. To maximize pec recruitment you should flare your elbows and let the bells fall out somewhat, as if you are about to do flies.

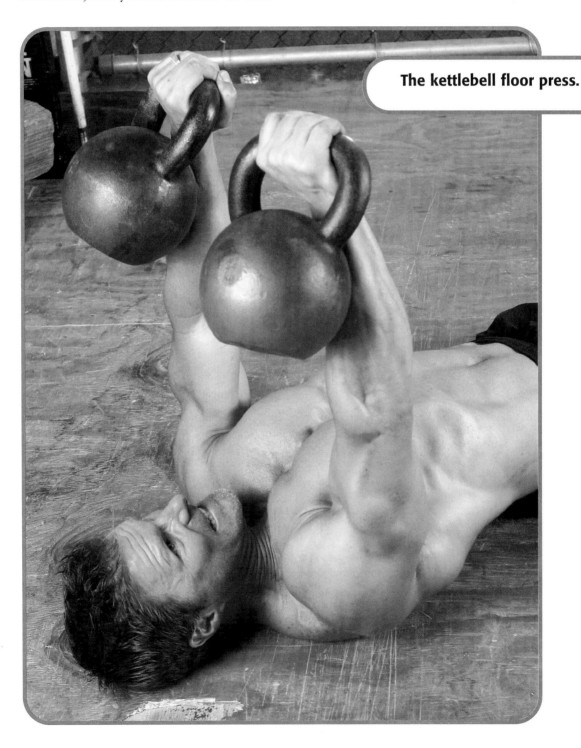

The kettlebell floor press.

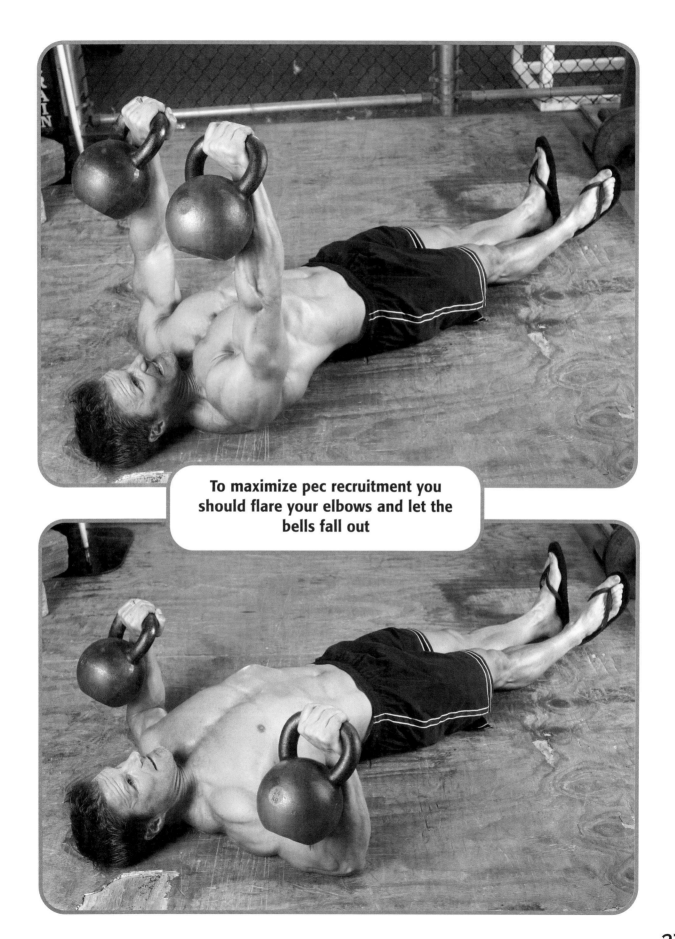

To maximize pec recruitment you should flare your elbows and let the bells fall out

Stay tight and push back up in a wide arc. You may perform the floor press with your palms facing forward as in the barbell bench press or with the palms facing each other. Naturally, you can do floor flies as well.

If you like to get a good pec stretch – although not necessary, it is conducive to muscle growth – do modified one arm floor presses. If you are pressing with your left, stick your slightly bent right arm under a couch, palm up, to anchor yourself. Both of your feet will be facing the couch as if you are walking. The feet should be spread as wide apart as your flexibility allows, the left leg atop the right one and closer to the couch.

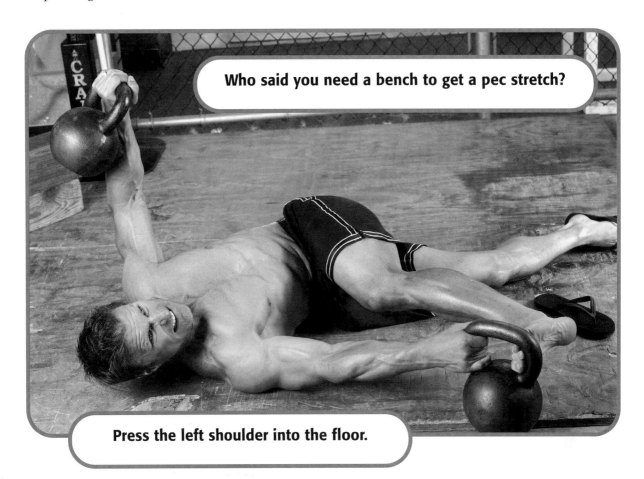

Who said you need a bench to get a pec stretch?

Press the left shoulder into the floor.

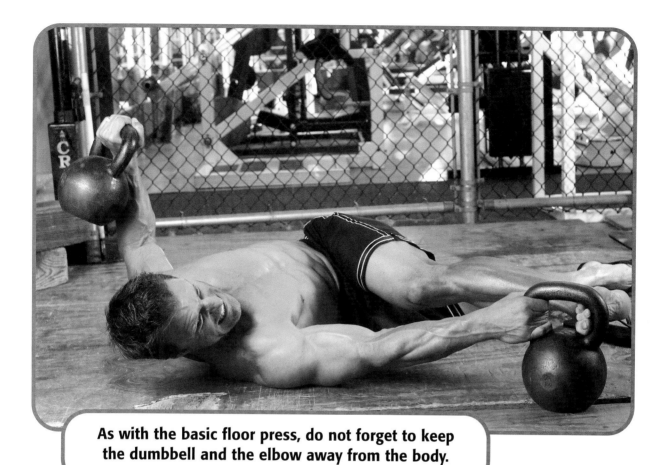

As with the basic floor press, do not forget to keep the dumbbell and the elbow away from the body.

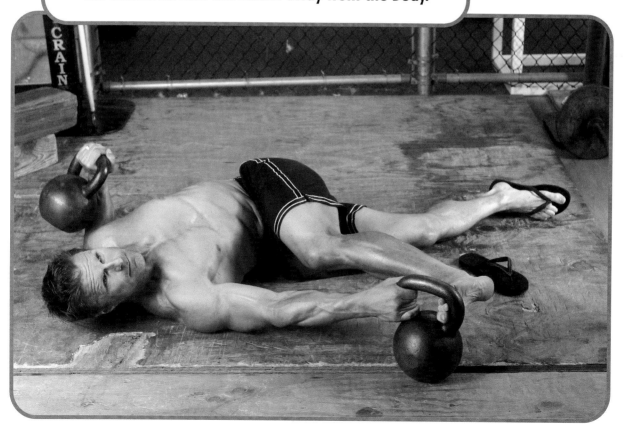

HAVING A HARD TIME RECRUITING YOUR PECS? — WE'LL FIX IT!

Question: I don't feel my pecs when I am benching! What am I doing wrong?

First, position yourself on the bench properly. Force your chest out, spread your collarbones out, pinch your shoulder blades together, and press your shoulders towards your feet, away from your ears. Do not lose that alignment throughout the set.

Pausing for a second with the bar touching your chest will help you recruit those pecs. Stay tight and do not let the bar sink into your chest; it is barely brushing your rib cage. Flex your bis. Do not try to bend your elbows, which is counter-productive, but flare the biceps as if you are posing. Thanks to the recruitment relationship between the pectorals, the biceps, and the triceps – and the fact that one of the biceps heads is directly involved in pressing – you WILL feel your pecs! Or else.

It is a dirty little secret of bodybuilding, but in addition to blasting the pecs, benching this way builds big pipes better than curls. Try it!

THE POWERLIFTING SECRET OF PEC POWER

Question: I have a hard time feeling my pecs when I am bench pressing. What am I doing wrong?

Bench press record breaker George Halbert offered a first-rate tip on how to recruit your pecs to the max when benching, in an issue of *Powerlifting USA* (a must have, immediately call (800) 448-7693 to subscribe).

Instead of pressing the barbell straight up, grip it tight, flare your elbows, and imagine that you are *trying to bring your hands together*. In other words, you are trying to compress or shorten the bar with your chest power. Incidentally, you may employ the same technique with wide grip pushups. You will have a hard time believing you can get such a great pec pump with lowly pushups.

"Although we are not bodybuilders," says Halbert, "we can use their exercises and put a power spin on them." Do not forget that it works both ways in the iron community.

SECTION EIGHT

NAKED WARRIOR

STRONG ANYWHERE, ANYTIME WITH BODYWEIGHT EXERCISES

CONTENTS

Articles

POWER TRAINING CONTENTS

Questions and Answers

THE RUSSIAN SPECIAL FORCES LADDER TO POWER

Time and time again, I have made the point: the ticket to muscles and might is to increase the training volume while staying relatively fresh.

One powerful approach to boosting the loading volume was practiced in the Soviet Special Forces. The Spetsnaz requirement of eighteen dead hang pullups with ten kilos, or twenty-two pounds, of body armor demanded smart training. So between the classes – firearms training, foreign languages, and less friendly 'special disciplines' – we would file out to the pullup bars and perform what we called 'ladders'. I do a pullup, you do one. I do two, you match me, etc. until one of us cannot keep up. Then, if we still had time, we started over. 1, 2, 3, 4, 5, 6, 7, 8, 9, 10... 1, 2, 3, 4, 5, 6, 7... 1, 2, 3, 4, 5. We totaled hundreds of pullups almost daily without burning out. And the extreme PT tests of our service became a breeze.

Since the Evil Empire went out of business I have been training various elite military units and law enforcement agencies in the US. The ladders have been delivering the goods just as reliably as they did on the other side of the old Iron Curtain. A Recon Marine, and vet of the first Gulf War, boosts his impressive twenty pullups to thirty-five.... A Texas SWAT cowboy goes from twenty-five pullups to forty.... A boy fresh out of high school climbs the ladder all the way to the coveted Navy SEAL trident... Naturally, people who are not in spec ops shape do even better. Improving from ten to twenty pullups in a couple of months is typical.

The ladder enables the trainee to maximize the volume without burning out, because only the top sets of each ladder are tough. You get a respite by starting over on the bottom rung. For that reason it is important that once you have climbed to the top you start over on the bottom, e.g. 1, 2, 3, 4, 5, 1, 2... rather than work down: 1, 2, 3, 4, 5, 4, 3, 2, 1. The pyramid approach rapidly builds up the fatigue and compromises the volume. The ladder, on the other hand, enables the strong man or woman to' grease the groove' of his or her chosen feat with extraordinary volume. 1+2+3+4+5 = 15. Repeat this series eight times – not a great feat unless you are a heavyweight – and you have totaled 120 pullups! Try to stuff that many in a workout with any other structure and you will fail miserably (for example, the popular approach of doing as many sets to the limit as it takes to get the target number, say 12,10, 9, 7, 7, 5, 4, 2, 1, 1, 1,).

THE TWO TYPES OF LADDERS

There are two types of ladders: competitive and preset. The former terminates when you or your partner cannot top the last set. The rest intervals are naturally timed: you go whenever the other comrade jumps off the bar. Two or more comrades can compete. If you train alone, time your breaks by imagining that you are competing with one or more other guys.

The preset ladder requires you to work up to the specified number of reps, e.g. five if you could have made it to seven, and start all over. Although not as much fun, this variation generally delivers more reliable progress because your odds of burning out are lower. You could follow the preset ladder format when you train by yourself and sprint up the competitive ladder when joined by your training buddy.

Although the classic ladder is primarily a strength endurance and muscle building technique, some Russian experts such as Bondarchuk state that the cumulative effect of many low intensity sets has a somewhat similar effect to that of a heavy load. In other words, expect that your strength will go up with your strength endurance and muscle mass. Indeed, ladders in 'uniform two', or the boots plus the fatigue pants, noticeably improved our pulling strength with weapons and gear on the obstacle course. But you will do even better strength wise if you choose a more direct approach. Take a 5-6RM weight and perform series of 1, 2, 3 reps. Take one-minute breaks and keep up the sequence till fatigue.

There is no law that says you must go up one rep at a time. With higher rep exercises, you can jump a few of the steps every set, for instance 5, 10, 15, and 20 pushups for a comrade who can do fifty or 3, 6, 9, 12, 15 for someone who can do twenty-five.

The ladder is highly adaptable to any trainee and definitely is not limited to pullups. The number of sets and series is up to you. So is the training frequency, the weight, and the exercises. You may climb the ladder daily or take a day or two off between the sessions. It goes against my totalitarian nature, but you have the freedom to design your own ladder workout. I will outline a sample workout though to make your task easier.

Here is a competitive ladder workout made up of pullups and dive-bomber pushups done in a circuit. Keep going from one exercise to the next, resting no longer than it takes your training partner to do his set. When you have petered out on one drill, rest a minute and start over. Let us presume that you max out at 10 pullups and 20 dive-bombers. This calls for single rep jumps on pullups and two-rep steps on pushups. Hit the deck!

A SAMPLE LADDER WORKOUT

Ladder #	Pullups	Dive-bomber Pushups
1	1	2
2	2	4
3	3 (hard)	6

When you have not made the required reps on one of the exercises or you are certain that you will not make it on the next step, rest for a minute and start over from the bottom:

4	1	2
5	2	4
6	3 (very hard)	6

Rest again.

7	1	2
8	2 (you know that you will not make 3)	4

Rest.

9	1	2
10	2 (hard)	4

Rest.

11	1	2
12	1 (could not get 2)	4

You are smoked! If you cannot get more than a single on the second set, the gig is up. Go stretch and rest. The competitive ladder pushes you to the limit so you will need to rest two days before hitting it again or do a very light workout the day after. You get the idea. The ladder is a power cycle compressed from twelve weeks to twelve minutes. Periodization, miniaturized to fit into a single workout. And best of all, you do not need to be a Russian Special Forces operator or a Recon Marine to up your strength and mass with ladders. It is as simple as one-two-three.

THE EVIL RUSSIAN'S 'HIT THE DECK'! PROGRAM

Before the bench press was a twinkle in some early powerlifter's eye, the pushup was the measure of a man. One hundred separated the men from the boys. Still does. How will you rate?

Pretty good, if you follow my program.

Where heavy resistance training builds the contractile proteins, high volume low intensity loading such as pushups kicks into growth other wheels of the muscle machinery. The volume of sarcoplasm, muscle cell jello-like filler, goes up. Mitochondria, the muscle cells' energy plants, get buff. Capillaries spread their tentacles throughout the muscle.

Even though capillaries, the muscle's 'plumbing', make up but a fraction of the muscle's girth, they serve a VIP function in bulking your myofibrils, or 'real muscle', when you get back to heavy training. Here is how it works.

A British study by Schott et. al (1995) concluded that greater exposure of muscle cells to various metabolites, or 'muscle engine exhaust fumes', leads to greater gains in strength and mass. It has been suggested by some experts that the more extensive a muscle's vascularity, the more the muscle will be soaked in intra-muscular metabolites and growth factors. And the more it will grow.

At least, up to a point. According to Soviet research (Zalesskiy & Burkhanov, 1981), vascular network development generally cannot keep up with muscle hypertrophy. So if you want to keep on growing beyond the easy first gains, you must find a way of developing your vascular network.

This is where super high reps come in. Lüthi et. al (1986) discovered that heavy training has no effect on capillarization. Tesch et. al (1984) added that Olympic weightlifters and powerlifters, athletes who favor low rep training with long rest periods, display capillary density that is even lower than that of untrained subjects! And Sjøogard (1984) stated that enhanced capillarization is the result of endurance training (could this explain why your legs gain mass so much easier than your arms?). So hit the deck, Comrade!

THE EVIL RUSSIAN'S 'HIT THE DECK!' PROGRAM

	Relative intensity	Set frequency
Monday	100% (test); 30%	60 min
Tuesday	50%	60 min
Wednesday	60%	45 min
Thursday	25%	60 min
Friday	45%	30 min
Saturday	40%	60 min
Sunday	20%	90 min
Monday	100% (test); 35%	45 min
Tuesday	55%	20 min
Wednesday	30%	15 min
Thursday	65%	60 min
Friday	35%	45 min
Saturday	45%	60 min
Sunday	25%	120 min
Monday	100% (test)	

**Don't follow this or any other routine blindly and use your judgment!
If this is too much – back off and build back up slowly!**

The program is self-explanatory. Just drop and give me a specified percentage of your last PR at given time intervals throughout the day. For instance, if you managed fifty pushups on your test, do twenty-five on the day that calls for 50% relative intensity. On Mondays test yourself for one set and do easy sets for the rest of the day.

Time the breaks between your sets but do not have a fit if you missed your date with the concrete here and there. Make it up if you can; do not sweat it if you cannot. Do your sets from the time you get up until an hour before your bedtime. Naturally, most comrades with real jobs will have a couple of gaps in their day when they cannot drop and pump out pushups. Do not worry about it; just get back on schedule when the boss looks the other way.

Note that you are supposed to go to the limit only once a week. High rep sets to exhaustion are a lot more dangerous then they look. The tension in the stabilizing muscles is not enough to protect the joints and the connective tissues; the latter really get it in the shorts. So do not mess with the outline; stay well within your ability except on the test days! Do not worry, you will make great gains without doing a jackhammer on the last rep, dripping sweat, and making macho faces.

The prescribed regimen requires that you say no to any other upper body work with the exception of pullups or chinups. Either of these military favorites will hit the muscles missed by the pushups and balance out your shoulders. The choice of a pullup regimen is up to you.

A word on pushups for reasons other then getting buff or becoming one of the few good men. Pushups are no good for strength unless you can barely manage a couple. The old faithful are useful however for developing shoulder endurance for select sports such as boxing. Prizefighters are traditionally fond of pushups; they believe that this exercise improves their punching power. Indeed it does, although not in the manner they believe it does. Relaxed shoulders are critical to fluid transmission of power from the hip into the fist. Anyone who has put on a pair of gloves and climbed into the ring knows that holding your guard up and punching for a few rounds exhausts the shoulders. A fatigued muscle is a tight muscle. Punches deteriorate into pushes when the delts get tired. Which is why the last rounds of a professional boxing bout look like an amateur brawl. And which is why prizefighters ought to faithfully stick with their tried and true pushup.

Whether you are training for the boxing ring or something else, proper pushup technique will amplify your gains.

Place the weight near the bases of your palms rather than closer to the fingers. If the traditional technique hurts your wrists you have a couple of options. The yuppie choice is a set of pushup handles or a pair of hex-shaped dumbbells. The manly alternative is to do your pushups the karate way, on your knuckles. If you do not plan on kicking butt in the near future you may do your pushups on the full surfaces of the fist (shame on you). But the proper martial arts knuckle pushup calls for resting your weight only on two knuckles of each fist, those of the index and the middle fingers for bare-knuckle fighters. You will find that this manly technique will strengthen your wrists in a hurry. No, your forearms will not look any better, but your bench will go up because your noodle thin wrists will stop screaming for mercy and wraps.

In the Soviet Special Forces we knocked off knuckle pushups on concrete, but you would be wiser to do your knuckle pushups on a surface that has some give, for instance grass or a rubberized gym floor. Make sure that the floor is clean; dirt particles can do a number on your baby soft skin.

The grip width is up to you; you may vary it from set to set.

Keep your butt tucked under; this will make your pushups look crisp and protect your back from sagging and hurting.

Do not constrict your chest; keep it wide open. The range of motion will be slightly reduced, the pecs will be pre-stretched for more power, and you are less likely to hurt our shoulders that way.

Synchronize your breathing with your movement. Failing to do so in an endurance event is the kiss of death. Under the circumstances it is most natural to inhale on the way down and exhale on the way up. Imagine how your breath or 'Chi' flows out of your stomach into your arms. Do not underestimate the power of such visualization. There is plenty of evidence that the choice of a breathing pattern has a profound effect on performance.

Try to rest your muscles on the way down; a good endurance athlete knows how to let his limbs recover between strides. Find your rhythm ASAP and stick to it. Rhythmical activity takes a lot less energy than a non-rhythmical one, thanks to something called 'the central pattern generators' in your nervous system.

Take advantage of the elastic rebound on the bottom. This is not a bench press meet; you will not get red-lighted if you fail to pause.

When you are almost at the end of the rope – this applies only to your 100% test sets! – it is time to pull out the heavy artillery of the 'High-Tension Techniques' explained in my book *The Naked Warrior*. These HTT are so powerful that the elite military and law enforcement personnel I train routinely add 10-15 reps to their very impressive pushup maxes in just one or two days.

I repeat, these nukes are supposed to be deployed only during your test sets! Or for very difficult, low rep exercises. If you are trying to master the one-arm pushup or an out of shape friend of yours is struggling with regular pushups, the high-tension techniques will save the day.

If you do not wear a uniform and don't box, do not stay on a pushup diet too long. Two weeks is about right. Why risk a shoulder injury from overuse? Besides, according to Russian scientists Nikityuk & Samoylov (1990), repetition lifting of a submaximal weight promotes sarcoplasmic hypertrophy (fake muscle) while breaking down the contractile protein (real muscle). Can't have that.

One of the best approaches that will enable you to have your cake and eat it too, is alternating two-week cycles of pushups with two-week low rep strength cycles. This Russian rotation schedule is superior to doing everything at once, e.g. doing your pushups as back off sets following your bench presses and dips. Mixing up high tension and high rep stimuli in one workout confuses the body; the muscles are not certain what they should adapt to. The new approach enables you to shock your muscles into specific adaptation with a laser focus and then hit them from the flank with a fresh stimulus when they expect it the least.

Eventually you may opt for a more rigorous routine such as the one outlined below or build your own based on it. The rules are simple:

- Never come close to failure except when testing your max.
- Vary the reps and the rest periods between the sets daily.
- Adjust the load to your recovery ability.
- Build up cumulative fatigue.
- Taper down before a peak.

285

THE EVIL RUSSIAN'S 'DROP AND GIVE ME 100 PUSHUPS!' PROGRAM

	Relative intensity	Set frequency
Monday	100% (test), 40%	60 min
Tuesday	50%	30 min
Wednesday	70%	45 min
Thursday	40%	60 min
Friday	80%	60 min
Saturday	55%	90 min
Sunday	20%	90 min
Monday	90%	120 min
Tuesday	45%	60 min
Wednesday	20%	10 min
Thursday	65%	90 min
Friday	75%	60 min
Saturday	30%	90 min
Sunday	15%	120 min
Monday	100% (test)	

Here you have it, Comrade, your complete guide to pushup excellence. Put it to work and fill out your shirt before the month is up! In one of his famous courses Charles Atlas promised that you will add at least an inch to your chest in just ten days of practicing pushups without strain every morning and evening. This advice may not sound trendy in our age of hi-tech machines, 'total muscle failure', and training once in a blue moon, but it will work its magic for you just the same.

Hit the deck, trooper! Gimme a hundred!

THE NASA PUSHUP PROGRAM

Once in a blue moon I come across a training program that is simple, effective, soundly rooted in science, and easily adaptable to anyone. The NASA Pushup Program is one of these few.

The following routine is aimed at maxing out one's pushups, but don't turn that dial if your goals lie elsewhere! The author, Laurence Morehouse, Ph.D. helped design the conditioning programs for US astronauts. Grasp his logic and you will become a better strength coach. And if the only athlete you coach is yourself, so what?

If you had to learn only one thing from this article, let it be this – traditional progressive overload does not work. Or rather, it works only up to a point. "...you can't keep adding one more repetition a day," explains Dr. Morehouse, the founding director of the Human Performance Laboratory at UCLA. "The day comes when you can't do more. The big mistake in any kind of training is to set a number and try to achieve that number and assume that, if you do, you've done your training. You may by chance be getting just the right training effect – but you are probably getting either too much of a strain or too little training effect."

And even if the workout is perfect for you, it is not going to work forever. The physiological law of accommodation states that an organism stops adapting to a training stimulus after a period of time, usually 2-6 weeks. Your body figures, "Hey, it hasn't killed me, why bother to adapt?" At this point a change in the program is called for.

You can tinker with the three basic components of overload: *volume*, *intensity*, and *density*.

Volume is the total number of repetitions in a workout. For instance, you have done 10 sets of 20. The volume equals 10 x 20 = 200.

Intensity, in the context of high rep pushups or girevoy sport, is a percentage of your best result. If 40 reps is your max, then 20 reps corresponds to 50% intensity.

Density refers to the amount of work done in a unit of time. Doing one set of 20 pushups every fifty minutes is a denser workout than 1x20 every hour.

"Ideal training involves changing just one of many variables, until that variable reaches a constant," writes Dr. Laurence Morehouse. "Then you change another, and then another until you reach your goal."

Dr. Morehouse did design one pushup program that makes use of all three of the overload variables. A student, at Dr. Morehouse's class on conditioning for maximum performance, made a bet that in two month's time he would be able to do 100 consecutive pushups, 40 being his ceiling at the time.

Every day the trainee would do 200 pushups, twice as many as his target number. He started with sets of 20 pushups, or 50% of his current maximum. He did one set every hour.

If you cannot do that many each hour, adjust the repetitions to your abilities while keeping the daily total at 200. It might take you longer than ten hours to reach the daily goal. It is OK. Add a pushup to each set every day until you can do ten sets of 20.

Then start reducing the time between the sets, say five minutes every hour, until you cannot recover sufficiently between sets to pump out your 20 reps. It is a signal to increase the time between sets slightly and start gradually adding more reps.

Repeat the process until you have reached your goal. Test your max occasionally after a day or two of rest.

NASA PUSHUP PROGRAM SAMPLE SCHEDULE

Day 1, every hour for 10 hours:
x15, 15, 15, 15, 15, 15, 15, 15, 15, 15
Day 2, every hour:
x16, 16, 16, 16, 16, 16, 16, 16, 16, 16
Day 3, every hour:
x17, 17, 17, 17, 17, 17, 17, 17, 17, 17
Day 4, every hour:
x18, 18, 18, 18, 18, 18, 18, 18, 18, 18
Day 5, every hour:
x19, 19, 19, 19, 19, 19, 19, 19, 19, 19
Day 6, every hour:
x20, 20, 20, 20, 20, 20, 20, 20, 20, 20 – Reached 10x20.
Start reducing the rest intervals between sets by 5 min a day.

Day 7, every 55 min:
x20, 20, 20, 20, 20, 20, 20, 20, 20, 20
Day 8, every 50 min:
x20, 20, 20, 20, 20, 20, 20, 20, 20, 20
Day 9, every 45 min:
x20, 20, 20, 20, 20, 20, 20, 20, 20, 20
Day 10, every 40 min:
x20, 20, 20, 20, 20, 20, 20, 20, 20, 20
Day 11, every 35 min:
x20, 20, 20, 20, 20, 20, 20, 19, 19, 19 – Can't keep up 10x20.
Time to increase the rest intervals by 10 min and concentrate
on adding reps.

Chart continued next page

NASA PUSHUP PROGRAM SAMPLE SCHEDULE

Day 12, every 45 min:
x21, 21, 21, 21, 21, 21, 21, 21, 21

Day 13, every 45 min:
x22, 22, 22, 22, 22, 22, 22, 22, 22

Day 14, every 45 min:
x23, 23, 23, 23, 23, 23, 23, 23, 23

Day 15, 16: rest

Day 17: max test: 1x47. Continue the progression the next day.

Day 18, every 45 min:
x24, 24, 24, 24, 24, 24, 24, 24, 24

Day 19, every 45 min:
x25, 25, 25, 25, 25, 25, 25, 25, 25

Day 20, every 45 min:
x26, 26, 26, 26, 26, 26, 26, 25, 25, 25 – Can't keep up adding a rep every day. Back off on the reps a little and start cutting time.

Day 21, every 40 min:
x25, 25, 25, 25, 25, 25, 25, 25, 25, 25

Day 22, every 35 min:
x25, 25, 25, 25, 25, 25, 25, 25, 25, 25

Day 23, every 30 min:
x25, 25, 25, 25, 25, 25, 25, 24, 24, 23 – Can't keep up 10x25. Increase the rest intervals by 10 min and add reps.

Day 22, every 40 min:
x26, 26, 26, 26, 26, 26, 26, 26, 26, 26

Day 23, every 40 min:
x27, 27, 27, 27, 27, 27, 27, 27, 27, 27

Day 24, every 40 min:
x28, 28, 28, 28, 28, 28, 28, 28, 28, 28

Day 25, every 40 min:
x29, 29, 29, 29, 29, 29, 29, 29, 29, 29

Day 26, 27: rest

Day 28: max test:
1x50. Continue the progression the next day.

**"Ideal training involves changing just one of many variables,
until that variable reaches a constant.
Then you change another, and then another
until you reach your goal."**

Repeat this until your memorize it.

GRIP-UPS, SPIDER-UPS, AND PINCH GRIP PUSHUPS

In this day and age owning a set of decent pipes and defined abs announces that one is 'in shape'. In shape for what, I would like to know? Call me old-fashioned, but I refuse to give the 'in shape' designation to anyone with soft hands and a weak grip. Hand strength is a hallmark of a physical culturalist who has arrived.

Any road warrior can figure out some sort of pushup for the upper body, an abs move, and something for the legs. But can you smoke your forearms and steel your fingers anywhere, anytime? Now you can.

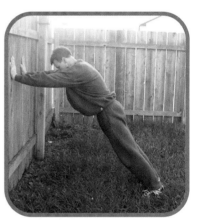

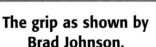

**The grip as shown by
Brad Johnson.**

*Photos courtesy
ExtremeBodyweightTraining.com*

This move comes highly recommended by S. Bogdasarov, Distinguished Coach of the USSR. Stand one step away from a wall. Keeping your legs and torso straight, lean on it with your locked arms, your palms flush on the wall. Now come up on your fingertips by gripping the surface of the wall and moving your hand towards the inside of your wrist. The movement of the hand is identical to that in a barbell wrist curl. The major difference is the involvement of the fingers. Move slowly. Increase the difficulty by shifting your feet further from the wall and/or using one arm at a time. Do not overdo it; give your tendons time to get conditioned.

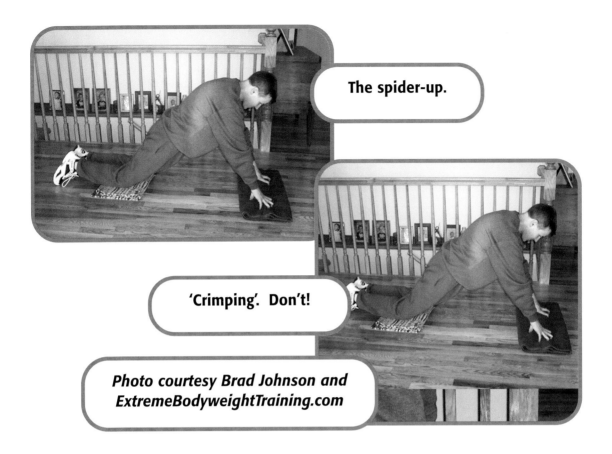

The spider-up.

'Crimping'. Don't!

Photo courtesy Brad Johnson and ExtremeBodyweightTraining.com

I learned the next two drills from ingenious fanatic of bodyweight strength training, Brad Johnson. "Place a cloth on a hard, smooth floor and get into fingertip push-up position. Begin with your fingers in a wide claw position and then pull all of your fingers toward the center until they meet each other. Return to starting position... Be careful to keep your fingers bent at the first joint to reduce the chances of injury."

Let us face it: unless you are a kung fu master, you are a long way from doing the spider in the pushup position. So rest most of your weight on your knees and your free hand, and work one arm at a time. You will be able to give yourself exactly the right amount of resistance by shifting your weight forward or back. And if things suddenly get hairy, you can quickly unload your fingers by leaning towards your free hand.

Brad employs the 'pivot point variation' technique extensively to customize the resistance of bodyweight exercises. PPV "refers to the age old technique of dropping your knees to the ground in order to reduce the load in a push up," explain Rick Osbourne and Brian McCaskey in their book *Pull Your Own Weight*. "With the old standard method, you have two potential pivot points: 1) your knees, and 2) your feet. And, strangely enough, it can be a long ways from your knees to your feet when you're ready to make progress... simply use a small bench that can be placed under your body at any point between your hips and your feet. When the bench is moved toward your hips, resistance is reduced. As your strength increases, the bench should gradually be moved toward your toes. Eventually, of course, the idea is to eliminate the PPV bench altogether..."

One more time: do not do hyperextend your fingers and thumb! Rock climbers have learned the hard way that 'crimping', as they call this type of cheating, will do your joints no good. Keep your digits slightly flexed, as if you are gripping a ball. It is much harder and safer this way.

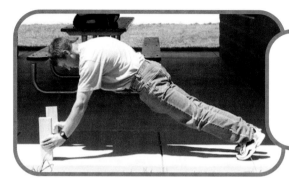

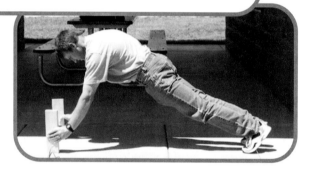

Fanatic of bodyweight strength training does a pinch grip pushup.

Photos courtesy ExtremeBodyweightTraining.com

If you know a thing or two about the old time physical culture, you must have heard about pinch gripping. Lifting two forty-five pound York Barbell plates sandwiched together with their smooth surfaces outward with one hand is a classic test of pinch grip strength. But what if no plates are handy? As usual, veteran gymnast Brad Johnson has the answer. The man got a couple of short 2x4s (about six inches) and laid them on the floor. He pinch gripped both boards hard between his thumbs and fingers and started doing pushups. Ingenious.

Grip like a vise, so your fingers do not slip and do not cheat by resting your weight on your palms. And make sure to start in a very easy position, e.g. off your knees. There is no dishonor in starting on the wall so even less of your weight is on your fingers. That way you will not even need a board; just pinch grip a narrow doorway with one hand and spot yourself with the other. The further you move your feet away from your working hand, the harder the exercise.

Do not extend your elbow completely; as your body becomes nearly vertical the pressure on your fingers falls off. Better do short, slow half reps with your chest close to your hand. Pinching an open door is even more challenging, just beware of the risks of training in an unstable environment.

Attention! The above exercises will load your fingers, thumbs, and wrists in a manner you are not accustomed to. Novelty is good because it means explosive new muscle growth. But it is also a double-edged sword that could get you injured. So start by doing just a couple of very easy low rep sets of all three drills, e.g. four sets of four. Practice almost every day and build up slowly enough to avoid any joint soreness or pulled tendons. Iron claws will be your reward.

THE DRAGON WALK

I do not care for lunges. Never have, never will. First, they are never done right. Second, they have a lightweight, 'aerobics, spinning, and toning', kind of reputation. Can't have that.

Enter the evil alternative to the lunge: the Dragon Walk. It is a Chinese Chi Kung exercise that I learned from my friend and author of *The Five Animal Frolics* videos, John Du Cane. John knows a thing or two about training on the road and in unfamiliar places. Born in South Africa, he soon moved with his parents to Sierra Leone and then to a boarding school in England. When studying in Cambridge, Du Cane drove a VW bus to the Middle East, places like Afghanistan and Iran. He lived in a yoga community in India for five years and in a few other exotic places after that before landing in the US. All along, in environments most unfriendly for staying in shape, John has been consistently improving his terrific physique reminiscent of Mikhail Baryshnikov or Bruce Lee. The dragon walk has been one of his secrets.

Ideally, practice outdoors. Go barefoot or wear thin-soled flat shoes common among martial artists. Turn your palms up, bend your elbows to about forty-five degrees, and hold your hands out to your sides slightly above your shoulders. This alignment is supposed to help you accumulate the mysterious 'Chi' energy. Even if you do not believe in that sort of thing, still stick to the recommended arm position. It will aid you in keeping your chest open, your shoulders down, and your back upright.

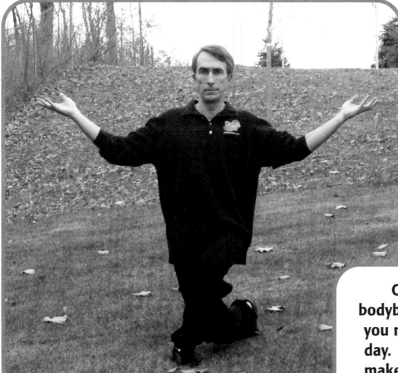

Let your shoulders relax away from your ears and imagine that your head is suspended from the ceiling by a string, the neck long and loose. Keep your back ramrod straight and upright for the duration of the drill! If you bend over, you are not a dragon but a smaller and weaker mythological critter. A leprechaun comes to mind.

Contrary to the bodybuilding mythology, you may practice every day. Just make sure to make some days much easier than others.

293

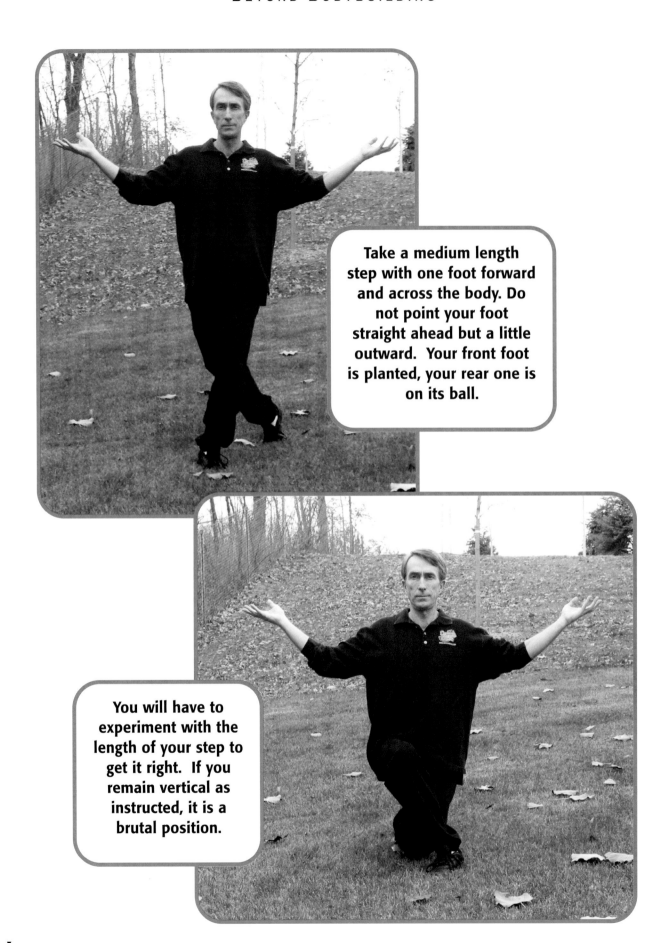

Take a medium length step with one foot forward and across the body. Do not point your foot straight ahead but a little outward. Your front foot is planted, your rear one is on its ball.

You will have to experiment with the length of your step to get it right. If you remain vertical as instructed, it is a brutal position.

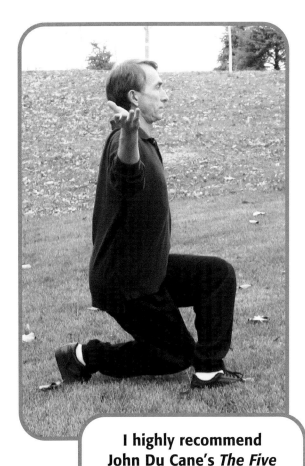

I highly recommend John Du Cane's *The Five Animal Frolics* and *Qigong Recharge* DVDs.

Take a medium length step with one foot forward and across the body. Do not point your foot straight ahead but a little outward. Your front foot is planted, your rear one is on its ball. Make sure that your knees are always tracking your feet. Sink down – stay upright! – and let your rear knee come down to within an inch of the ground. Touching the deck is cheating.

Now comes the interesting part. The knee that is catching up must end up exactly outside your leading ankle. You will have to experiment with the length of your step to get it right. If you remain vertical as instructed, it is a brutal position. Pause there for a moment to drive the point home.

Be sure to study the photos. Now walk! Expect to stumble around for a while until you find the groove. Trust me, it is worth the trouble. Look straight ahead. If you cannot help bending over, squeezing your glutes and driving your hips forward will help.

It will not take you long to find out that this martial arts secret exercise delivers cut and muscular legs with staying power. And makes you a better man or a woman in the process. To give you something to shoot for, John Du Cane can dragon walk for an hour straight! John also happens to be the man who had the rare honor of teaching a Chi Kung seminar at the Arnold Schwarzenegger Fitness Expo. So plan to dedicate years to work up to his level. Your best bet is to build up the load in the rest-pause fashion. Take a few steps. As soon as you feel that the next rep might be not up to the draconian standard, stop. Relax and shake the tension out of your legs as if you are shaking water off, then carry on.

Contrary to the bodybuilding mythology, you may practice every day. Just make sure to make some days much easier than others. And if you decide to incorporate the dragon walk into a standard bodybuilding routine, do it instead of leg extensions and similar silliness as a 'finisher'.

Enjoy the pain!

SLOW KICKS

Full contact fighters are known for their outstanding strength, conditioning, and physiques. Which is why many of the exercises featured in the *Naked Warrior* series come from martial arts and this technique is no exception. Slow kicks over a chair have been made popular by kickboxing legend Bill 'Superfoot' Wallace. Way into his fifties, Superfoot is still a formidable fighter with a cut to ribbons body. It is almost comical how Bill, who lives on a steady diet of hamburgers (hold the cheese!) and fries, puts ephedra-popping kids young enough to be his grandchildren to shame with his abs.

The kickboxing champion practices super slow kicks in order to enhance his power, precision, and flexibility. The side effect of his training is highly defined legs and hips. It would be unrealistic to expect you to emulate Superfoot's state of the art moves from the get go. Instead we shall apply his drill's basic principle to two of the most basic kicks, front and back. You need to learn how to crawl before flying; you can always get Wallace's videos from Superfoot.com once you get hooked.

The front kick. Practice barefoot. Hold the back of a chair for balance – something you should part with eventually, like a bike's training wheels – and raise your knee as high as your solar plexus. Keep the knee of the leg you are standing on slightly bent and tracking the foot. Turn the foot out at an approximately forty-five-degree angle to the direction of the kick.

Slowly extend your airborne leg and 'kick' an imaginary target with the ball of your foot or the entire surface of your foot. Pull your toes back. Tense your whole body when you have connected with the virtual target, then slowly return your foot to the ground by retracing its path back. Relax momentarily and repeat on the other side.

Performance pointers. Don't turn your hips but keep them square to the target. Pinching an imaginary coin with your cheeks will help. Press hard into the deck with your stationary foot and imagine that you are wedging yourself in between the target and the ground.

Reread the last sentence; it is extremely important.

Tense your abs hard. Don't lean back or forward. One subtle karate tip that never fails to make a huge difference in my military and law enforcement courses is to point your belly button slightly up by shortening your 'lower abs'. You will not get all these subtleties at once; it is alright, just be persistent in your practice. Eventually do your slow kicks over an elevation; work up to the back of a chair. Naturally, this type of active flexibility will not come overnight.

Strength, height, and precision are the goals of this drill. Which means do not keep cranking out mindless sloppy reps. Do one kick at a time and rest for as long as necessary to make the next one perfect. Shoot for the total of twenty-five reps per leg every other day. Stretch your hip flexors afterwards.

The back kick. You have been 'attacked' from behind and you kick back like a mule. Look over your right shoulder and raise your right knee until your heel is pointing at the 'target'. Your kicking foot should be angled approximately forty-five degrees down and flexed toward its knee. Your stationary foot is pointing straight away from the target and the knee is slightly bent.

Slowly kick back and lean forward at the same time. The back kick is very powerful and it generates a lot of recoil; the lean helps you counter it and generate even more power. Keep your eyes on your target, which should be knee to waist high. Eventually you may practice high back kicks, not very useful in a real trouble but great for competition and conditioning.

At the point of impact 'wedge' yourself between the deck and the 'attacker'. Tense your both glutes as hard as possible and drive your hips forward. Retrace your kick back to the ground. Superset your front and back kicks with the same leg. Between the two of them, these kicks will work your hips and thighs very thoroughly.

More sophisticated kicks – side, round, hook, axe, crescent, and reverse crescent – may be practiced in the same fashion: slow, tight, with the abs locked on 'impact'. However, I would prefer that you learned these from a martial arts instructor. You would have to go out of your way to hurt yourself with slow front and back kicks; this is not the case with the rest.

For instance, during the roundhouse kick the knee of the base leg must be protected from the torque by either a pivot until the heel points at the target or by a counter rotation of the torso. If it sounds complicated, it is. And failing to learn these subtleties is what hurt many folks during the cardio kickboxing craze a few years ago. So knock on your local dojo's door if you want to go an extra mile. Otherwise just stick to the front and back kicks.

Slow kicks are far from being the only powerful and innovative moves in Bill Wallace's strength and conditioning arsenal. Even if you are not a martial artist, you will do yourself a favor if you pick up a copy of his book *Dynamic Stretching & Kicking* from Superfoot.com.

THE "LIZARD"

There is a term in the military, 'individual movement technique'. Only movie actors and third world insurgents stand tall and shoot from the hip; professional soldiers eat dirt, keep a low profile, and make the other guy die for his country.

The Russian Spetsnaz uses five types of low IMT. Move on all fours behind low cover such as tall grass, otherwise crawl on your belly. Stay on your side when dragging a wounded comrade or a prisoner. Flip on your back in a ravine, when expecting an ambush, or when covering a leaving team. Finally, there is 'the Lizard'.

Unique to the former Soviet spec ops community, the lizard is the fastest, the most silent, and the hardest low movement technique. It is used to approach a sentry. The operator slings his AK on his back, assumes a low pushup position, and quickly runs like a lizard over to the enemy with a knife in his teeth. Why am I telling you all this? – Because this deadly maneuver also happens to be an excellent exercise for your upper body and waist. Tactical efficiency alone would not explain the glee in the DIs' eyes. The drill is evil!

Hit the deck and let us start. With your elbows bent at ninety degrees take a step forward with your left arm. Then a step with your left foot. Bring your knee forward far enough to twist your waist like a reptile's. Repeat the sequence with your right arm and then your right leg. At any point your weight should be supported by three points: arm-arm-leg, or arm-leg-leg. Move! Lizards do not drag their bellies or hind paws like overfed crocs; they run! And don't even think about lifting your head or semi-straightening out your elbows! At a Russian Special Forces training base you would be punished with a painful whip of a thin metal rod. Right where it counts.

Don't expect to succeed at once; the lizard takes practice. But it is well worth it as your painfully pumped pecs, arms, and waist will soon find out. Don't count the reps; go for distance instead. Belly flop and rest, like a reptile in cold weather, between spurts.

THE DECK SQUAT

Repetition bodyweight squats are the mainstay in martial artists' conditioning. They build leg and cardiopulmonary endurance, burn fat, and toughen one up. Unfortunately, not every pair of knees can handle them.

Not any more. Enter the 'deck squat' or 'rock-up squat', a recent rage among Brazilian Jiu Jitsu players, mixed martial artists, and Recon Marines.

To work up to a deck squat start by sitting on a curb, your hips pushed as far back as possible, your body folded over, and your arms reaching forward for counterbalance. Touch down, rock back, immediately rock forward, and get up without hesitation.

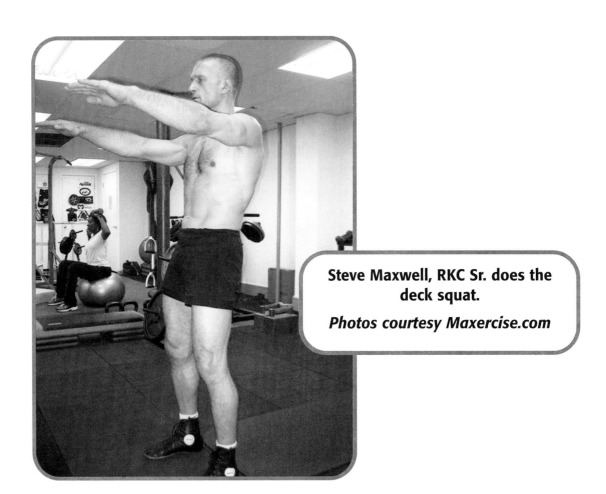

Steve Maxwell, RKC Sr. does the deck squat.

Photos courtesy Maxercise.com

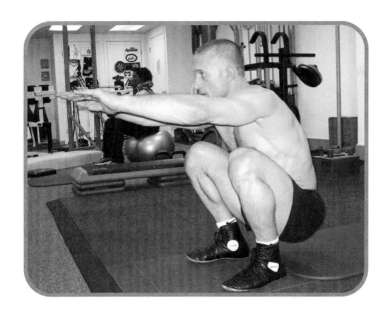

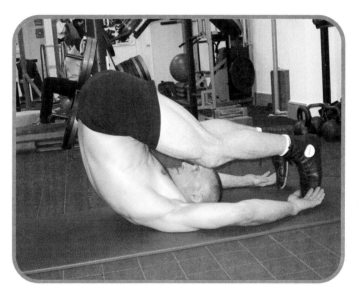

Do not move your feet underneath you or cross them. Do not let your knees bow in either. Finally, do not let your knees slip forward and try to keep your shins vertical. This is the secret to unloading your knees while working the rest of your body hard. The patella tendon is not smashing the kneecap into the joint. Besides, the knee is further protected from the rear by hamstring tension when the shin is vertical.

The deck squat is to the regular bodyweight squat what the box squat is to the standard barbell squat. Coached by Louie Simmons, powerlifter Matt Dimel who blew out his patella tendons with conventional power squats rehabbed himself by squatting to a box and went on to lift over a thousand pounds!

If you are a big fellow or gal, hold a light weight such as a five pound plate in front of you for counterbalance. And do not be afraid to use momentum; this is not a strength exercise.

Crank up your reps. Your legs will get shaky and you will feel like coughing up a hairball. When you have had it, walk around to let your heart rate come down and come back for more punishment.

After a couple of workouts try the deck squat proper – to the deck. BJJ world champion Steve Maxwell, MS, RKC Sr. explains the drill succinctly. "The rock-up squat is one of my favorite exercises for my martial arts classes… It's like combining a pullover, a situp, and a squat all in one move. Done in high sets… it is a tremendous cardio movement."

If you are wondering what does the pullover have to do with the deck squat, Steve brings the kettlebell behind his head on the bottom of each rep, then pulls it forward, sits up, and finally rocks up.

Practice on a surface that gives a little, such as a wrestling mat, grass, or a thick carpet. Use your momentum and keep moving or you will not get up. Holding a weight for a counterbalance is almost a must in the beginning.

Once you do enough reps you are likely to cut corners on the negative and literally fall and roll. Do not slow down, relax and go with the flow as long as you land softly rather than slam on your rear end. Do not worry; you will get enough work on the way up. Here is your opportunity to learn how to fall properly while getting conditioned.

Some comrades will have to stick with the curb or box rock-up squat as the repeated 'tucking the tail in' of the deck squat would not agree with their backs. (Repeated flexion may jack up the discs.) Even if you are not one of them, it is a good idea to do a few back bends between your sets.

THE RUSSIAN LAUNDRY

Russian life is hard and it produces hard people. Many conveniences Americans take for granted are rare luxuries in the countries of the former Soviet Union. Washing machines and dryers, for instance. Most Russian women still wash and wring out their laundry by hand! They usually do not get much help from their husbands unless their husbands are Sambo players.

Sambo stands for SAMOzaschita Bez Oruzhiya, 'self-defense without weapons', a Russian martial art and sport similar to judo. Its practitioners are not better husbands; they have a selfish reason. They know that twisting wet clothes, especially the tough jackets they train and compete in, develops a vise-like grip. Besides, you cannot help using the rest of your upper body muscles, especially the abs, the pecs, and the lats. The result is a body of stone.

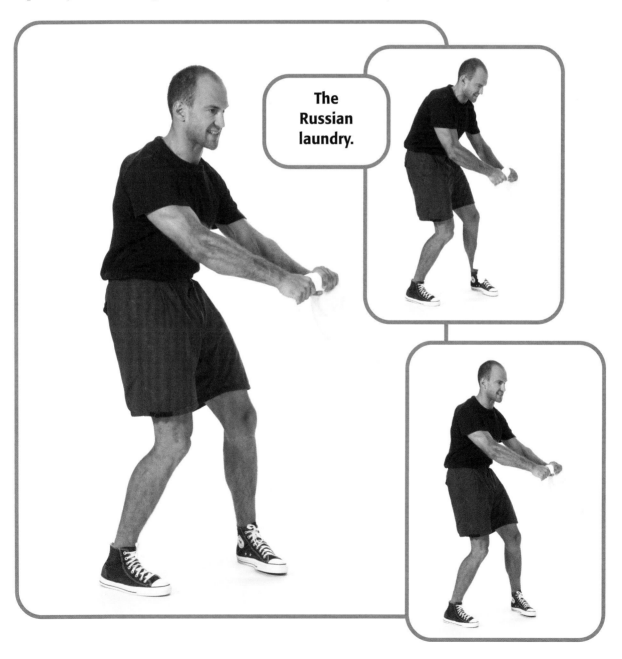

The Russian laundry.

I do not really see any of you doing laundry by hand, but you can find a towel anywhere, wet it, and wring it out. Somehow it is more fun when it is not a household chore. Fold a wet towel, the more times the harder. Start wringing it out. Forcefully exhale as you twist the towel. Pretend that the air flows through your hands. Don't let the pressure go to your head. Turn your toes slightly in and keep your legs tense as bowstrings. Tuck in your tailbone and tense your glutes. Flex your abs, but do not suck them in. Note how your torso muscles tense and your body 'winds up'. Pay attention to how the action starts in your lower abdomen and spirals through your armpits, the pecs and the lats, into your arms. Press your shoulders down away from your ears and do not let your elbows flare. Feel incredible overall tension.

Rest briefly, rewet your towel, and wring it out in the opposite direction. Try to get every bit of water out of the towel. Do as many sets as you wish, until your muscles from the waist up feel thoroughly worked. Remember that the more times you fold the towel and the drier you wring it the greater the overload. In a pinch this exercise will work with a dry towel, but not quite as well.

Make sure to practice *Fast & Loose* style relaxation exercises between sets. 'Shake water' off your limbs, jog loosely in place, etc. Such moves are an essential part of all Russian athletes' regimens. It is a fact that improving your relaxation skills will make you a more efficient animal. Also relax briefly between each twist. You should not feel any pressure in your head or get dizzy.

For variety you can wring out the towel behind your back, over your head (you had better be on the beach), hold it vertically rather than horizontally, etc. A more localized variation of the drill is drying out a washcloth and eventually a hand towel with one hand. Gather it up into a progressively smaller ball into your hand. Behold the power pump in your forearms!

This out of the box Russian exercise offers a number of unexpected benefits in addition to a thorough upper body workout anywhere, anytime. It teaches you good body mechanics for max strength.

Russian military hand-to-hand combat instructors mention three important principles of power generation: 'summation', 'wave', and 'corkscrew'. The first two refer to the essential skill of initiating any effort from the core and then dynamically passing it into the striking limb while adding force from every muscle on the way. If any muscle along the power route fails to kick in, you have, in the words of boxing coach Steve Baccari, RKC of PowerBehindthePunch.com a 'power leakage'. The strength goes down the drain. It is as true in the bench press as it is on the boxing ring or the wrestling mat.

Mangling a towel will teach you to seamlessly 'chain' the effort of all your muscles together. This will pay off in many strength exercises. Not only will you get stronger, your training will also become safer. In addition to robbing you of strength, 'power leakages' also create weak links where injuries are likely to occur. Say no to the 'leakage'. Say yes to the 'linkage'.*

The third principle of martial power is the 'corkscrew'. A threaded firearm is superior to a smooth-barreled one. Rotation or spiral tension increases the stability and power of almost any action. This is the essence of the corkscrew principle. Gripping the rifle while isometrically twisting both hands in opposite directions made a dramatic difference for bayonet fighting in the Marine Corps Martial Arts Program. The Marines' thrusts became more powerful and harder to deflect.

The same is true for gym exercises. Try 'breaking' the bar when benching and your BP will go up, once you get the hang of it, because the corkscrew action engages more muscles and makes the weight more stable. You have, in effect, created your own Smith machine. The Russian sambo drill will teach you how to apply this corkscrew.

Because the towel wringing drill does not have an eccentric component it will not make you too sore and you can practice it almost every day. And when you leave the Russian laundromat dripping with sweat, your torso will look like Bruce Lee's during his striking pauses in the middle of fight scenes.

THE TIGER BEND PUSHUP

Comrade, have you heard of the 'tiger bend'? It is a superman variation of the handstand pushup that makes you press up from an elbow stand, where your parallel forearms and palms are planted flat on the floor while your body is in up the air. "The tiger bend is... a terrific strength feat," promises Bob Hoffman's old magazine. "... The movement develops exceptional triceps, the only fault however, you must be a good balancer to perform it."

Indeed, unless you are a mutant, you have a snowball's chance in hell of eking out even a single tiger bend. Fortunately, you can improvise a much easier version of this triceps killer in your hotel room. Dennis 'the Yukon Hercules' Weis (DennisBWeis.com) recommends it in one of his excellent books.

Do a pushup off your forearms planted parallel about four inches apart, your fingers pointed forward. Tighten up and push up so your elbows clear the deck. Lock out without letting your elbows flare out. Lower yourself in the same groove until your elbows rest on the floor under your body. Do not fall through the last inch or two; this tough portion of the range of motion is most productive! Unless you have weak elbows – enjoy!

You can vary the effect of the exercise slightly by placing your elbows underneath you and bending your arm almost to the point where your forearms touch your bis or planting them further forward and reducing the elbow flexion. Experiment!

Beware: rocking forward to start a rep is a forced rep at best; you will build more muscle if you press up without cheating.

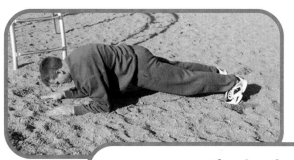 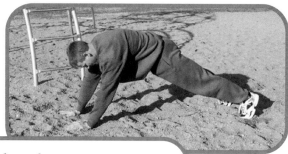

The tiger bend pushup

Photos courtesy ExtremeBodyweightTraining.com

The tiger bend pushup can be customized for different levels of strength. Elevate your feet if you can hack it; elevate your hands if the floor version is too hard. You can also practice off your knees.

The toughest variation of the tiger bend pushup calls for using only one arm. You may point your fingers slightly in and your elbow slightly out but do not let your elbow flare out any more when it clears the deck.

As if that was not hard enough, you can shift more of your weight to your hand and almost overbalance forward. You can also make the one arm tiger bend pushup easier by lifting your hips and rocking back on your feet. And easier yet by pushing up from your knees. Calisthenics, or 'cals' as they are known in the military, are very versatile.

In any type of the tiger bend pushup, keep you reps under five per set (not that you are likely to manage more anyway). Since your elbows are not used to the intense overload of the tiger bend, start out with the total of ten reps per workout and gradually build up the volume. It is imperative that you employ the high-tension techniques for maximum safety and performance: tense your glutes and abs, squeeze your thighs together, etc.

Go get 'em, tiger!

QUESTIONS & ANSWERS:

HOW TO MAKE BODYWEIGHT NECK BRIDGES HARDER

Question: What is the best way to make neck bridges harder?

For back bridges, old-timers held a weight on their chests, which is one option. Here is another that works even better. Lie on your back and get ready to bridge. Raise your arms overhead and hold on to a stationary object such as an upright of a power rack or a heavy kettlebell. Bend your elbows slightly and bring them closer together as if you are about to do a pullover. Pull your feet towards you and start back bridging, that is, push down with the back of your head until the top of your head rests on the mat.

Here is the wrinkle: as you are extending your neck, perform a low intensity isometric pullover. This is a self-resistance exercise; you can give your neck as much or as little resistance as you want which makes for a very thorough and safe workout.

For front bridges instead of using extra weight move your feet further back and rest your weight on your forehead rather than the top of your head. Spot yourself with your hands. To get a stronger contraction 'flare' your neck.

GYMNASTIC RINGS FOR BODYBUILDERS

Question: I've been told that exercises on the rings are largely responsible for gymnasts' awesome strength and built. I'm way too heavy for iron crosses and such; could I still benefit from ring training?

You bet. The first exercise that comes to mind is the pushup, your feet up on a bench and the rings set up a few inches off the ground. Strength coach extraordinaire Ethan Reeve has his athletes at Wake Forest University in North Carolina combine these with Power Breathing for a greater contraction. Mr. Olympia Larry Scott (LarryScott.com) used to do flies on the same type of rig – an unbelievably powerful and challenging pecs exercise!

Rings are great for pullups and chinups and they are a lot kinder to the elbows than the straight bar. All of the ring drills have a fun, athletic feel to them and are brutal on the prime mover and stabilizer muscles alike. The great variety of ring exercises is limited only by your imagination.

There are many ways to customize the difficulty of ring exercises to any level. You could incline or decline your body. You could extend or flex your arms. You could hang one ring higher than the other. And these are just a handful of many possibilities.

Competition gymnastic rings are pricey and you don't need them anyway. I like the rings made by RingTraining.com. They are light enough to throw into your gym bag and you can hook them up to a power rack or basement rafters and take them down in seconds. The above website also offers plenty of free ring training advice for athletes who are not gymnasts.

JACK LA LANNE'S PIKE PUSHUP

Question: What is a good exercise to build strength for handstand pushups? I wouldn't mind building my delts at the same time.

The following unique incline pushup from the gymnasts' arsenal has been practiced by great Jack La Lanne. Put your feet up on a chair, but instead of keeping your body in a straight line jackknife it at the hips so your hips are way up in the air. La Lanne instructs to keep your legs rigid and to place your hands as close to the chair as possible. In other words, as close as your strength allows. The nearer your hands are to your feet, the more jackknifed is your body. The pec involvement decreases and your delts have to work extra hard, almost as if you are doing a handstand pushup.

You can also vary the difficulty of the drill by redistributing the weight between your feet and hands. Once you get pretty good, shift weight so much on to your hands that you come close to overbalancing and making a forward tumble. Be careful.

In order to work your delts hard do not look at the floor but rather touch it with the crown of your head. It is a very important fine point!

If you manage the basic incline jackknife pushup with ease, try putting your feet up on a Swiss ball or an office chair on wheels for extra excitement. You can also increase the range of motion by elevating your hands on stools. Put up your feet even higher than before, if you go this route.

The La Lanne pushup is guaranteed to fill out your shoulders and build your overhead pressing strength – fast.

ACE THE MARINE PULLUP TEST WITH THE 'RUSSIAN REST-PAUSE'

Question: I am trying to ace the USMC pullup test with 20 but I am stuck at 17. My grip gives out first; how should I train?

Rock climbers know that once your forearms get pumped, you are toast. Incidentally, the jarhead who holds the USMC pullup record is a climber. During his record attempt he would periodically hang on one arm while shaking out and resting the other. Following is a technique we used in the Russian military to build our pullup specific grip strength.

The technique is a variation of the rest-pause, although the 'no rest pause' would be a more appropriate name. Do a pullup, then hang for a specified period of time, usually five to ten seconds, and do another rep. Hang some more, do a pullup, etc. Incredibly simple and highly effective.

The Russian rest pause works with most high rep exercises. Kettlebell lifting competitors sometimes purposefully slow down their jerk tempo to five reps a minute in training. Even if the grip is not an issue, a special type of isometric fatigue builds up in extended sets. Improving your specific endurance in holding, say, the pushup lockout will improve your pushup numbers. Do five or ten pushups and pause in the top position without sagging for fifteen seconds, then do another ten, and keep on going.

Add a day of Russian rest pause training to your regular pullup week and you will score 100% on that PFT test. Or else.

S.W.A.T. DIPS: SAFER AND HARDER

Question: I heard that you teach a special kind of parallel bar dip to S.W.A.T. teams. I am curious, what is different about it and is there any reason for a bodybuilder to do it?

As demonstrated in my *Rapid Response* video set, the S.W.A.T. dip to the regular dip is what the bench press from the power rack pins set at the chest level is to the regular bench. Safer and harder.

Without any extra weight, slowly lower yourself as deep as your shoulders find comfortable. Straighten out your legs and note how close your feet are to the ground. Get out and rig up a box or some other sturdy object to support you exactly at that level.

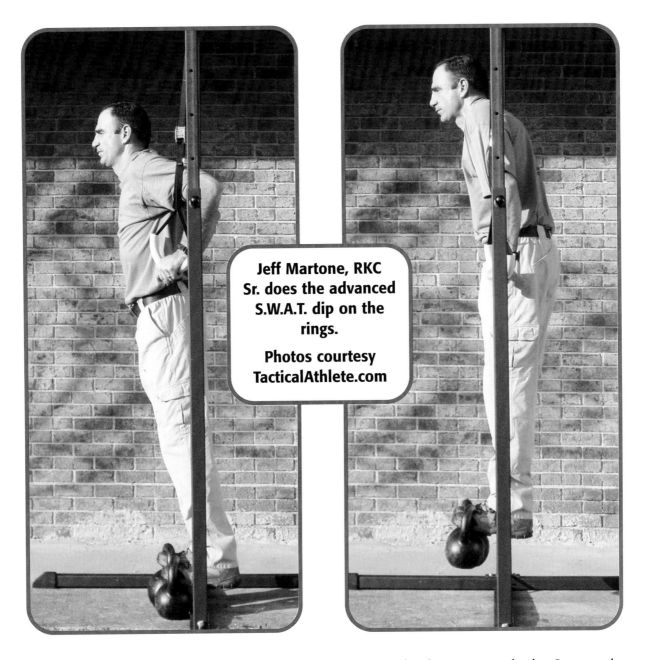

Jeff Martone, RKC Sr. does the advanced S.W.A.T. dip on the rings.

Photos courtesy TacticalAthlete.com

Climb on the box, place your hands on the bars. Inhale and tighten up your body. Squeeze the bars and straighten out your arms. Make sure not to cheat by jumping; keep your knees locked and your feet flat.

Lock out and move up as high as possible by pressing your shoulders away from your ears by tensing your lats and pecs. Lower yourself under control, keeping your legs straight and your feet parallel to the deck. Touch down lightly and relax completely before the next rep. You will quickly realize that overcoming a dead weight without a pre-stretch and a bounce is a real bear. Like a squat from the low pins.

Once you get the groove down pile on weight. No more sore shoulders and stretch marks. Hello, powerful and healthy shoulder girdle!

THE ROLLING NECK BRIDGE

Question: Should I work my neck directly?

If you want to build a neck so muscular that you have to turn your whole torso as a gun turret to face someone go get yourself a neck harness and go nuts on heavy shrugs. If the prospect of ordering custom made dress shirts does not excite you and you are satisfied with the size you are getting from your regular routine, you should still include the following exercise into your regimen.

The rolling neck bridge will strengthen your neck from every direction and make you a lot more injury proof. Besides, it feels awesome when your traps are fried from heavy deads and shrugs. Really gets those kinks out.

Start with an easier version of the drill. Stand a couple of feet away from the wall and lean against it with your forehead while keeping your body rigid. You may wear a hat if the wall is too rough or you have a thing against greasy spots on your wallpaper.

Move your feet in place and slowly rotate, so first the side of your head presses against the wall, then the back, etc. until you make a full circle. Spot your self with your hands.

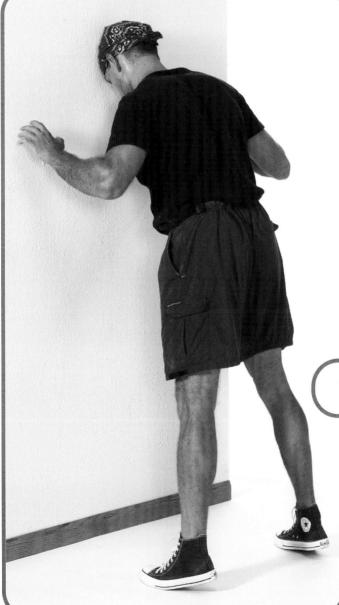

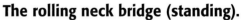

The rolling neck bridge (standing).

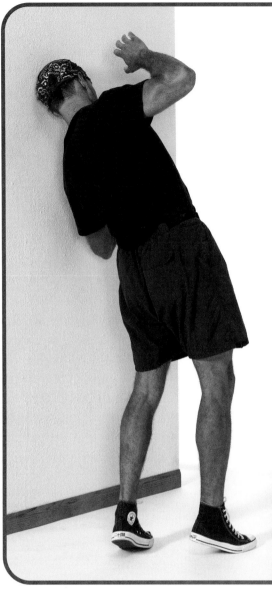

Make a very smooth transition of the load from muscle to muscle as you are spinning. It is not as easy as it sounds. What will help is tightening other muscles on the side of your body that faces the wall. The key word here is 'linkage'! When you face forward, flex your abs and thighs. When you face away, tense your back, glutes, and hams. Tighten your obliques, etc. when you are sideways. Keep your head fairly neutral throughout.

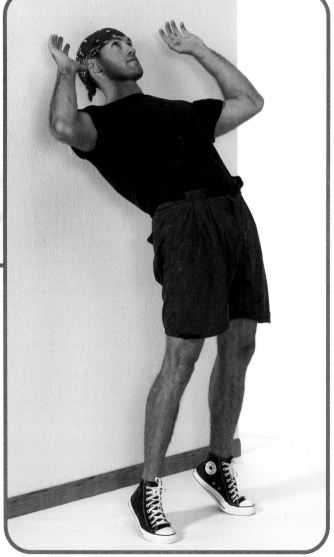

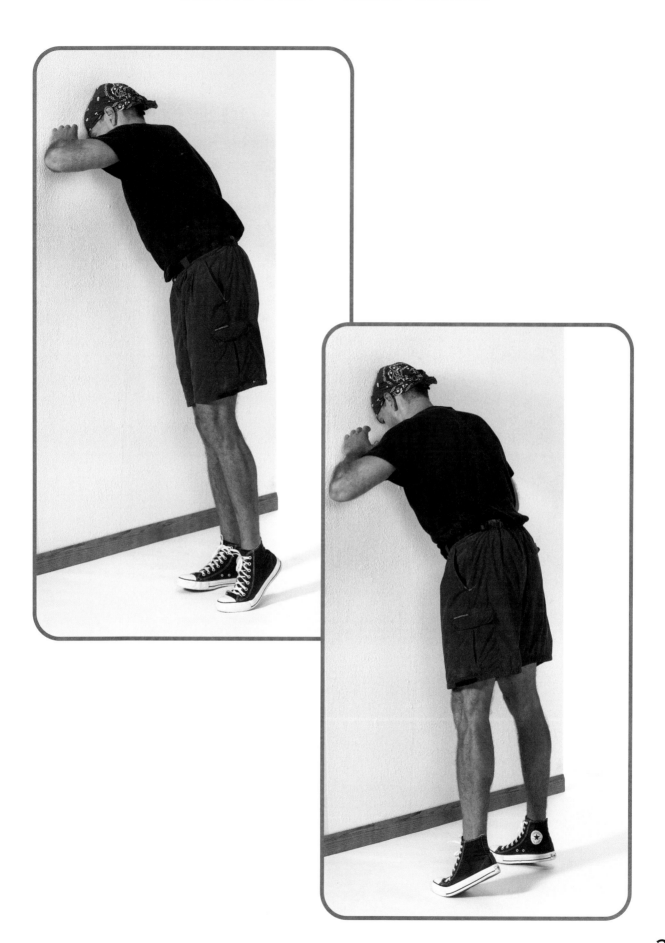

When you feel ready, try the same on the floor. You will have to keep your body semi-bridged unless your neck strength is truly freaky. Do not confuse this drill with the true wrestler's bridge that hyperextends and hyperflexes the neck; keep your head almost in line with your body! Do not think this will make the exercise easier; just the other way around!

One more time: keep your body tensed and semi-bridged!

Carefully spot yourself with your hands at all times; breaking your neck is not on the agenda. You will find that your shoulders are also helping by unloading your neck as they roll on the ground. That is fine, at least until wrestlers start asking you what have you been doing for your neck.

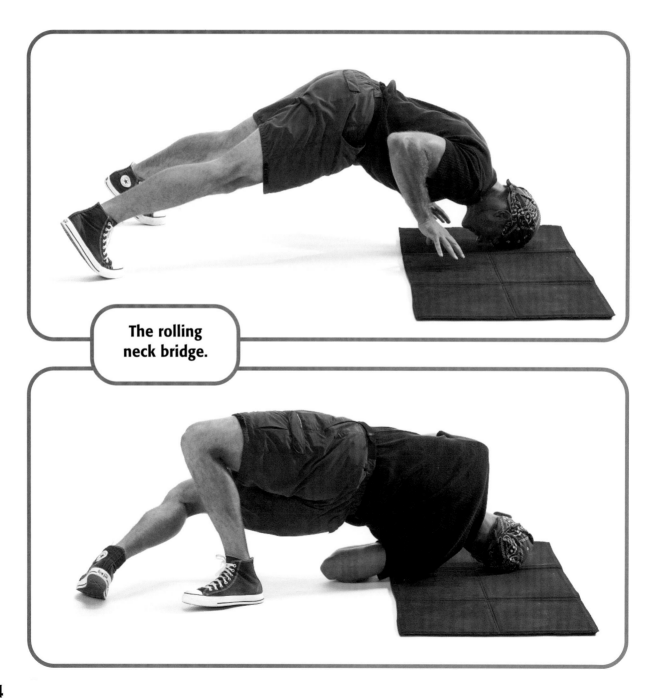

The rolling neck bridge.

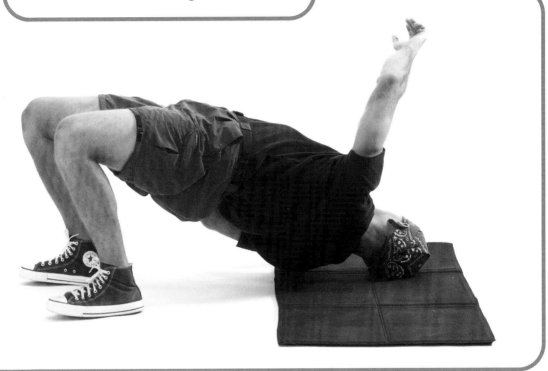

Carefully spot yourself with your hands at all times; breaking your neck is not on the agenda.

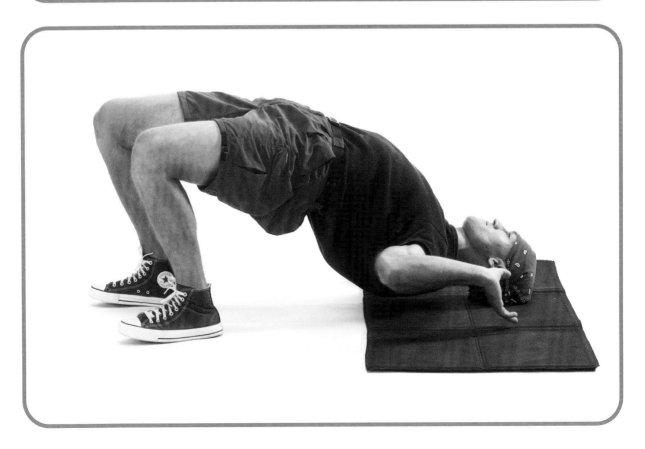

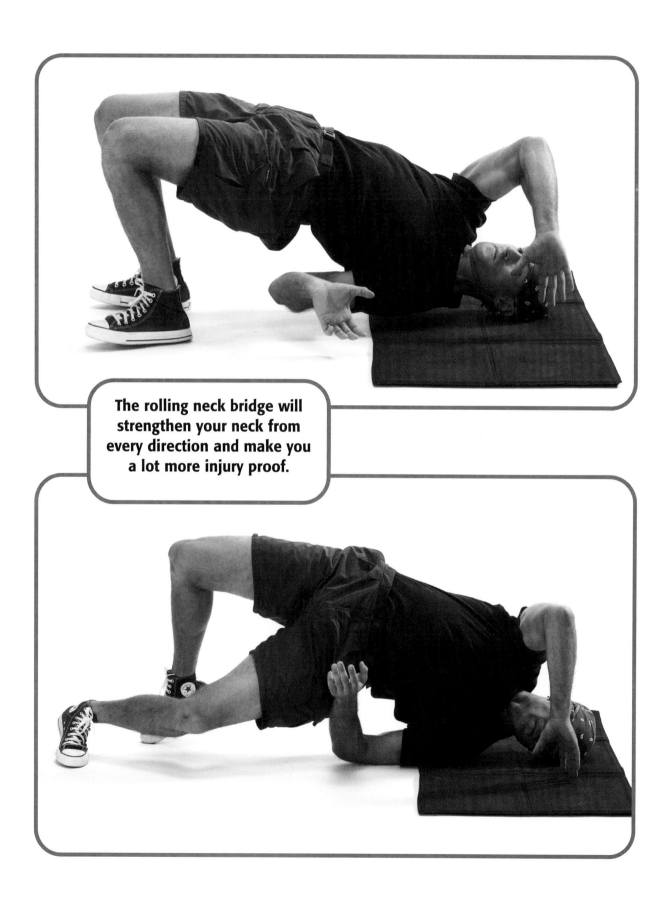

The rolling neck bridge will strengthen your neck from every direction and make you a lot more injury proof.

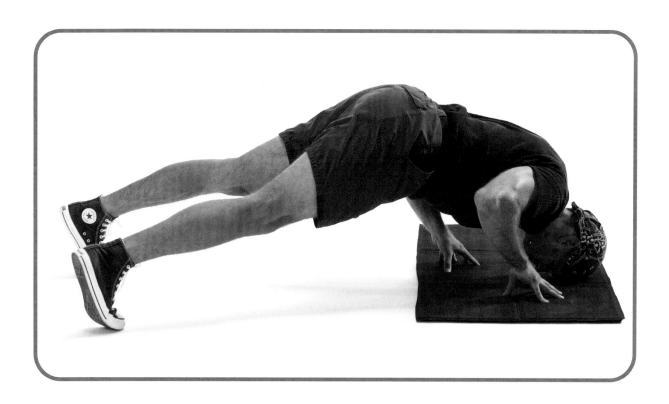

SHOULD I DO WEIGHTED PULLUPS TO UP MY BODYWEIGHT PULLUPS REPS?

Question: You mentioned that in Russia a bodybuilder is considered a raw beginner until he can do twenty pullups. I have decided to achieve the 20 mark, hell or high water. Should I add weight to my pullups to get there faster?

Yes, if you already can do at least ten pullups and the extra weight is light. 'Light' is the secret. While hanging a heavy kettlebell on your waist will build absolute strength, it might not make an impression on your high rep efforts. Yes, you will fly through your first few reps once you take off the weight belt but you will wilt shortly afterwards. Specificity, comrades. Ten to twenty-five pounds of extra poundage is about right. If, for instance, you can do fifteen unweighted pullups, a quarter will bring you down to below ten but not as low as five. Alternating pullup workouts with and without extra weight will bring about the greatest gains.

SUPER STRICT PULLUPS — THE HARD WAY

Q: *You have convinced my training partner and myself to do pullups from a dead hang. It works, my armpits are finally chafing! Is there a way to make the exercise even stricter and more brutal?*

For a Tactical Strength Challenge competition hosted by Maxercise gym in Philadelphia, evil genius Steve Maxwell, RKC Sr., MS rigged up a pullup bar suspended on chains. The chains enforced ultra strict performance; any attempt to jerk or cheat made the competitor swing, get out of the groove, and sometimes slam into the wall! To give you an idea of the increased difficulty, Level 2 runner-up John Allstadt can crank out 14 dead hang, neck to the bar pullups with a 70-pound kettlebell on a stationary bar. The Maxercise bar stopped him at 8! Definitely consider this type of rig for your home gym; a plumbing pipe, a couple of chains, and the fittings to hold it all together and attached to the rafters is all you need. At the club you can suspend a barbell from chains hooked to the top of the power rack with carabiners. Or you could buy the Dual Suspension System from MilitaryFitness.org. Enjoy the pain!

INDEX

Q

Quad exercises/training, 85, 120–121

R

Rader, Peary, 204
Radley, Alan, 246
Randall, Bruce, 70–72
Random practice, 51–52
Reading, Jim, 171
Reape, Jack, 64, 105, 111
Reeve, Ethan, 307
Remer, Jason, 249
Renegade lunges, 169–176
Reverse grip presses, 240, 242
Rigert, David, 87, 112, 212
RKC ladder program, 54
Rodionov, V. I., 46–47
Rolling neck bridges, 311–317
Roman, Robert, 25, 50, 217
Rotator cuff exercises/training, 217, 238. *See also* Neck and shoulder exercises/training
Rowing exercises, 148
Russian barbell calf raises, 177. *See also* Calf exercises
Russian bodybuilding programs
    Bench press training, 30–37
    Fatigue cycling, 18–21
    Growth of, 18, 137–138
    Intensity and, 13
    Volume and, 13
Russian farmer walk (exercise), 178. *See also* Calf exercises
Russian laundry (exercise), 303–305
Russian military/special forces
    Fatigue cycling by, 21
    Kettlebell training by, 13–15, 21, 267. *See also* Kettlebell techniques/methods
    Ladder technique, 48–49, 279–281
    Training by, 106, 217, 260, 267, 279, 281, 284, 299, 304, 309
Russian National Powerlifting Team
    Bench press training and, 30–37, 48, 114
    Layoffs by, 110
    Pyramid workouts and, 48, 165
Russian squat assault, 21–25

S

Saddle deadlifts, 178, 185
Sale, Digby, 93–94

Sandow, Eugene, 80, 242, 270
Saxon, Arthur, 2, 39, 77
Schwarzenegger, Arnold, 86, 151, 295
Scialpi, Steve, 56
Scott, Larry, 307
Seated barbell military press, 88
Secondary exercise/drill combinations, 5, 6
See-saw presses, 209–211
Self-esteem (bodybuilding and), 3
Sequential development, 106–107
Sheyko, Boris, 30–37, 165
Shoes (weightlifting and), 27–29. *See also* Extensor reflex training
Shoulder exercises/training. *See also* Neck and shoulder exercises/training
    Arnold press, 88
    Injury prevention, 192–193, 209–211, 213
    Seated barbell military press, 88
    See-saw presses, 209–211
    Sots presses, 205–206
    Twenty-rep squat routine, 204–205
Shrug techniques/methods, 67–69
Siff, Mel, 58–59, 91, 102, 104, 108, 149, 176
Simmons, Louie, 50, 55, 85, 131, 253, 301
Singles routines, 44–45. *See also* Bench pressing techniques/methods
Sisco, Peter, 115
Sissy deadlift, 85
Situps, 82
Sivokon, Alexey, 30, 31, 33, 114
60% Rule, 103
Skill strength, 1, 39
Skinner, Todd, 226
Slow kicks, 296–298
Smirnov, Victor, 63
Smith machines, 87, 253
Smith, Charles, 204
Smolov, S. Y., 21, 55, 117
Sommer, Chris, 99
Sonnon, Scott, 247
Sots, Victor, 205
Sots presses, 205–206
Soviet military. *See* Russian military
Spider-ups, 291
Split routines, 99, 100–101, 113
Squat techniques/methods
    Active negatives and, 63–64
    Arm development and, 249
    Belt squats, 178
    Breathing and, 75
    Cycling and, 104
    Dead squats, 73–74

ABOUT PAVEL

Pavel Tsatsouline, Master of Sports, is a former Soviet Special Forces physical training instructor who has been called **"the modern king of kettlebells"** for starting the Russian kettlebell revolution in the West.

In 1998 Pavel introduced the ancient Russian strength and conditioning tool to the American public in his subversive article, *Vodka, Pickle Juice, Kettlebell Lifting, and Other Russian Pastimes.* The article was published by *MILO*, a magazine for tough hombres who bend steel and lift rocks. When Pavel started getting mail from guys with busted noses, cauliflower ears, scars, or at least Hell's Angels tattoos his publisher took notice.

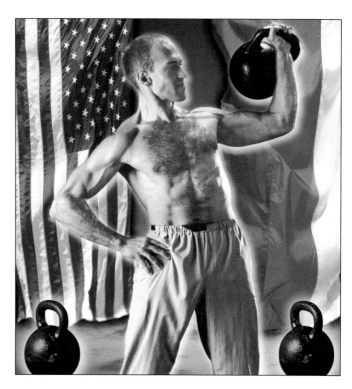

In 2001 Dragon Door published Pavel's groundbreaking book *The Russian Kettlebell Challenge* and forged the first US made Russian style cast iron kettlebell. RKC™, the first kettlebell instructor course course on American soil, kicked off.

Several years later Dragon Door published Pavel's book *Enter the Kettlebell!* which became the golden standard in kettlebell instruction. It was followed by *Return of the Kettlebell* which introduced the most advanced Russian strength and muscle building techniques.

Pavel is a subject matter expert to the US Marine Corps, the US Secret Service, and the US Navy SEALs. A kettlebell in his fist, he was voted the 'Hot Trainer' by *Rolling Stone* and appeared in media ranging from *Pravda* to *Fox News*. Dr. Randall Strossen, one of the most respected names in the strength world, stated, "In our eyes, Pavel Tsatsouline will always reign as the modern king of kettlebells since it was he who popularized them to the point where you could almost found a country filled with his converts..."

To further develop your kettlebell knowledge and skills base and to possibly receive direct feedback from Pavel, visit Dragon Door's forum at **RussianKettlebells.com**.

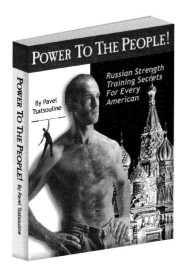

"I used the strength building secrets from *Power to the People* for one week and my max deadlift went up 18%."

—Larry Scott, 1st Mr. Olympia, author of *Loaded Guns*

Power to the People!

Russian Strength Secrets for Every American **Book** By Pavel Tsatsouline

Paperback 124 pages 8.5" x 11"

#B10 $34.95

"I have gained 25 lbs. in my bench and 40 lbs. in my deadlift in six weeks. All this improvement and I would spend only 20 minutes a day in the weight room and not one day was I ever sore. If you are serious about strength, you are not doing everything you can if you don't purchase this book."—ALEX RODRIGUEZ, Redondo Beach, Ca

"I've been lifting for eight years, and *Power to the People!* is the most functional strength training system that I have ever tried. In four short months, I went from being able to deadlift 165 for five reps to being able to dead 405 for a single. All without putting on a pound of weight, but by making my nervous system more effective. Though, to be honest... I seem to have replaced some of my fat with muscle.... My ex-girlfriend told me: "You're so buff now.... I hate you." My new girlfriend told me: "They should make a statue out of you." The difference? Pavel."
—DAN MCVICKER, Boulder, CO

"I started using the PTP program about 6 weeks ago, and the results for me have been phenomenal....50 lbs. on the deadlift and 35 lbs. on the bench press."
—WYLDMAN, Kansas City, KS

"A good book for the athlete looking for a routine that will increase strength without building muscle mass. Good source of variation for anyone who's tired of doing standard exercises."
—JONATHAN LAWSON, *IronMan* Magazine

"I learned a lot from Pavel's books and plan to use many of his ideas in my own workouts. *Power to the People!* is an eye-opener. It will give you new—and valuable—perspectives on strength training. You will find plenty of ideas here to make your training more productive."
—CLARENCE BASS, author of *Ripped 1, 2 &3.*

"This is the best of the best, and you owe it yourself to try it. You will experience a surge of strength you never thought possible. My personal experience has been a two-fold increase in my pulling strength and a 70% increase in my presses. Unlike my previous experiences with weight training, these gains were functional. I now run faster, jump higher, and hit harder."
—TYLER HASS, Pullman, WA

"I've been a student of the martial arts for over 15 years... I've added 30 pounds to my bench press with only 6 training sessions in 1 month. My deadlift has also gone up 100 pounds too. All of this without gaining additional bodyweight. I definitely recommend this book to anyone who is serious about their Martial Arts training."
—ICHIBAN, Columbus, OH

"I have increased my deadlift by 150% and have doubled my snatch and power clean. My workouts now take less than half the time they did before. And now I'm strong! Best of all, I've regained the strength in my leg that I had lost after a botched knee surgery. Power to the People! will teach you how to gain true real-world strength to move your couch, heavy boxes, your piano, etc. in a 15-20 minute workout you can do at home. It also explains why most popular American workouts are useless or dangerous or both. I can't recommend PTP enough."
—DAVID COOKE, Atlanta, GA

"I have been a training athlete for over 30 years. I played NCAA basketball in college, kick boxed as a pro for two years, made it to the NFL as a free agent in 1982, powerlifted through my 20's and do Olympic lifting now at 42. I have also coached swimming and strength athletes for over 20 years.I have never read a book more useful than **Power to the People!** I have seen my strength explode like I was in my 20's again—and my joints are no longer hurting."—CARTER STAMM, New Orleans, LA

"I personally added 120 pounds to my deadlift following *Power to the People!* principles -going from 300 lbs. to 420 lbs. in a little over six months -at a bodyweight of 160 pounds. This book is worth its weight in gold."
—JOHN QUIGLEY, Hazleton, PA

"I have been following a regimen I got from *Power to the People!* for about seven weeks now. I have lost about 17lbs and have lost three inches in my waist. My deadlift has gone from a meager 180lbs to 255 lbs in that short time as well."
—LAWRENCE J. KOCHERT

"I had very little previous experience with deadlifting (or much of any type of lifting for that matter) when I purchased *Power to the People!*. I found the information to be most interesting, and well written. The book is now tattered, coffee-stained, and beat up from usage a year later, and my deadlift max is 100lbs higher than when I began. The techniques and cycles are simple to understand and undeniably effective. PTP is a must-read for the individual looking to truly get stronger." —JIM WISSING, dragondoor.com review

"I finally broke the double bodyweight DL barrier, 1 year ago I damaged my back to the point of not being able to move let alone bend over with out being in major pain and today I pulled over 2xBW destroying my previous PR by about 50lbs. So much here from dragondoor has been immensely helpful, from the material to the people this place is a huge resource. Next up is the RKC in less than a week and I can't wait."—KEVIN PERRONE, dragondoor.com forum

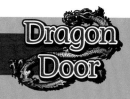

How to Instantly Increase Your Biceps Strength With the *Successive Induction* Technique

Successive induction is another one of the Sherrington Laws exploited to the max by unscrupulous Commies. According to this law, a contraction of a muscle—say, the triceps—makes its opposite number—in our case, the biceps—stronger than usual. In the early eighties scientists suggested that this maneuver has a disinhibition effect. In non-geek terms, when your triceps powerfully contract, they send the neural centers controlling the biceps a message that your bis do not have to hold back out of fear of an injury; if things get out of hand the tris are strong enough to stop them!

A year later the same group of researchers determined that a strength training program which employs antagonist pre-tensing, or successive induction, is more effective than a conventional one. The benefits of antagonist pre-contraction do not stop at immediate performance improvement, but include lasting changes in your strength.

Let the basic one-arm curl be the testing range of the effects of successive induction. Perform a set of strict curls with a weight that allows about five solid reps and make sure that your elbow stays at your side and does not drift back. Note how many reps you have done in good form.

Rest for five minutes and do another set of curls with the same weight, but employ the new trick. Instead of lowering the barbell with the braking strength of your biceps, try to "push" the weight down and away from you with your triceps. Imagine that you are doing a triceps cable pushdown with a reverse grip.

You are guaranteed to squeeze out an extra rep or two with this technique! And these reps will be super strict because now you have two "motors" to control the weight instead of one.

Power to you!

The Power Points – what you'll get with Pavel's *Power to the People!*:

- How to get super strong without putting on an ounce of weight

- OR how to build massive muscles with a classified Soviet Special Forces workout

- Why high rep training to the 'burn' is like a form of rigor mortis — and what it really takes to make your muscles stand out in bold relief

- Why it's safer to use free weights than machines

- How to design a world class body in your basement — with $150 worth of basic weights and in twenty minutes a day

- How to instantly up your strength with Pavel's High-Tension Techniques™

- How to become super strong and live to tell about it

- How to dramatically amplify your power with the proprietary Power Breathing TM techniques (and why everything you know about breathing when lifting is wrong!)

- How to feel energized and fantastic after your strength workout — rather than dragging and fatigued

- How to get brutally strong all over — with only two old-school exercises

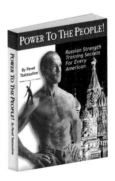

Power to the People!
Russian Strength Secrets for Every American
By Pavel Tsatsouline
Paperback 124 pages
8.5" x 11"

#B10 $34.95

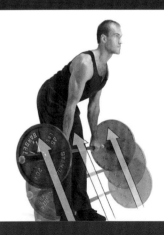

"If there was only one book I could recommend to help *you* reach your ultimate physical potential, this would be it."

—Jim Wright, Ph.D., Science Editor, Flex Magazine, Weider Group

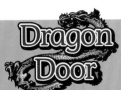

How to Develop a
"POWER PRESENCE"

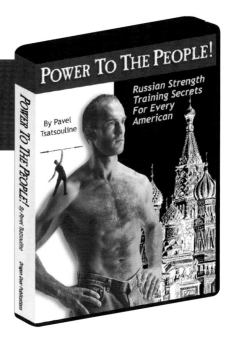

Turn on Pavel's *Power to the People!* DVD
and watch in amazement as you rapidly increase your strength by 20, 30, even 50 percent!

Do you have a "power presence"?
The quiet strength of a man with whom, as Russians say, 'you would go on a recon mission'. The bearing of an old warhorse who does not need his campaign ribbons to show that he has been around. That look of a hand-to-hand combat expert whose efficiency in violence is advertised, rather than hidden, by his serene composure.

You can't fake it!
You can't fake it with a tough grimace from a cheesy action flick or vain flexing of virtual muscles pumped up with Barbie weights. It must be earned.

The look comes from cultivated power
So stop being a mirror-gazing sissy and get strong. And strength has never been so quick to achieve. Just pop in your copy of *Power to the People!: Russian Strength Training Secrets for Every American* and hit 'Play'!

Start deadlifting!
The deadlift separates the serious students of strength from the wannabes.

Any weenie can answer the question, "How much can you bench?" Ask the poser how much he deadlifts and he will run for cover.

No other exercise will work more muscles in five reps of concentrated agony. Your back will fill with strength and vitality. Your legs will harden into powerful pistons. Have you seen photos of strongmen in the pre-squat days? No chafing, just wiry power. Your forearms will demand an outlet for their new, claw-like power.

No other exercise will give you more functional strength. 'Functional' implies 'a function'. Does your life require balancing on rubber balls and performing weird circus tricks? I didn't think so. Do you have to lift things? I rest my case.

Start side pressing!
Learn the barbell Side Press, a classic exercise from the days when broad shoulders rather than breast-like pecs were it.

This lift will fill your lats, shoulders, and arms with power and give you that awesome V-look. Due to the unique nature of this exercise, your obliques will be smoked. Back to the old-time strongmen. One-arm overhead lifts like the Side Press is the cause of their gladiator midsections.

What else? –
'Instant strength techniques.'
It is not just the exercises themselves but how you do them. *Power to the People!* teaches Pavel's patented Power Breathing™ and High-Tension Techniques™. These secrets make an amazing, often instant difference in strength. Once Pavel had a Marine deadlift 70 pounds over his previous best in just an hour. Such gains aren't exactly typical, but you get the idea.

Did Pavel invent the 'instant strength techniques'? — No. All top strength athletes use them, some consciously, others not. These elite specimens figured these things out after years of practice. But for one reason or another they generally choose to keep it to themselves. When Pavel mentioned one of these obscure moves to a world champion powerlifter, the latter thought for a moment and said, "I already do that."

Now, you don't have to be an elite lifter with decades of experience to take advantage of these incredibly powerful ways of aligning your body for maximum power. Hit 'Play'!

Power to you!

Power to the People!
Russian Strength Secrets for Every American **DVD**
With Pavel Tsatsouline
Running Time 47 Min
DVD **#DV004 $29.95**

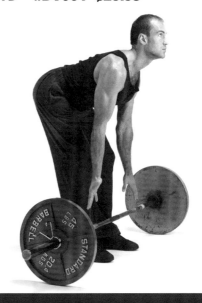

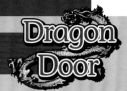

Discover New Keys to Superior Athletic Achievement

In his strength books Pavel emphasizes the importance of learning to maximally tense the muscles. Because tension IS strength. But strength/ tension is only half of the total performance package. The other half is relaxation. The body of a karate expert will freeze in total tension at the moment of impact, but will remain totally loose before and after.

Mastery of relaxation is the hallmark of an elite athlete. Soviet scientists discovered that the higher the athlete's level, the quicker he can relax his muscles. The Soviets observed an 800% difference between novices and Olympians. Their conclusion: total control of tension = elite performance.

If you can master your muscular tension, a new dimension of athletic excellence opens to you. New achievements. New heights of performance. Some genetically-endowed superstars seem to possess this ability from birth. But according to former Soviet Special Forces trainer, Pavel, a SKILL–SET is available that can transform *anyone's* current physical limitations.

Now, for the first time, Pavel reveals these little known Soviet performance secrets, so you too can become the master of your body — not its victim. From years of research and experience, Pavel has selected these *Fast & Loose* techniques as the best-of-the-best for practical and quick results.

Mandatory for the serious fighter "I've spent the last couple of years desperately trying to recover the speed I've been losing by inches. Before I'd even finished watching this DVD, it became clear what I'd really lost. Years ago, I used to 'snap' strikes in. As I've become a more serious fighter, I've succumbed to trying to 'drive' them in (karateka can read this as misunderstanding what it really means to train "with kime"). It's ironic that the fact that I'm trying so much harder is what has been slowing me down all along. I credit Pavel for explaining this so clearly & demonstrating drills that deliver rapid results. If you're a serious competitor looking for that extra edge, you *must* add these drills to your routine. Thank you, Pavel, for another excellent product. OSU!!" —B, Boston – MA

Fast & Loose
Secrets of the Russian Champions: Dynamic Relaxation Techniques for Elite Performance
with Pavel
#DV021   **$29.95**

2 Mid-Level

DVD Running time: 27 minutes

3 Advanced

Fast and Loose + Rough and Tough = Deadly Force

Invest in the "Deadly Force" set of Pavel's *Fast and Loose* DVD with Pavel's *The Naked Warrior* DVD and book— and SAVE...

Item #DVS008
$94.85

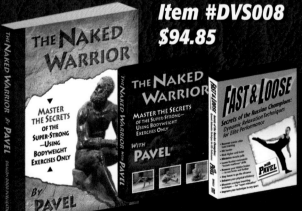

- **Recover sooner after hard training**
- **Kick higher and faster**
- **Hit harder**
- **Minimize muscle pulls**
- **Stay loose to go the distance**
- **Improve your technique in any sport**
- **Enhance your physical efficiency**
- **Remove your hidden brakes — to run faster and further**
- **Learn Russian commando "instant readiness" drills**
- **Discover a unique breathing technique — for "super-relaxation"**

"*Fast & Loose* is another amazing tool from Pavel... Everyone knows that once you really start pushing the envelope on your current abilities, you need those subtle yet all-important tools to move from average to elite performance. They can seem insignificant to the untrained observer, but are better than gold to those who have the faculties to incorporate them. Pavel delivers as always."
—Mark Hanington, Huntington Beach, CA.

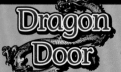

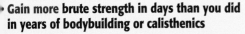
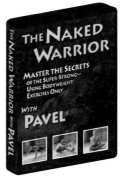

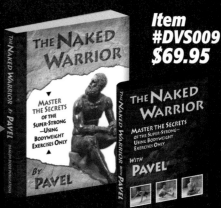
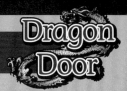

Highlights Of What You Get With Pavel's *The Naked Warrior*

Chapter 1
The Naked Warrior Rules of Engagement

'The Naked Warrior', or why strength train with bodyweight? The definition of strength...strength classifications...examples of the three types of strength...the only way to build strength...high resistance and mental focus on contraction ...tension generation skill...a powerful instant-strength mix...**The Naked Warrior Principles** ...the six keys to greater strength...**How do lifters really train?**...'best practice' secrets of powerlifters and Olympic weightlifters...**How do gymnasts get a good workout with the same weight?**...five strategies for making 5-rep exercises harder...how gymnasts achieve super strength...how to customize the resistance without changing the weight.

Chapter 2
The Naked Warrior Workout

"Grease the groove," or how to get superstrong without a routine...the secret success formula...**Some GTG testimonials from the dragondoor.com forum**...how does the GTG system work?...turning your nerves into superconductors...avoiding muscle failure... strength as a skill—the magic formula..."The Pistol": the Russian Spec Ops' leg strengthener of choice...how to do it—the basics...**The one-arm/one-leg pushup: "an exercise in total body tension"**...what gymnastics has to teach us...another advantage of the one-arm pushup...GTG, the ultimate specialization program.

Chapter 3
High-Tension Techniques for Instant Strength

Tension. **What force is made of**...the relationship between tension and force...high-tension techniques...'Raw strength' versus 'technique' ...the power of mental focus...**Low gear for brute force**...speed and tension...putting explosiveness in context..."Doesn't dynamic tension act like a brake?"... a dirty little secret of bodybuilding ...the dangers of mindless lifting...**The power of a fist**...the principle of irradiation...Accidental discharge of strength: a tip from firearms instructors...interlimb response and your muscle software...Power abs = a power body...the relationship between abs tension and body strength... he 'back-pressure crunch'...the source of real striking power...**A gymnast instantly gains 40 pounds of strength on his iron cross with the three techniques you have just learned**...The "static stomp": using ground pressure to maximize power...a secret of top karatekas and bench pressers...how the secret of armpit power translates into paydirt for one-arm pushups, punches, and bench presses..."The corkscrew":

Another secret of the karate punch...the power of rotation and spiral...the invisible force...**Bracing: boost your strength up to 20% with an armwrestling tactic**...when to brace...the advantage of dead-start exercises...'Body hardening'—tough love for teaching tension...the quick and hard way to greater tension control...Beyond bracing: "zipping up"...taking your pretensing skills to a new level...**Wind up for power**...the art of storing elastic energy for greater power...the reverse squat.

Chapter 4
Power Breathing: The Martial Arts Masters' Secret for Superstrength

Bruce Lee called it "breath strength"...cranking up your breath strength...your body as a first-class sound system—how to make it happen... definition of true power breathing...**Power inhalation**...the mystery breathing muscle that's vital to your strength...amping up the compression...when and why to hold your breath...**Reverse power breathing: evolution of the Iron Shirt technique**...the pelvic diaphragm lock...two crucial rules for maximal power breathing...**Power up from the core, or the 'pneumatics of Chi'**...two important principles of power generation...how to avoid a power leakage...the "balloon" technique for greater power.

Chapter 5
Driving GTG Home

Driving GTG home: focused...skill-building— why "fewer is better"...the law of the jungle...**Driving GTG home: flawless**...how to achieve perfection—the real key...the five conditions for generating high tension...the significance of low rep work...**Driving GTG home: frequent**...the one great secret of press success...Driving GTG home: fresh...the many aspects of staying fresh for optimal strength gains...staying away from failure...the balancing act between frequency and freshness...**Driving GTG home: fluctuating**...how to avoid training plateaus..."same yet different" strategies... 'waviness of load'...countering fatigue...training guidelines for a PR...backing off and overtraining.

Chapter 6
Field-Stripping the Pistol

Box Pistol...how to go from zero to hero...the box squat—a champions' favorite for multi-muscle strength gains...making a quantum leap in your squats...various options from easier to eviler...the rocking pistol...how to recruit your hip flexors...how to avoid cramping...**One-Legged Squat, Paul Anderson style**...Airborne Lunge...Pistol Classic...mastering the real deal...**Negative-Free Pistol**...the three advantages

of concentric-only training...Renegade Pistol ...Fire-in-the-Hole Pistol ... Cossack Pistol ...Dynamic Isometric Pistol...combining dynamic exercise with high-tension stops...multiple stops for greater pain...taking advantage of your sticking points...easier variations...three reasons why adding isos to dynamic lifting can increase effectiveness by up to 15%...protecting yourself against injury...**Isometric Pistol**...holding tension over time...the art of "powered-down" high-tension techniques...**Weighted Pistol**...working the spinal erectors.

Chapter 7
Field-Stripping the One-Arm Pushup

The One-Arm Pushup, floor and elevated...how to shine at high-intensity exertion...change-ups for easy and difficult...the authorized technique...developing a controlled descent... Isometric One-Arm Pushup...The One-Arm Dive Bomber Pushup...The One-Arm Pump...The One-Arm Half Bomber Pushup...Four more drills to work up to the One-Arm Dive Bomber...The One-Arm/One-Leg Pushup...the Tsar of the one-arm pushups.

Chapter 8
Naked Warrior Q&A

Are bodyweight exercises superior to exercises with weights?...the advantage of cals...what cals enforce...the biggest disadvantage of bodyweight exercising...the advantage of barbells...the advantages and disadvantages of dumbbells...the advantages of kettlebells...**Why is there such an intense argument in the martial arts community as to whether bodyweight exercises are superior to exercises with weights?**...confusions explained ...what a fighter needs...**Can I get very strong using only bodyweight exercises?**...Should I mix different strength-training tools in my training? ...How can I incorporate bodyweight exercises with kettlebell and barbell training?...Can the high-tension techniques and GTG system be applied to weights?... Can the high-tension techniques and GTG system be applied to strength endurance training?...I can't help overtraining. What should I do?...Can I follow the Naked Warrior program on an ongoing basis?...Can I add more exercises to the Naked Warrior program?...Will my development be unbalanced from doing only two exercises?...Is there a way to work the lats with a pulling exercise when no weights or pullup bars are accessible?...door pullups...door rows...Where can I learn more about bodyweight-only strength training?...Low reps and no failure? This training is too easy!...Will I forget all the strength techniques in some sort of emergency?...Isn't dedicating most of the book to technique too much?...why technique is crucial...moving from ordinary to extraordinary.

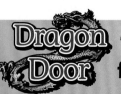

How to Instantly Increase Your Upper Body Strength With the *Irradiation* Technique

Hit the deck and give me five pushups, Comrade! Only five, but of a challenging variety, for instance with your feet up or on one arm. When you are done with five you should be able to grind out another couple but no more than that.

Note the difficulty of your first set. Rest briefly. Do another fiver but with one difference: on the way up grip the deck hard with your fingertips. Don't go up on your fingertips; just grip the floor so your fingertips turn white. Only on the way up. All the way up or just at the sticking point. You will have to experiment whether you will get the best results by gripping throughout the lift or just at the sticking point.

You cannot help noticing that your arms have suddenly gotten a jolt of extra energy, as if your tensing forearms have sent some juice up into your triceps. Which is exactly what has happened. Whenever a muscle contracts, it irradiates "nerve force" around it and increases the intensity of the neighborhood muscles' contraction. The effect is strongest in your hands.

Make a fist. A tight fist. A white-knuckle fist! Note that as you grip harder the tension in your forearm overflows into your upper arm, and even your shoulder and armpit. You will increase your strength in any upper body exertion, bodyweight or not, by strongly gripping the floor, the bar, etc.

Power to you, Naked Warrior! Anywhere, anytime.

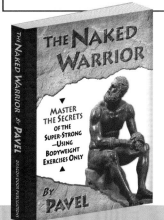

Extraordinary Praise for Pavel's Enter the Kettlebell! Book and DVD

Pavel has done it again!
Rated 10 out of 10

"Pavel's has taken the Art of the Kettlebell to a new level of Zen simplicity. A more detailed sequel to the tersely written original *Russian Kettlebell Challenge* (the book that started it all) *Enter the Kettlebell* streamlines the process of using the KB as a serious stand alone fitness training method.

The book is the KB equivalent to the Pavel's outstanding treatise on barbell strength training *Power to the People!*, taking the same simple (but not easy) approach to KB training that he took to getting strong with just two barbell exercises.

Cutting through the myriad of possible movements to the most important Pavel teaches how to organize and progress the fundamental movements of the RKC system for real progress with real training over the long haul. Focusing on movement mastery by going deeper into the lifts Pavel shows what the martial art of strength training is all about. *Enter the Kettlebell* is a must read for all KB aficionados and anyone who is serious about the most efficient fitness system around."
—*Mark Reifkind, RKC, Owner Girya Kettlebell Training, CA*

Essential Pavel!!!!!
Rated 10 out of 10

"Answers the question: 'If I could only get one Kettlebell book, which one should it be.'...... THIS ONE!!!!! Pavel once again 'brings home the bacon' to the Kettlebell Nation. Direct, honest, no-fluff instruction boiled down to its most essential form. Enjoy the read.......then enjoy the pain!" —*Craig T. O'Connell, RKC - HQ / FDLE, Tallahassee, FL*

The complete idiots guide to kettlebell super strength
Rated 10 out of 10

"Take a system that is too simple to screw up, add the fine points that makes Pavel such an effective instructor, and you get the next perfect evolution of *Power to the People!*. Simple and sinister is the most accurate description of the program. I am adding this to

the training of our deployed troops, and you should do it too." —*SSgt Glass - Okinawa, Japan*

Pavel again proves his genius and brilliance with "Enter The Kettlebell"   Rated 10 out of 10

"Is there a more influential strength author in the US over the past 30 years than Pavel? In a few short years he seems to have revolutionized strength and fitness in this country for those of us lucky enough to discover him. After lifting and competing (powerlifting) over the past 20+ years I am stronger, more muscular, and more fit than anytime previous all as a result of Pavel's routines and genius. Now Pavel does it again with the companion book to *The Russian Kettlebell Challenge*. After giving up powerlifting and concentrating solely on KBs, I thought I had read it all and tried it all. As I tell my students sometimes, 'just when you think you know the answer, I change the question'. Pavel again has changed the question with his new book, *Enter the Kettlebell*. As brilliant as *Power to the People* (the first Pavel book I ever bought) 'Enter the KB' makes KB training simple but so effective with his push/pull routine. He also leaves nothing to chance by giving you the formula for success with routines and can't miss workouts. With this book there is no more excuses, as Pavel would say 'enjoy the pain—but I would also add 'enjoy the results'! 2 thumbs up!" —*Patrick "Phil" Workman, RKC - Fort Worth, Texas*

Tremendous book and DVD!
Rated 10 out of 10

"For the last 4 years I've increased the percentage of kettlebell exercises in the training programs of my elite athletes, regular folks, and high school students. Hockey, volleyball, basketball, football, soccer, boxers and other athletes, have all benefited greatly from their kettlebell training. In addition to being thrilled with their outstanding results, everyone I train actually ENJOYS the kettlebell practices. In a recent example, I put a group of male and female Provincial Rugby players (Manitoba Buffalo) through twice weekly training

sessions for 4 months (and continuing). Their programs emphasized kettlebells. The test results: A dramatic loss of bodyfat, more muscularity, far more strength and power, a big increase in rugby specific endurance measured in various shuttle runs, and an increase in 'mental toughness'.

Now that the season has started, my Kettlebell trained players stand out in their ability to get around the pitch (field) and make play after play. They're hitting harder, they're quicker, and far more enduring. I thank Pavel for putting kettlebells, and all his (and other RKC's) great kettlebell books and DVDs into my hands. I've helped develop champions since the 1970s; Pavel has helped me take my instruction to a whole new level. This is very rewarding and exciting.

Pavel's *Enter The Kettlebell* book (and DVD) are the newest additions to my coaching and (own) training arsenal. Quite simply, they are GREAT! Comprehensive, step by step guides for the beginner or the advanced practitioner (and everyone in between). I've read and re-read *Enter The Kettlebell*. Each time something 'new' jumps out at me. Replaying the DVD does likewise. I encourage everyone interested in improving themselves and/or their athletes, to purchase *Enter The Kettlebell*." —*Cole Summers: Team Canada Strength Coach - Winnipeg, Canada*

I went from 124 to 162 snatches in one month! Rated 10 out of 10

"Another classic from Pavel. I'm following the Rite of Passage program and went from a previous best 124 snatches in ten minutes that was VERY difficult to 162 and it wasn't as bad. That was after one month! I'm planning on hitting 200+ reps within 3 months of starting this program. I recommend both the book and DVD to anyone who wants to get started training with kettlebells. Follow the programs and you will become a better man for your effort." —*Joe Pavel RKC - Cottage Grove, MN USA*

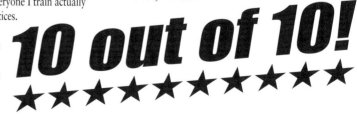

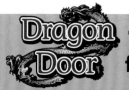

1·800·899·5111 24 hours a day
fax your order **(866)-280-7619**

Enter The Kettlebell! Highlights

Foreword by Dan John

Preface: A Step to the Left and I Shoot
"Do it this way!"... the no-more-guesswork, failure-is-not-an-option, quick-start guide to kettlebell success... *Power to the People!* for kettlebells.

Introduction: When We Say "Strength," We Mean "Kettlebell." When We Say "Kettlebell," We Mean "Strength."

How the Kettlebell Has Bred Weakness Out of the Russian Gene Pool
The Russian recipe for doubling or tripling your strength ... kettlebells as the backbone of Russian military strength training... why Soviet scientists gave the kettlebell two thumbs-up... the Voropayev study—kettlebells boost pull-ups, jumping, and running... the Vinogradov & Lukyanov study—kettlebells improve fitness across the board... the studies by Luchkin and Laputin... the Soviet armed forces strength training manual—kettlebell training "one of the most effective means of strength development potential"... the Shevtsova study... the Gomonov study—consistently low body fat in kettlebell lifters.

Chronicle of the Russian Kettlebell Invasion of America
Kettlebells and the American iron men of old... rise of the machines... kettlebells change the face of exercise in America.

Chapter 1: Enter the Kettlebell!

Which Kettlebells Should I Start With?
Choosing the correct size of kettlebell for

Save Money with the Enter The Kettlebell! Quick Start Kits

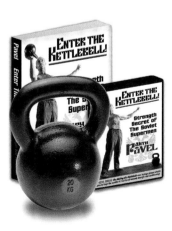

men and women of differing backgrounds, strength and skills... understanding your goals with kettlebells.

How to Make Your Hips, Back, and Shoulders Speak Russian Body Language
Developing flexibility in the hip flexors for greater power... the kettlebell preschool test... the kettlebell Sumo Deadlift checklist... how to make the fastest gains... the Halo for looser shoulders... the Pump Stretch.

"It's Your Fault": Kettlebell Safety 101
Ten key tips to have your strength and your health too... practicing safety to make safety permanent.

Safety as a Part of, Not the Opposite of, Performance
Nine secrets for guaranteeing greater strength and reduced risk of injury in your kettlebell training.

Chapter 2: The New RKC Program Minimum

Practice Before Workout: The Break-in Plan
The two staples of the Russian Kettlebell Challenge program—Swing and Get-up... building skill by practicing, not working out.

The Swing—for Legs and Conditioning That Won't Quit
The single most effective strength and conditioning exercise in the world?... mechanics of a good and a bad Swing... the three essential standards for a perfect Swing ... Swing mastery, Steps 1 through 4.

The Get-up—for Shoulders That Can Take Punishment and Dish It Out
Miraculous shoulder comebacks... developing shoulder mobility and stability... pressing heavier... the six essential standards for a perfect Get-up... Get-up mastery, Steps 1 through 4.

The New RKC Program Minimum
For the most important and immediate concerns: world-class conditioning, rapid fat loss, a steel back, muscular, flexible, and resilient shoulders—and a skill base for the rest of the RKC drills... "simple and sinister" S&C routine.

The Next Step
What to do next, once you are rocking on the RKC Program Minimum.

Chapter 3: The RKC Rite of Passage

The RKC Proven Formula: Low-Rep Grinds + High-Rep Quick Lifts

The priority in RKC-style training... the value of "slow strength" training... a counter-intuitive and rarely revealed secret of Russian athletic might... the advantages of slow strength for a fighter... definition of power...mastering the natural athletic rhythm of tension and relaxation... a killer one-two combination for the gym and the ring.

A Pull and a Press—Sound Familiar?
A PTP format for kettlebells... pulls to build backs... a dramatic way to reduce back injuries... building stronger abs... forging a vice grip... why kettlebell presses rule... how to go from regular guy to hard guy—a set of goals... and a set of goals for women.

The Clean—Crisp Like a Punch
Defining the RKC Clean... the six essential standards for a perfect Clean... Clean mastery, Steps 1 through 4.

The Press—for a Classic Torso
The five essential standards for a perfect Press... Press mastery, Steps 1 through 5.

The Snatch—for Android Work Capacity and the Pain Tolerance of an Immortal
The Tsar of kettlebell lifts... snatches for military and law enforcement... physical and mental benefits of the Snatch... The six essential standards for a perfect Snatch... Snatch mastery, Steps 1 through 6.

Chapter 4: A Step-by-Step Guide to Becoming a Man Among Men

Have Your Borsch and Eat It Too: The Hazards of Variety and How to Dodge Them
A system for the really ambitious man... constructive corrections and waving the loads... the function of variety days... working your "in-between strength"... schedules for the RKC Right of Passage.

The RKC Ladder to Pressing Power
The intensity and volume equation... the "ladder," for highly effective strength building... the perfect rest interval between sets... the role of density in your strength training... George Hackenschmidt's regimen ... compressed rest periods... Pull-ups as a great addition to your Presses.

Rest Less, Snatch More
The kettlebell rules for conditioning... when to do your high-rep kettlebell pulls... the heavy-light-medium template... how to log your workouts... warning for shoulders and elbows in your first year of kettlebelling... how to get the same results for different fitness levels with the same workout... the Russian science of periodization in your kettlebell training...

high-intensity intervals—the new Rx for heart health.

From Boy to Man
Testing yourself for progress in the RKC Rite of Passage... the United States Secret Service kettlebell Snatch rules... the RKC Rite of Passage training plan summary... how to measure a man's true character.

Chapter 5: FAQ

Is kettlebell training a fad?

What makes the kettlebell superior to other weights and fitness equipment?

Should I train with the kettlebell as a stand-alone tool or mix it up with a barbell and dumbbells?

How can I combine kettlebell training with *Power to the People!* and *The Naked Warrior*?

How can I incorporate *Bullet-Proof Abs* exercises into my kettlebell regimen?

I have a bad back. Can I train with kettlebells?
The top five reasons RKC kettlebell training is great for your back.

What diet do you recommend?

Will kettlebells help my sport-specific strength?
The pros and cons of sports-specific training... the kettlebell "what-the-hell effect" for improving at things you have not practiced... how to truly excel at a certain exercise... when to do "special strength" training.

Why are your exercise descriptions so detailed? Come on, kettlebells are not rocket science!
Reverse-engineering what the greats do naturally... learning how to move like the elite... refining the basics.

Can I substitute the . . . with the . . .?

Once I have put up the RKC Rite of Passage numbers, where do I go next?

If Russian stuff is so tough, why did the USSR lose the Cold War

Chapter 6: The Making of a Kettlebell

The kettlebell pattern... pressing the kettlebell mold... crucible for a hot kettlebell... pouring the kettlebell molds... shaking out the kettlebell... hammer and kettlebell... sandblasting the kettlebell... grinding the kettlebell.

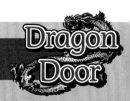

"Kettlebell Training...The Closest Thing You Can Get to Fighting, Without Throwing A Punch"

—Federal Counterterrorist Operator

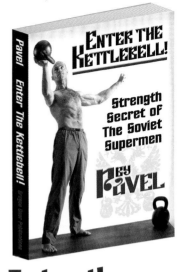

The kettlebell. AK-47 of physical training hardware. Hunk of iron on a handle. Simple, sinister, brutal—and ferociously effective for developing explosive strength, dramatic power and never-say-die conditioning. The man's man's choice for the toughest, most demanding, highest-yield exercise tool on the planet. Guaranteed to forge a rugged, resilient, densely-muscled frame—built to withstand the hardest beating and dish it right back out, 24/7.

Once the prized and jealously-guarded training secret of elite Russian athletes, old-school strongmen and the military, the kettlebell has invaded the West. And taken no prisoners—thanks to former **Soviet Special Forces** physical training instructor and strength author, *Pavel Tsatsouline's* 2001 publication of *The Russian Kettlebell Challenge* and his manufacture of the first traditional Russian kettlebell in modern America.

American hardmen of all stripes were quick to recognize what their Russian counterparts had long known—nothing, nothing beats the kettlebell, when you're looking for a single tool to dramatically impact your strength and conditioning. A storm of success has swept the American S & C landscape, as kettlebell "Comrades" have busted through to new PRs, broken records, thrashed their opponents and elevated their game to new heights of excellence.

With *Enter the Kettlebell!* Pavel delivers a significant upgrade to his original landmark work, *The Russian Kettlebell Challenge*. Drawing on five years of developing and leading the world's first and premiere kettlebell instructor certification program, and after spending five years of additional research into what really works for dramatic results with the kettlebell—we have *Enter the Kettlebell!*

Pavel lays out a foolproof master system that guarantees you success—if you simply follow the commands!

- **Develop** all-purpose strength—to easily handle the toughest and most unexpected demand
- **Maximize** staying power—because the last round decides all
- **Forge** a fighter's physique—because the form must follow the function

Enter the kettlebell! and follow the plan:

1. The New RKC Program Minimum

With just two kettlebell exercises, takes you from raw newbie to solid contender—well-conditioned, flexible, resilient and muscular in all the right places.

2. The RKC Rite of Passage

Jumps you to the next level of physical excellence with Pavel's proven RKC formula for exceptional strength and conditioning.

3. Become a Man Among Men

Propels you to a Special Forces level of conditioning and earns you the right to call yourself a man.

When you rise to the challenge—and *Enter the Kettlebell!*—there will be no more confusion, no more uncertainty and no more excuses—only raw power, never-quit conditioning and earned respect.

Enter the Kettlebell!
Strength Secret of The Soviet Supermen
by Pavel #B33 $34.95
Paperback 200 pages 8.5" x 11"
246 full color photos, charts, and workouts

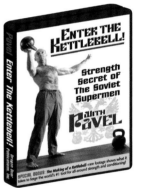

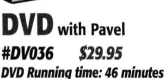

DVD with Pavel
#DV036 $29.95
DVD Running time: 46 minutes

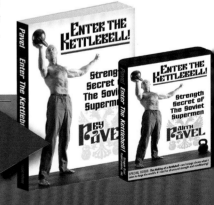

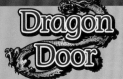

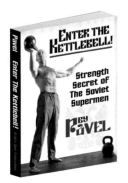

"Pavel's *Enter the Kettlebell!* helps you weed out weakness... develop explosive power, strength and never-quit endurance—with his PROVEN system for rapid, spectacular and across-the-board gains in physical performance"

The kettlebell has proved its worth many times over since Pavel has introduced it to America. Elite athletes, fighters, special operators, and regular hard Comrades swear by the extraordinary strength and conditioning delivered by this ancient Russian tool. Now, it is YOUR turn to *Enter the Kettlebell!*

For a kettlebell novice, the hardest part is knowing where to begin. And what you really need to do to get off to a **quick—yet rock-solid—start.** Pavel delivers.

For the Comrade who's already put in a year or two of kettlebell time, it's easy to hit a plateau after explosive early gains. Pavel knocks him out of his sophomore slump and helps him take his game to a higher level.

Then there's the grizzled KB vet who's been around the block and got too arrogant to practice his fundamentals (or never learned them in the first place). Pavel **hammers the fundamentals** because "it is the mastery of the basics that separates the elite from the rest."

With *Enter the Kettlebell!* Pavel has done all the work for you—honing a masterplan of essential training secrets that guarantee to make you powerful, resilient, and enduring—if you simply follow the proven guidelines.

Lift Your Kettlebell Like a Pro...

- **Are you** making these beginner's mistakes in your training?
- **Nine secrets** of greater strength and reduced injuries
- **Get the most** technique improvement with the least instruction
- **How to stop** fighting your body and get stronger
- **These two** movements will give you the biggest bang for your KB buck
- **Discover** a "simple & sinister" routine for killer conditioning and muscular shoulders
- **A common cause** of back pain after workouts—you would never guess what it is!—and how to avoid it
- **How to stretch your back after training**—everyone does it wrong
- **One style** of breathing will weaken you and make your back vulnerable—the other style of breathing gives you the explosive power of a trained fighter... know which is which

- The top five reasons RKC kettlebell training is great for your back
- **You have been misled:** sucking your stomach in does not protect your back but makes it more vulnerable! How to really protect your back when lifting
- **Reducing the odds** of arthritis—with ballistic loading
- A surefire **shortcut** to loosening stuck shoulders
- How to temper your shoulders for sports that trash them
- **A great visualization** for resilient elbows and shoulders
- **Why** cool-downs are important to your heart health
- **What you must know** about your heart rate and kettlebell training

- The **new prescription** for a power pump heart and great body composition
- **This little-known drill guarantees** improvement in your squatting depth, flexibility, technique and power

- **How to** make a simple towel your kettlebell coach—and reach your training goals faster
- **Get this one** foundational drill down—and most of the remaining exercises will be a piece of cake to learn and master
- **Why** most Comrades should choose pulls over squats
- **How to strengthen** your legs and hips without blowing them up

- **How to time** the hip movement for maximum explosive power
- **How to be** the indisputable master of the force you generate
- **Understand** the crucial value of "slow strength" training—the counterintuitive and rarely revealed secret of Russian athletic might
- **What it takes** to be more resilient in the ring
- **A simple way** to increase an experienced fighter's punching power
- **How to master** the natural athletic rhythm of tension and relaxation
- **A killer one-two combination** for the gym and ring
- **The key characteristics** of a kettlebell pro's press
- **Master this skill** and you will wield awesome pressing power
- **How to** make the heaviest kettlebell feel like a toy in your hand
- **Prof. Verkhoshansky's secret** for improving your strength by up to twenty percent
- **How** amateurs "leak" strength from their knees—and how pros fix the drain
- **How to get the most** out of your press while putting the least amount of stress on your shoulders
- **A unique** isometric drill to improve your pressing power
- **Where to look**—and not look—when pressing

- **An unexpected** assistance exercise for achieving a one-arm pull up
- **Smoke** your abs and obliques the old fashioned way
- A foolproof method for accelerating the curve on snatch mastery

- **The snatch** is a three-stage rocket—how to finesse the stages
- **How to avoid** bruising the forearm when snatching
- **A crucial warning about** shoulders and elbows in your first year of snatches
- **How to accomplish** the USSS Counter Assault Team 10-min snatch test—and be a man among men
- **How to keep** your training targeted while still having fun with new exercises
- **How to idiot-proof** your kettlebell workout—for consistently powerful gains

- **The little-understood but crucial** value of "in-between-strength"
- **Russian research** finds the day of the week when you are strongest—and it is not Monday
- **Work harder?** Or do more work?
- **The "ladder" method** for highly effective strength building

- **The kettlebell rules** for conditioning
- **A gambler's method** for deciding your high-rep workout
- **How to** log your workouts for optimal results
- **How to use** timed sets—for a foolproof and flexible practice

- **What** makes the kettlebell superior to other weights and fitness equipment?
- **Should you** train with the kettlebell as a stand-alone tool or mix it up with a barbell and dumbbells?
- **How to get superior** gains in athletic performance without sport specific training
- **The kettlebell "what the hell effect"**—for improving at skills you have not practiced

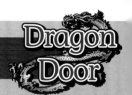

The World's #1 Handheld Gym For Extreme Fitness

RUSSIAN KETTLEBELLS

Use Kettlebells to:

- **Accelerate your all-purpose strength**—so you can readily handle the toughest demands
- **Hack away your fat**—without the dishonor of dieting and aerobics
- **Boost your physical resilience**—to repel the hardest hits
- **Build your staying power**—to endure and conquer, whatever the distance
- **Create a potent mix of strength-with-flexibility**—to always reach your target
- **Forge a fighter's physique**—so form matches function
- **Be independent**—world's #1 portable gym makes you as strong as you want to be, anywhere, anytime

Kettlebells Fly Air Force One!

"There's a competitive reason behind the appearance of kettlebells at the back doors and tent flaps of military personnel. When Russian and US Special Forces started competing against each other after the Soviet Union broke up, the Americans made a disturbing discovery. "We'd be totally exhausted and the Russians wouldn't even be catching their breath," says… [a] Secret Service agent… "It turned out they were all working with kettlebells."

Now, half the Secret Service is snatching kettlebells and a set sometimes travels with the President's detail on Air Force One."—*Christian Science Monitor*

Pavel's Kettlebell FAQ

What is a 'kettlebell'?

A 'kettlebell' or girya (Russ.) is a traditional Russian cast iron weight that looks like a cannonball with a handle. The ultimate tool for extreme all-round fitness.

The kettlebell goes way back – it first appeared in a Russian dictionary in 1704 (Cherkikh, 1994). So popular were kettlebells in Tsarist Russia that any strongman or weightlifter was referred to as a girevik, or 'a kettlebell man'.

"Not a single sport develops our muscular strength and bodies as well as kettlebell athletics," reported Russian magazine Hercules in 1913.

"Kettlebells—Hot Weight of the Year"—Rolling Stone

Why train with kettlebells?

Because they deliver extreme all-round fitness. And no single other tool does it better. Here is a short list of hardware the Russian kettlebell replaces: barbells, dumbbells, belts for weighted pullups and dips, thick bars, lever bars, medicine balls, grip devices, and cardio equipment.

Vinogradov & Lukyanov (1986) found a very high correlation between the results posted in a kettlebell lifting competition and a great range of dissimilar tests: strength, measured with the three powerlifts and grip strength; strength endurance, measured with pullups and parallel bar dips; general endurance, determined by a 1000 meter run; work capacity and balance, measured with special tests.

Voropayev (1983) tested two groups of subjects in pullups, a standing broad jump, a 100m sprint, and a 1k run. He put the control group on a program that emphasized the above tests; the experimental group lifted kettlebells. In spite of the lack of practice on the tested exercises, the kettlebell group scored better in every one of them! This is what we call "the what the hell effect".

Kettlebells melt fat without the dishonor of dieting or aerobics. If you are overweight, you will lean out. If you are skinny, you will get built up. According to Voropayev (1997) who studied top Russian gireviks, 21.2% increased their bodyweight since taking up kettlebelling and 21.2% (the exact same percentage, not a typo), mostly heavyweights, decreased it. The Russian kettlebell is a powerful tool for fixing your body comp, whichever way it needs fixing.

Kettlebells forge doers' physiques along the lines of antique statues: broad shoulders with just a hint of pecs, back muscles standing out in bold relief, wiry arms, rugged forearms, a cut-up midsection, and strong legs without a hint of squatter's chafing.

Liberating and aggressive as medieval swordplay, kettlebell training is highly addictive. What other piece of exercise equipment can boast that its owners name it? Paint it? Get tattoos of it? Our Russian kettlebell is the Harley-Davidson of strength hardware.

"Kettlebells—A Workout with Balls"—Men's Journal

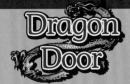

Who trains with kettlebells?

Hard comrades of all persuasions.

Soviet weightlifting legends such as Vlasov, Zhabotinskiy, and Alexeyev started their Olympic careers with old-fashioned kettlebells. Yuri Vlasov once interrupted an interview he was giving to a Western journalist and proceeded to press a pair of kettlebells. "A wonderful exercise," commented the world champion. "...It is hard to find an exercise better suited for developing strength and flexibility simultaneously."

The Russian Special Forces personnel owe much of their wiry strength, explosive agility, and never-quitting stamina to kettlebells. *Soldier, Be Strong!*, the official Soviet armed forces strength training manual pronounced kettlebell drills to be "one of the most effective means of strength development" representing "a new era in the development of human strength-potential".

The elite of the US military and law enforcement instantly recognized the power of the Russian kettlebell, ruggedly simple and deadly effective as an AK-47. You can find Pavel's certified RKC instructors among Force Recon Marines, Department of Energy nuclear security teams, the FBI's Hostage Rescue Team, the Secret Service Counter Assault Team, etc.

Once the Russian kettlebell became a hit among those whose life depends on their strength and conditioning, it took off among hard people from all walks of life: martial artists, athletes, regular hard comrades.

"I can't think of a more practical way of special operations training... I was extremely skeptical about kettlebell training and now wish that I had known about it fifteen years ago..."

—*Name withheld, Special Agent, U.S. Secret Service Counter Assault Team*

Am I kettlebell material?

Kettlebell training is extreme but not elitist. At the 1995 Russian Championship the youngest contestant was 16, the oldest 53! And we are talking elite competition here; the range is even wider if you are training for yourself rather than for the gold. Dr. Krayevskiy, the father of the kettlebell sport, took up training at the age of forty-one and twenty years later he was said to look fresher and healthier than at forty.

Only 8.8% of top Russian gireviks, members of the Russian National Team and regional teams, reported injuries in training or competition (Voropayev, 1997). A remarkably low number, especially if you consider that these are elite athletes who push their bodies over the edge. Many hard men with high mileage have overcome debilitating injuries with kettlebell training (get your doctor's approval). Acrobat Valentin Dikul fell and broke his back at seventeen. Today, in his mid-sixties, he juggles 180-pound balls and breaks powerlifting records!

"... kettlebells are a unique conditioning tool and a powerful one as well that you should add to your arsenal of strength... my experience with them has been part of what's led me to a modification in my thoughts on strength and bodyweight exercises... I'm having a blast training with them and I think you will as well."

—Bud Jeffries, the author of *How to Squat 900lbs. without Drugs, Powersuits, or Kneewraps*

How do I learn to use the kettlebell?

From Pavel's books and videos: *The Russian Kettlebell Challenge* or *From Russia with Tough Love* for comrades ladies. From an RKC certified instructor; find one in your area on RussianKettlebell.com. Kettlebell technique can be learned in one or two sessions and you can start intense training during the second or even first week (Dvorkin, 2001).

"...I felt rejuvenated and ready to conquer the world. I was sold on the kettlebells, as the exercises were fun and challenging, and demanded coordination, explosion, balance, and power... I am now on my way to being a better, fitter, and more explosive grappler, and doing things I haven't done in years!"

—Kid Peligro, *Grappling* magazine

What is the right kettlebell size for me?

Kettlebells come in 'poods'. A pood is an old Russian measure of weight, which equals 16kg, or roughly 35 lbs. An average man should start with a 35-pounder. It does not sound like a lot but believe it; it feels a lot heavier than it should! Most men will eventually progress to a 53-pounder, the standard issue size in the Russian military. Although available in most units, 70-pounders are used only by a few advanced guys and in elite competitions. 88-pounders are for mutants.

An average woman should start with an 18-pounder. A strong woman can go for a 26-pounder. Some women will advance to a 35-pounder. A few hard women will go beyond.

"Kettlebells are like weightlifting times ten."

"Kettlebells are like weightlifting times ten. ...If I could've met Pavel in the early '80s, I might've won two gold medals. I'm serious."

—Dennis Koslowski, D.C., RKC,
Olympic Silver Medalist in Greco-Roman Wrestling

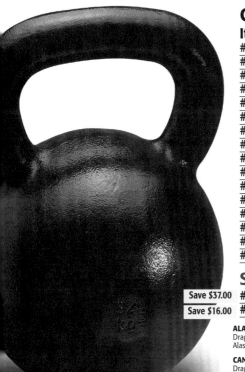

Classic RKC Kettlebells (Cast Iron/E-Coated)

Item	Weight		Price	MAIN USA	PUERTO RICO	AK&HI	CAN
#P10N	10 lb		$41.75	S/H $14.00	$47.00	$53.00	$35.00
#P10P	14 lb		$54.95	S/H $16.00	$51.00	$57.00	$41.00
#P10M	18 lb		$65.95	S/H $22.00	$65.00	$71.00	$46.00
#P10T	10 kg	(22 lb)	$71.45	S/H $25.00	$73.00	$79.00	$52.00
#P10G	12 kg	(27 lb)	$76.95	S/H $28.00	$80.00	$86.00	$58.00
#P10U	14 kg	(31 lb)	$87.95	S/H $34.00	$93.00	$99.00	$64.00
#P10A	16 kg	(35 lb)	$96.75	S/H $38.00	$104.00	$110.00	$72.00
#P10S (Women's)	16 kg	(35 lb)	$96.75	S/H $38.00	$104.00	$110.00	$72.00
#P10H	20 kg	(45 lb)	$107.75	S/H $44.00	$123.00	$122.00	$85.00
#P10B	24 kg	(53 lb)	$118.75	S/H $49.00	$141.00	$139.00	$94.00
#P10J	28 kg	(62 lb)	$142.95	S/H $53.00	$162.00	$157.00	$107.00
#P10C	32 kg	(70 lb)	$153.95	S/H $55.00	$186.00	$193.00	$121.00
#P10Q	36 kg	(80 lb)	$175.95	S/H $58.00	$203.00	$209.00	$134.00
#P10F	40 kg	(89 lb)	$197.95	S/H $64.00	$223.00	$229.00	$148.00
#P10R	44 kg	(97 lb)	$241.95	S/H $69.00	$241.00	$247.00	$160.00
#P10L	48 kg	(106 lb)	$263.95	S/H $75.00	$261.00	$267.00	$175.00

SAVE! ORDER A SET OF CLASSIC KETTLEBELLS & SAVE $$$

			Price				
Save $37.00 #SP10	Classic Set—35, 53 & 70 lb.		$332.50	S/H $142.00	$431.00	$450.00	$287.00
Save $16.00 #SP11	Women's Set—10, 14 & 18 lb.		$146.37	S/H $52.00	$163.00	$181.00	$122.00

ALASKA/HAWAII KETTLEBELL ORDERING
Dragon Door now ships to all 50 states, including Alaska and Hawaii, via UPS Ground.

CANADIAN KETTLEBELL ORDERING
Dragon Door now accepts online, phone and mail orders for Kettlebells to Canada, using UPS Standard service. UPS Standard to Canada service is

guaranteed, fully tracked ground delivery, available to every address in all of Canada's ten provinces. Delivery time can vary between 3 to 10 days.

IMPORTANT – International shipping quotes & orders do not include customs clearance, duties, taxes or other non-routine customs brokerage charges, which are the responsibility of the customer.

- KETTLEBELLS ARE SHIPPED VIA UPS GROUND SERVICE, UNLESS OTHERWISE REQUESTED.
- KETTLEBELLS RANGING IN SIZE FROM 4KG TO 24KG CAN BE SHIPPED TO P.O. BOXES OR MILITARY ADDDRESSES VIA THE U.S. POSTAL SERVICE, BUT WE REQUIRE PHYSICAL ADDDRESSES FOR UPS DELIVERIES FOR THE 32KG AND 40KG KETTLEBELLS.
- **NO** RUSH ORDERS ON KETTLEBELLS!

For more information visit: www.dragondoor.com

www.dragondoor.com

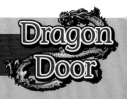

Dragon Door

Proven, "Best Practice" Methods To Take Your Genetic Destiny by the Throat and Force-Feed Greatness Upon It...

Gang-Tackle Your Weakness, Elevate Your Game, And Rip Out New PRs— When You Hook-Up with the Best in the Biz!

Two "masters of the art" reveal key, but little-known and often surprising strategies to dramatically enhance your performance...

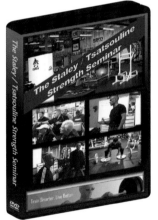

**The Staley/
Tsatsouline
Strength
Seminar**
By Charles Staley and
Pavel Tsatsouline
#DVS014 $247.00
2-DVD set
Running time: 6 hours

Charles Staley is creator of the now-legendary EDT system, which has helped athletes worldwide achieve remarkable success in every imaginable sport. Pavel Tsatsouline's landmark classics like *Power to the People!*, *The Naked Warrior* and *Enter the Kettlebell!* have been redefining our fitness landscape for the last decade.

What more can you ask for than to have both these greats combine their knowledge and skills into one information-packed training?

Charles and Pavel have made it a life-long quest to wrestle free the real nuggets from the morass of half-truths masquerading out there as "strength training". Each man, in his very different way, makes actual, realizable results the bottom line in his quest for superior physical performance.

Put the two men's knowledge and experience base onto the same team—and you're guaranteed methods that have been proven over and over again where it really counts—the trenches.

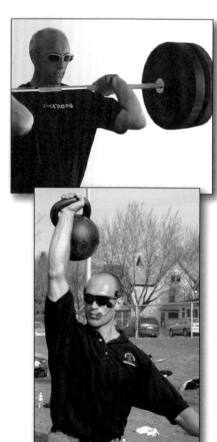

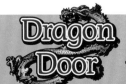

1·800·899·5111 24 hours a day
fax your order (866)-280-7619

Just some of what you'll discover from Pavel:

▶▶ **How to cultivate the skill of strength by** CORRECTLY applying the master principle of "linkage"—not one in a thousand trainers understand or know how to apply this key method!

▶▶ **Understand the finer points** of **slow** and **explosive** strength

▶▶ **The best methods** for developing **starting** and **absolute** strength.

▶▶ **The importance and applications of** absolute strength as a foundation for all your strength programs.

▶▶ **What it really takes to** generate and apply massive tension—AT THE RIGHT MOMENT—get this timing and application science wrong and you'll be trapped in mediocrity for the rest of your days…

▶▶ **How to build an impregnable foundation using** the method of "easy strength"—a guerilla tactic that hands you an instant unfair advantage in your training.

▶▶ **How to combine** tension with relaxation drills to avoid injury and sub-par performance.

▶▶ **When to employ the** Russian secret of **specialized variety**, to get a dramatic edge over your competitors.

▶▶ **How to significantly** finesse the skills of your sport by practicing them isometrically.

▶▶ **How to clean up your technique and** jump in proficiency using **neurological erasure**.

▶▶ **How to walk away from your** practice feeling stronger than when you started—rather than a wiped-out rag!

▶▶ **How to recruit your breath for** even greater power—guaranteed

▶▶ **How to use the** subtle but extremely important **wedge** method to enhance your strength and power.

▶▶ **How to avoid "leaking away"** your hard-earned strength—get this right and save yourself from a world of frustration and sub-par results.

▶▶ **How to release the** little-known, but deadly "parking brake" within your body that could be dooming your performance to constant failure.

And from Charles Staley discover:

▶▶ **The single biggest obstacle** to success in the weight room—and how to overcome it, every time!

▶▶ **The worst possible formula** for strength training—and why you want to ALWAYS do the very opposite…

▶▶ **The magic rep number** that yields the greatest power output—zero in on and fully employ this one secret in your training and you'll transform your practice, guaranteed…

▶▶ **How to avoid floundering** around and correctly evaluate "success" in your workout.

▶▶ **How to pack** maximum strength benefits into minimum time.

▶▶ **How to manipulate** the variables in your training to trick your body into greater strength gains.

▶▶ **The cornerstone principle** in all strength training—and how to make it work even better for YOU.

▶▶ **A hobbled horse is** a useless horse…how to dramatically reduce the chance of injury in your training—and radically extend your athletic career.

▶▶ **You're sick of hearing the** cliché: "Worker smarter, not harder"—I know—but here's the secret to "spending" less yet "making" more in your training… (Don't be a chump and ignore this golden advice).

▶▶ **If you can't SUSTAIN your** program, then what on earth's the point and how far do you think you're ever going to get? Stop this madness! Learn how here…

▶▶ **The counter-intuitive secret that could** rock your world and turn it upside down: how to make your workout EASIER—yet GAIN MORE STRENGTH!

▶▶ **Your limbic system can be** your best friend—or betray you into mediocrity…learn what it takes to "manage" this potential monster.

▶▶ **How to identify the** "sweet spot" when activating your nervous system—for optimal gains in your workout.

▶▶ **The real yardstick** you need when measuring your recovery needs—anything else and I see a glue factory in your future…

▶▶ **How to properly use these** "key indicators" to measure your real progress.

▶▶ **How to achieve your** desired strength outcome—while still safeguarding your health.

▶▶ **Why, for most of us, knowing how** to time our "activations" is way more important than figuring out correct rest periods.

▶▶ **It's one of the crucial differences between** an elite and average athlete: understand what it really takes to engage your full physical capabilities—for true success on the court or field.

▶▶ **How to eliminate redundancy from** your workouts—and watch your effectiveness grow by leaps and bounds.

▶▶ **Why it's so important and** what it means to "preferentially train the higher qualities."

▶▶ **How to control and** manage your fatigue, instead of becoming its victim.

▶▶ **Understand and utilize the** key principles of variability and specificity—by correctly exploiting the benefits and minimizing the drawbacks.

▶▶ **Why extension-based exercises can be** crucial for balance in your training program.

▶▶ **How to utilize the** principle of "conscientious participation" to enhance your workout results.

▶▶ **How to cycle EDT and** the 3-to-5 method, for a superlative surge in your athleticism.

▶▶ **It's certainly the most unpopular—but is** this also the world's MOST EFFECTIVE therapy for muscle recovery?

▶▶ **What "percent of capacity" you need to** operate at—for the best workouts of your life…

▶▶ **"Auto-regulatory training"**—the often-slighted, often-ignored yet absolutely vital strategy for long term, significant strength gains…

▶▶ **The magic power of** "predetermined time-limits"—and how to become a wiz at manipulating time to your own infinite advantage…

Amazing instruction

"I attended this seminar and it was nothing short of awesome. Pavel and Staley really took the time to blow apart age-old beliefs and practices in strength training. I recommend this set to anyone wanting to work on strength development." —Jay Bell, Phoenix, AZ

Two phenomenal Coaches in one DVD

"Well worth the price. I had already read and tried EDT from Charles' book, *Muscle Logic*. The reason I bought it was because of Pavel's testimonial on the back. I have to admit, I never tire of hearing/seeing Pavel teach. Both Charles and Pavel are great instructors; those of you who have seen him know what I mean. Seeing the two present their ideas on strength and conditioning was just great. This will be an excellent DVD to study and apply to my classes." —Pete Diaz, RKC, Sacramento, CA

Serious Strength

"There is a staggering amount of information, not only in quantity, but also in QUALITY. I found myself taking notes while watching, which is something that rarely happens.

We begin with Charles Staley's thoughts on training principles and an enlightening look at what is really going on within a set of a given exercise. Charles also talks at length about program design and his own Escalating Density Training system, demonstrating it with a dumbbell snatch.

Then it is Pavel's turn. Pavel has a gift for taking complex subject matter and presenting it in a way that anyone can understand. This product is no exception. He explains the physics behind strength and tweaks technique to improve performance ad enhance safety. An excellent product." —David Whitley, Senior RKC, Nashville, TN

How to stay informed of the latest advances in strength and conditioning
VISIT HTTP://KBFORUM.DRAGONDOOR.COM/

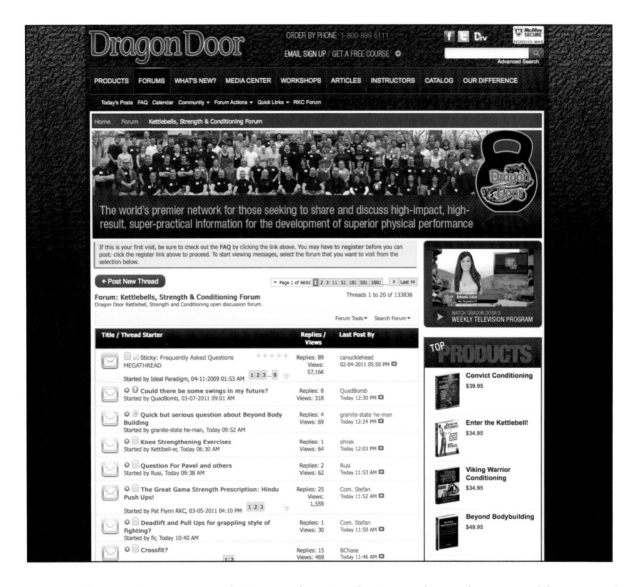

Visit **www.dragondoor.com** and sign up for Pavel Tsatsouline's free monthly e-newsletter, giving you late-breaking news and tips on how to stay ahead of the fitness pack.

Visit **http://kbforum.dragondoor.com/** and participate in Dragon Door's stimulating and informative **Strength and Conditioning** Forum. Post your fitness questions or comments and get quick feedback from Pavel Tsatsouline and other leading fitness experts.

Visit **www.dragondoor.com** and browse the **Articles** section and other pages for ground-breaking theories and products for improving your health and well being.

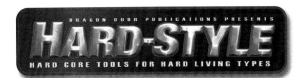

ORDERING INFORMATION

1·800·899·5111
24 HOURS A DAY
FAX YOUR ORDER (866) 280-7619

Customer Service Questions? Please call us between 9:00am– 11:00pm EST Monday to Friday at 1-800-899-5111. Local and foreign customers call 513-346-4160 for orders and customer service

100% One-Year Risk-Free Guarantee. If you are not completely satisfied with any product—we'll be happy to give you a prompt exchange, credit, or refund, as you wish. Simply return your purchase to us,

and please let us know why you were dissatisfied—it will help us to provide better products and services in the future. *Shipping and handling fees are non-refundable.*

Telephone Orders For faster service you may place your orders by calling Toll Free 24 hours a day, 7 days a week, 365 days per year. When you call, please have your credit card ready.

Complete and mail with full payment to: Dragon Door Publications, 5 East County Rd B, #3, Little Canada, MN 55117

Please print clearly

Sold To: A

Name _____

Street _____

City _____

State _____ Zip _____

Day phone* _____
* Important for clarifying questions on orders

Please print clearly

SHIP TO: *(Street address for delivery)* B

Name _____

Street _____

City _____

State _____ Zip _____

Email _____

Warning to foreign customers:
The Customs in your country may or may not tax or otherwise charge you an additional fee for goods you receive. Dragon Door Publications is charging you only for U.S. handling and international shipping. Dragon Door Publications is in no way responsible for any additional fees levied by Customs, the carrier or any other entity.

ITEM #	QTY.	ITEM DESCRIPTION	ITEM PRICE	A OR B	TOTAL

HANDLING AND SHIPPING CHARGES · NO COD'S
Total Amount of Order Add (Excludes kettlebells and kettlebell kits):

$00.00 to 29.99	Add $6.00	$100.00 to 129.99	Add $14.00
$30.00 to 49.99	Add $7.00	$130.00 to 169.99	Add $16.00
$50.00 to 69.99	Add $8.00	$170.00 to 199.99	Add $18.00
$70.00 to 99.99	Add $11.00	$200.00 to 299.99	Add $20.00
		$300.00 and up	Add $24.00

Canada and Mexico add $6.00 to US charges. All other countries, flat rate, double US Charges. See Kettlebell section for Kettlebell Shipping and handling charges.

Total of Goods
Shipping Charges
Rush Charges
Kettlebell Shipping Charges
OH residents add 6.25% sales tax
MN residents add 7.125% sales tax
TOTAL ENCLOSED

METHOD OF PAYMENT ❑ CHECK ❑ M.O. ❑ MASTERCARD ❑ VISA ❑ DISCOVER ❑ AMEX

Account No. *(Please indicate all the numbers on your credit card)*   EXPIRATION DATE

▢▢▢▢ ▢▢▢▢ ▢▢▢▢ ▢▢▢▢   ▢▢/▢▢

Day Phone: (   ) _____

Signature: _____ **Date:** _____

NOTE: *We ship best method available for your delivery address. Foreign orders are sent by air. Credit card or International M.O. only. For* **RUSH** *processing of your order, add an additional $10.00 per address. Available on money order & charge card orders only.*

Errors and omissions excepted. Prices subject to change without notice.

Do You Have A Friend Who'd Like To Receive This Catalog?

We would be happy to send your friend a free copy. Make sure to print and complete in full:

Name ....

Address ....

City .... State .... Zip ......

Do You Have A Friend Who'd Like To Receive This Catalog?

We would be happy to send your friend a free copy. Make sure to print and complete in full:

Name ....

Address ....

City .... State .... Zip ......

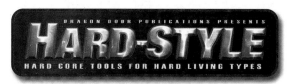

ORDERING INFORMATION

1·800·899·5111
24 HOURS A DAY
FAX YOUR ORDER (866) 280-7619

Customer Service Questions? Please call us between 9:00am– 11:00pm EST Monday to Friday at 1-800-899-5111. Local and foreign customers call 513-346-4160 for orders and customer service

100% One-Year Risk-Free Guarantee. If you are not completely satisfied with any product—we'll be happy to give you a prompt exchange, credit, or refund, as you wish. Simply return your purchase to us,

and please let us know why you were dissatisfied—it will help us to provide better products and services in the future. *Shipping and handling fees are non-refundable.*

Telephone Orders For faster service you may place your orders by calling Toll Free 24 hours a day, 7 days a week, 365 days per year. When you call, please have your credit card ready.

Complete and mail with full payment to: Dragon Door Publications, 5 East County Rd B, #3, Little Canada, MN 55117

Please print clearly

Sold To: **A**

Name_____

Street_____

City_____

State _____ Zip _____

Day phone*_____
* Important for clarifying questions on orders

Please print clearly

SHIP TO: *(Street address for delivery)*   **B**

Name_____

Street_____

City_____

State _____ Zip _____

Email_____

Warning to foreign customers: The Customs in your country may or may not tax or otherwise charge you an additional fee for goods you receive. Dragon Door Publications is charging you only for U.S. handling and international shipping. Dragon Door Publications is in no way responsible for any additional fees levied by Customs, the carrier or any other entity.

Item #	Qty.	Item Description	Item Price	A or B	Total

Do You Have A Friend Who'd Like To Receive This Catalog?

We would be happy to send your friend a free copy. Make sure to print and complete in full:

Name

Address

City   **State**   **Zip**

HANDLING AND SHIPPING CHARGES • NO COD'S
Total Amount of Order Add (Excludes kettlebells and kettlebell kits):

$00.00 to 29.99	Add $6.00	$100.00 to 129.99	Add $14.00
$30.00 to 49.99	Add $7.00	$130.00 to 169.99	Add $16.00
$50.00 to 69.99	Add $8.00	$170.00 to 199.99	Add $18.00
$70.00 to 99.99	Add $11.00	$200.00 to 299.99	Add $20.00
		$300.00 and up	Add $24.00

Canada and Mexico add $6.00 to US charges. All other countries, flat rate, double US Charges. See Kettlebell section for Kettlebell Shipping and handling charges.

Total of Goods	
Shipping Charges	
Rush Charges	
Kettlebell Shipping Charges	
OH residents add 6.25% sales tax	
MN residents add 7.125% sales tax	
Total Enclosed	

Do You Have A Friend Who'd Like To Receive This Catalog?

We would be happy to send your friend a free copy. Make sure to print and complete in full:

Name

Address

City   **State**   **Zip**

METHOD OF PAYMENT ❑ Check ❑ M.O. ❑ Mastercard ❑ Visa ❑ Discover ❑ Amex

Account No. *(Please indicate all the numbers on your credit card)*   EXPIRATION DATE

❑❑❑❑ ❑❑❑❑ ❑❑❑❑ ❑❑❑❑   ❑❑/❑❑

Day Phone: (   )_____

Signature: _____ **Date:** _____

NOTE: *We ship best method available for your delivery address. Foreign orders are sent by air. Credit card or International M.O. only. For **RUSH** processing of your order, add an additional $10.00 per address. Available on money order & charge card orders only.*

Errors and omissions excepted. Prices subject to change without notice.